Exercise: A Scientific and Clinical Overview

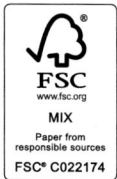

FSC
www.fsc.org
MIX
Paper from
responsible sources
FSC® C022174

Exercise: A Scientific and Clinical Overview

Dr Hugh J.N. Bethell and Professor David Brodie

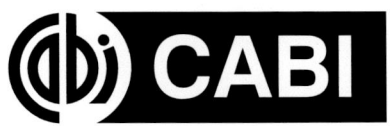

CABI is a trading name of CAB International

CABI
Nosworthy Way
Wallingford
Oxfordshire OX10 8DE
UK

CABI
200 Portland Street
Boston
MA 02114
USA

Tel: +44 (0)1491 832111
E-mail: info@cabi.org
Website: www.cabi.org

Tel: +1 (617)682-9015
E-mail: cabi-nao@cabi.org

A catalogue record for this book is available from the British Library, London, UK.

ISBN-13: 9781800621831 (paperback)
9781800621848 (ePDF)
9781800621855 (ePub)

DOI: 10.1079/9781800621855.0000

Commissioning Editor: Alexandra Lainsbury
Editorial Assistant: Lauren Davies
Production Editor: Shankari Wilford

Typeset by: SPi, Pondicherry, India
Printed and bound in the UK by Severn, Gloucester

Contents

About the Authors

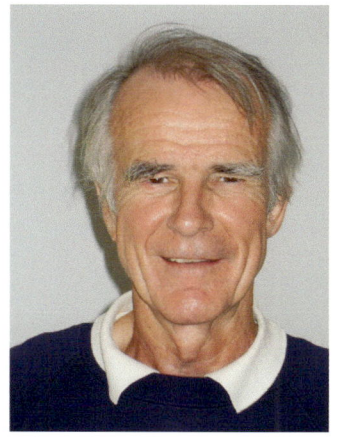

Dr Hugh J.N. Bethell MBE MD FRCP FRCGP qualified in medicine in 1966. His early career included a stint as a Cardiac Registrar at Charing Cross Hospital in London, where he first encountered the use of exercise for treating heart disease – a groundbreaking idea at the time.

In 1974 Hugh abandoned cardiology and entered general practice in Alton in Hampshire. There he set up an exercise programme in the Alton Sports Centre for patients recovering from heart attacks and other cardiac ailments and operations. Since then he has written extensively on exercise for heart disease, including two books, nine book chapters, 65 original scientific papers and 76 review articles. In the early 1990s he was the driving force in setting up the British Association for Cardiac Rehabilitation (now the British Association for Cardiac Prevention and Rehabilitation) and became its first President.

Over the past 12 years Hugh has expanded the Cardiac Rehab activities to embrace people with other problems, particularly those that increase the risk of coronary disease – high blood pressure, obesity, diabetes, etc. He has also become particularly interested in the exercise treatment of degenerative diseases, disability and frailty in later life, all of which are promoted by an inactive lifestyle. His aim is to encourage regular physical activity for all for disease prevention, increased longevity and, most of all, for a healthy and enjoyable old age.

For the last four years, Dr Bethell has written a weekly blog on many aspects of exercise and physical fitness, and this has reached a regular audience of health practitioners around the world. You can find it at https://www.cardiac-rehab.co.uk/blog/.

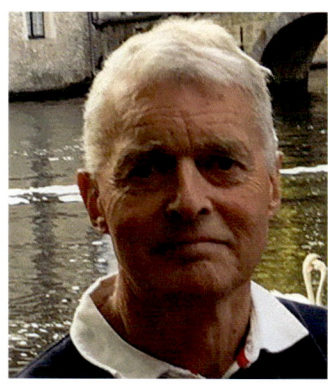

Professor David Brodie graduated from Loughborough University in 1969. Having taught for three years, he then moved into higher education, working at Saltley College, Leeds Metropolitan University and the University of Liverpool. At Liverpool, he was both Director of Physical Education and Professorial Head of the Department of Movement Science in the Faculty of Medicine. During this time, he established the first cardiac rehabilitation programme on the Wirral.

In 2001, he moved to Buckinghamshire New University, engaging in a research programme on cardiovascular health, particularly concentrating on physiological measures associated with heart failure.

He co-authored some 250 research papers and in 2010 was awarded a DSc from Coventry University for his research into body composition and cardiovascular health.

Since his retirement, David has published two novels and seven children's books, five of which have been republished in the Welsh language.

He has long been an advocate of the benefits of exercise and enjoyed physical activity all his life, including rugby, basketball, running and rowing, a sport he still enjoys weekly. He loves trekking and has recently returned from his seventh expedition to the Himalaya.

Preface

This book has perhaps never been more important than now. Life expectancy may now have plateaued (or be falling) in many wealthier countries, as non-communicable diseases take their toll. But these non-communicable diseases also shorten 'healthy' and disease-free life – adding a burden of suffering and also of cost. And this is not a cost which even the richest of societies will be able to bear in their 'disease treatment' services. Societal splits will widen as the poor become sicker, and unable to pay for care. Meanwhile, other urgent threats to health and survival – such as those due to climate change, or particulate pollution – have appeared. So what is to be done?

It is rare in medicine to find a panacea – a single 'thing' which will both prevent and treat multiple diseases and their causes. But exercise is that panacea, as this textbook shows. We learn just how woefully inactive we have all become. We learn of the harm that such sedentary lifestyles inflict. We learn of the powerful role which exercise has in the primary and secondary prevention of diverse diseases, across all age groups. And active transport, of course, also reduces fossil fuel emissions – meaning less particulate pollution and fewer greenhouse gases.

The contents of the book are comprehensive, covering the science of physical performance and how to measure it, through to its role across all elements of public health. As such, it is a book which sports scientists should read. But so, too, should all doctors: few will be aware of the data which they could deploy to the benefit of their patients.

But this is also a book which should be read by policy makers. Were they to take heed with systemic structural reform to facilitate physical activity (rather than simply 'encouraging individuals'), our society would be much the better. Many would live happier healthier lives. And our health systems – as well as our planet – would become that bit more sustainable.

Hugh Montgomery OBE FMedSci MBBS BSc FRCP MD FRSB FFICM FRI
Professor of Intensive Care Medicine, University College London

Introduction

There is no situation, there is no age and no condition where exercise is not a good thing.

Professor Sir Chris Whitty, Chief Medical Officer for England

This book is about all aspects of exercise. It explores what exercise is, how it affects the body, how it is measured and, most of all, what benefits it brings. It does not focus on any particular type of exercise. It will not cover specific exercise regimens related to different sports or to individual physical development. It will provide information about the science of exercise and how much it has to contribute to overall well-being. The book will provide a sound basis for the practitioner and ambassador of exercise, whether it is a clinician, student or coach. Our aim is that the reader will understand the issues of exercise and be armed with the knowledge to inform others. We want more people to exercise because they understand its true value.

The book starts with a brief history of exercise, then proceeds to a description of the physiology of the short- and long-term effects of exercise, a discussion of appropriate doses of exercise and a description of all the diseases and conditions that can be effectively prevented and/or treated by exercise.

The main message of the book is that exercise is essential for a long and healthy life. We both strongly believe that exercise is fundamental for the avoidance of the majority of degenerative diseases that assail us towards the end of our days. Heart disease, diabetes, osteoporosis, dementia and many other debilitating disorders can be prevented or reduced by regular exercise. These are the conditions that can make later life a misery and lead to the frailty and dependency that are such a burden in our later years.

The average time spent with some form of preventable disease towards the end of life is currently about 20% of total lifespan. With an active lifestyle, we believe this figure should be no more than 5%. Being physically fit extends lifespan, but more importantly and to an even greater extent, it extends 'healthspan'. It reduces the period of debility close to the end of life. It is no coincidence that the level of physical fitness in older people was a factor in the survival from infection with Covid-19. An alternative title for the book might be 'How Not to Kill Your Granny'.

The effects of exercise and its application to the prevention and management of disease are not usually taught as part of the curriculum of students of most medical and paramedical disciplines. Sport-related studies often focus on the fit and healthy, sadly a relatively small proportion of the population. There are few disease-risk scores that include exercise dose. Practising clinicians seldom take an exercise history from their patients and even more rarely prescribe exercise as prevention or treatment. Comparisons between the effects of drugs and exercise are rare. There are few publications to remedy these deficiencies. We believe this book will fill a gap and become essential reading for all those who advise and care for people's health. It will importantly be of value to those who would benefit from being more physically active – i.e. nearly everyone! It is particularly aimed at informing all health practitioners and also to help those who take too little exercise. Everyone needs to recognize the importance of becoming more active. We have aimed to set out clearly the dangers of inactivity and the huge benefits of physical engagement.

Exercise is medicine but its importance is too little recognized, and it is too little applied to the management of those with degenerative diseases and those at risk of such conditions. As a medical practitioner and health scientist, we have been using exercise as medicine for half a century. Yet the more we learn about the benefits of regular exercise and physical fitness for health, the more we realize that we should have been applying it to an even greater extent. The evidence for the importance of exercise rather than pills in the prevention of disease and the maintenance of a long and healthy life is growing by the day. There is now a medical group to represent this developing view – the British Association of Lifestyle Medicine. The recognition that lifestyle trumps medication is dawning on the medical profession and public alike – albeit rather slowly! This book is designed to accelerate and accentuate this critical process.

Dr Hugh J.N. Bethell
Professor David Brodie

1 A Brief Historical Context for Exercise

Animals need to move to survive and higher life forms, so-called vertebrates, have evolved muscles and bones for this purpose. These, together with tendons and ligaments, make up the musculoskeletal system. Each animal has developed to suit its own survival needs – the cheetah has a system designed for speed to enable it to catch its prey and likewise the antelope has a system designed for speed to escape being eaten by the cheetah. For other species strength may be more important than speed. The tiger, for example, has the strength to tear its prey limb from limb. For every animal there is a best possible, or 'optimal', mixture of speed and strength to enable it to survive and breed efficiently.

Evolution has given humans a musculoskeletal system of great versatility. We are neither immensely strong nor immensely fast – but we do have the greatest intelligence in the animal kingdom, and we use our brainpower to make the most efficient use of this versatility. Man evolved to be a highly efficient hunter-gatherer – to hunt animals and to gather edible plants for sustenance. For most of human history that has been the main function of our muscles. Primitive man took a lot of exercise because that is what he had to do to survive.

We do not know what prehistoric man did in the way of recreational exercise, though it is likely that during periods of relaxation he would have played and perhaps danced. There is evidence that in the Palaeolithic age (roughly 2.5 million–10,000 years BC) exercise played a part in social activities and inter-tribe visits (Boyd Eaton *et al.*, 1988). Hunting wild animals allowed the need for food and clothing to blend with recreational sport. Traces of this are seen today in the activities of some primitive Amazonian tribes who incorporate conversation and singing into their hunting rituals. In today's so-called developed world, the emphasis has been reversed. Fishing and shooting provide recreation first and food very much second, while in fox hunting the need to eat the famously inedible spoils of the hunt has been dispensed with altogether.

About 10,000 years ago, the development of a structured society with a more settled population and the growth of agriculture changed the pattern of human exercising to the more repetitive work associated with husbanding animals and sowing, growing and harvesting crops. With a more secure food source, there would have been more spare time for fun, with games and sports helping muscles to stay in shape even when not so vital for survival. Early forms of organized exercise would also have been used to keep the tribe in battle-ready physical shape. Games recorded by the ancient Egyptians and Greeks laid emphasis on activities that would have contributed to this. Egyptian pharaonic carvings and paintings show sports including javelin-throwing, running, swimming, wrestling, rowing and even a primitive form of hockey. Running is specifically recorded as one way of increasing readiness for battle and included distances of up to 96 km (60 miles). The original Olympic Games were staged in 776 BC and included running, jumping, discus-throwing, wrestling, boxing, chariot-racing and the first pentathlon. For the Greeks and Romans, exercise was also regarded as part of the culture of attaining physical perfection and as an aid to good education – *Mens sana in corpore sano* ('A healthy mind in a healthy body') (Juvenal, *c*.AD 100).

Although exercise at this time would have been a means to an end for contestants, it is likely that such sports would have mainly been pastimes of the strong, the fast and the talented. Even so, several early civilizations recognized exercise as an admirable pursuit, including China with tai chi and India with yoga. Running was a prominent feature of religious and daily life for the Kenyan Masai and the Native Americans. Several Greek physicians including Hippocrates (*c*.460–370 BC) and Galen (*c*.AD 129–210) extolled the preventive therapeutic

© H.J.N. Bethell and D. Brodie 2023. *Exercise: A Scientific and Clinical Overview* (H.J.N. Bethell and D. Brodie)
DOI: 10.1079/9781800621855.0001

benefits of physical activity: 'Eating alone will not keep a man well; he must also take exercise.' It was Hippocrates who claimed over 2400 years ago that 'walking is a man's best medicine'. The same could be said today! However, the idea of the general public taking exercise to maintain health and fitness is a relatively recent phenomenon. It is doubtful whether the average ancient Greek or Roman citizen would have performed recreational exercise as an aid to improving physical fitness.

The collapse of the Roman Empire in the 4th century AD and the arrival of the 'Dark Ages' saw an end to the culture of the body beautiful. The spread of Christianity brought a belief that the body is sinful – it was the mind and preparation for the afterlife that predominated – though physical fitness remained very much a necessity for the peasants who laboured in the fields and at their various crafts. Hunting was popular with the upper classes and was regarded as a form of work, bringing food to the table. If they exercised otherwise, it was to be prepared for the exertions of combat. As the Middle Ages advanced, jousting became another pastime for the rich. The common man, meanwhile, took to wrestling and early forms of ball games.

An illustration of the extent to which popular recreation expanded in the Middle Ages is to be found in Pieter Brueghel the Elder's painting of children at play, *Children's Games* (1560). More than 90 different children's games are depicted, including sledging, skating, leapfrog, archery and tug of war. Many medieval activities have survived. Among games with a modern equivalent was tennis, perhaps first played with the hand in the 12th century but which has been a racket sport since the 16th century. So called 'real' or 'royal' tennis was commonplace across the courts of Europe in the 1500s, but we know from Shakespeare's *Henry V* that it was played at least a hundred years before then. Football has been played since the 15th century and cricket since the 16th century.

The Renaissance brought not only a rebirth of academic and other cerebral pursuits, but, to a lesser extent, a recognition that the body was more than a mortal shell for the mind and soul. In 1553 a Spaniard, Cristóbal Méndez, published a book on gymnastics entitled *Libro del exercicio corporal y de sus prouechos* (*Book of Physical Exercise and Its Benefits*), while in 1569 an Italian, Girolamo Mercuriale, extended the uses of exercise into the management of disease by natural methods in his book *De Arte Gymnastica* (*The Art of Gymnastics*).

The next stage in the advance of recreational exercise came in the late 18th and early 19th centuries with the Industrial Revolution. Up to this time most of the population was still dependent on physical activity to earn their daily living. The mechanization of many manual tasks meant that, for the first time in history, a large proportion of the population no longer had to exercise as part of their gainful employment.

Over the ensuing two centuries, the lessening of necessary physical activity has progressed and, since the advent of the motor car and later the computer, has accelerated. Between 1995 and 2014 the proportion of less active occupations rose from 55 to 67%, while the proportion of more active occupations fell from 43 to 33%. 'Less active occupations' include managers, professionals, clerks, technicians, sales and service workers. 'More active occupations' include agriculture, construction, manufacturing, industry and labouring (ISCA Report, 2015). A survey of the nation's fitness carried out by Allied Dunbar in 1992 estimated that about 80% of men and 90% of women were in occupations that were neither vigorous nor even moderately active (Fentem *et al.*, 1994).

Today some 75% of jobs are sedentary or require only light physical activity. Figure 1.1 shows the inexorable reduction of exercise-based occupations in Westernized societies over the past five decades (Church *et al.*, 2011).

Since the Industrial Revolution there has been an increase in the number of organizations encouraging exercise for the sake of fitness. Initially, in both Europe and the USA, this was based on gymnastics. Competitive games and other sports followed and became increasingly popular – and in 1896 the Olympic Games were revived. Sports included were athletics, cycling, fencing, swimming, gymnastics, sailing, shooting, tennis, weightlifting and wrestling. More recently there has been a progressive increase in the provision of community exercise facilities, with gyms now being a standard facility of hotels and many clubs. At the same time, the cult of competitive sports has also grown, and the top players and clubs have attracted enormous devoted fan bases and equally enormous financial rewards.

Paradoxically, the populations of developed nations have become less and less fit, and fatter and

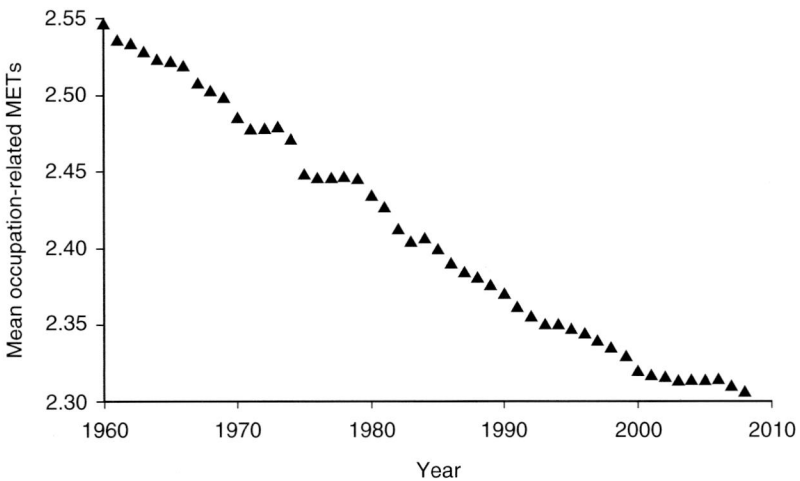

Fig. 1.1. Reduction in occupational energy expenditure over time from 1960 to 2010, plotted as mean occupation-related metabolic equivalents (METs). (From Church *et al.*, 2011.)

fatter. We have divided ourselves into those who exercise and those who spectate. The movement for exercise has certainly attracted many people, but it has failed to entrap the majority. Several population surveys have confirmed this sad fact. As one commentator put it: 'Today's interest in sport is more often vicarious than participatory. We idolize the elite athlete who performs for us, rather than the everyday athlete we could and should become' (Paffenbarger *et al.*, 2004).

Another factor in reducing physical activity in the population has been childhood behaviour. The exercise habit should start early in life. The young of all mammals have a tendency to play – they just frolic and frisk about for general enjoyment and the display of high spirits. This leads to the development of the exercise habit, which, because it is fun, influences how adults use their spare time later in life. There has been a dramatic change over the past few decades. First came motorized transport which relieved children of the need to walk or cycle to get to school and elsewhere. Then came the change in emphasis to more narrow academic demands at school, resulting in less playtime and leading to the scandal of playing fields being sold for building. The spread of television (TV) meant less outdoor play. The final nail in the coffin of the exercise habit has been the inexorable rise in the time that children spend on their 'screens' – those highly addictive devices that can occupy so much of their leisure time.

A fit and regularly exercising population would have tremendous benefits for the physical, mental, social and financial health of the nation. This will now be explored by examining the physiology of exercise, the effects of lethargy and exercise, the effects of physical training and the relationship of exercise to disease and longevity.

Summary

Humans have evolved to have versatile musculoskeletal systems. As people settled, they often turned to sports for recreation and competitions. Following the Industrial Revolution, individuals exercised less as part of their employment. In more recent times, the increase in the availability of television and other screens has resulted in a less active population. The benefits of exercise to many aspects of health are now recognized and this book will explore these in detail.

References

Boyd Eaton, S., Shostak, M. and Konner, M. (1988) *The Palaeolithic Prescription: A Program of Diet & Exercise and A Design for Living*. Harper Collins, New York.

Church, T.S., Thomas, D.M., Tudor-Locke, C., Katzmarzyk, P.T., Earnest, C.P., *et al.* (2011) Trends over 5 decades in US occupation-related physical activity and their associations with obesity. *PLoS One* 6, e19657. https://doi.org/10.1371/journal.pone.0019657

Fentem, P.H., Collins, M.F., Tuxworth, W., Walker, A., Hoinville, E., *et al.* (1994) *Allied Dunbar National Fitness Survey. Technical Report*. Allied Dunbar, Health Education Authority and Sports Council, London.

ISCA Report (2015) *The Economic Cost of Physical Inactivity in Europe. An ISCA/Cebr Report*. International Sport and Culture Association (ISCA), Copenhagen/Centre for Economics and Business Research (Cebr), London.

Juvenal (*c*.AD 100) *Satires, Book IV, Satire X: Wrong Desire is the Source of Suffering*, tr. G.G. Ramsay (Heinemann, 1928).

Paffenbarger, R.S., Morris, J.N., Haskell, W.L. and Thompson, P.D. (2004) An introduction to the Journal of Physical Activity and Health. *Journal of Physical Activity and Health* 1, 1–3.

2 The Muscles and Types of Exercise

This chapter describes the internal workings of the muscles and the broad principles of exercising them. The anatomical details may not seem particularly important for the average exerciser, but the effect of inheritance on different muscle types and how this determines the best exercise for the individual may be of interest to others.

The muscles are the body's engines – all movement depends on muscular contraction and relaxation. All joints and limbs are powered by muscular contraction and the physiology of muscle action – the way in which they work – is both beautiful and elegant.

Muscle Types

All muscles are divided into three distinct varieties:

1. *Voluntary muscles* – these are also called skeletal or 'striated' muscles, because of their striped appearance under the microscope (Fig. 2.1). Their movements are under our control. The biceps is an example. When a person decides to bend an arm, the nervous system goes into action immediately, contracting the biceps and bending the arm.

2. *Involuntary muscles* – these are also called 'smooth' muscles. They perform the vital activities of the body over which we have *no* control. They act without conscious thought, like the muscles of the gut, which labour away moving food down the gastrointestinal tract. Another example is the ocular muscles, which control the pupil: they respond to light but without any conscious thought process.

3. *Cardiac muscle* – the heart comprises a very specialized form of involuntary muscle, which is designed to allow both contractile and rhythmic elements.

This book is mainly concerned with the voluntary muscles, the muscles of movement. They have a main body, the belly of the muscle, and very strong fibrous cables called tendons that attach the muscle to our bones. Most movements depend on muscles contracting, bending or straightening the joints that connect the bones to which the tendons are attached.

Each muscle is made up of thousands of fibres, which in turn are made up of thousands of myofibrils. These are tubular structures extending the whole length of the cell. The myofibrils are made up of thick and thin filaments; the thick filaments are composed mainly of the protein myosin and the thin filaments of the protein actin. The basic contractile unit of a myocyte (muscle fibre) is known as a sarcomere. (Fig. 2.2).

Muscle contraction is stimulated by an impulse passing down the nerve supplying the muscle – the motor neuron, rather similar to the arrival of an electrical impulse. Each muscle is served by a large number of nerve fibres and the individual motor neuron plus the muscle fibres that it stimulates is called a motor unit. When an impulse reaches the muscle fibres of a motor unit, it stimulates a reaction between the actin and myosin filaments. This reaction results in the start of a contraction, which is achieved by the two different types of filaments sliding alongside each other causing the whole muscle to shorten. Contraction continues until the neuron stops stimulating the muscle, or until muscle fatigue sets in, which happens when the supply of energy that fuels contraction is exhausted.

Viewed under a microscope, the muscle fibres have a striped appearance – hence striated muscle. The striation is caused by the highly ordered arrangement of the actin and myosin within the fibrils and the similarly ordered arrangement of the fibrils within the muscle cell.

Striated muscles are made up of two distinct types of fibre – slow-twitch (Type I) and fast-twitch (Type II) fibres (which are further subdivided into Type IIa and Type IIb fibres). Slow-twitch fibres contract slowly and can maintain their shortening for long periods. They are the endurance-giving fibres and are particularly used during such activities

© H.J.N. Bethell and D. Brodie 2023. *Exercise: A Scientific and Clinical Overview*
(H.J.N. Bethell and D. Brodie)
DOI: 10.1079/9781800621855.0002

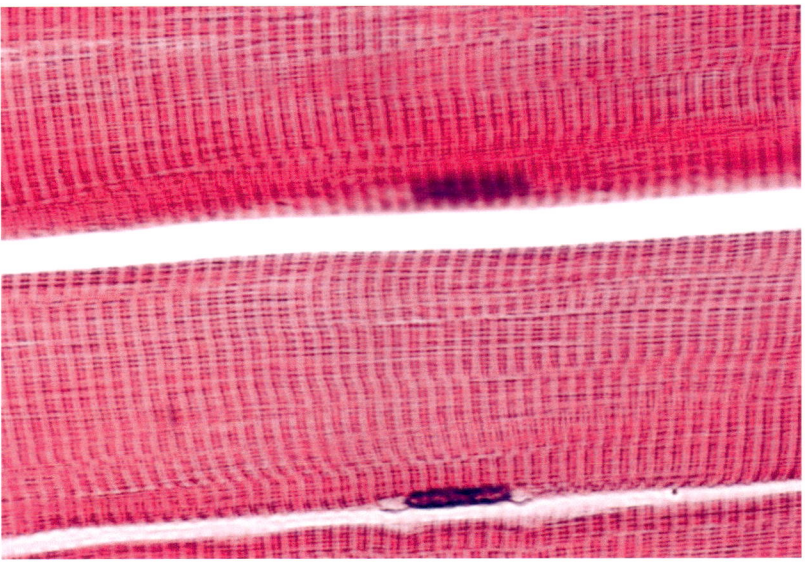

Fig. 2.1. Microscopic image of striated muscle.

as distance running and cycling. Fast-twitch fibres contract rapidly but tire quickly and are those most used by sprinters and weightlifters. Repeated contractions give speed to action.

A summary of the different fibre characteristics is shown in Table 2.1.

Most muscles consist of a combination of slow- and fast-twitch fibres, but one often predominates in particular muscles. For example, back muscles, which move little but contract continuously to maintain posture, are predominantly slow-twitch. Eye muscles, on the other hand, are almost all fast-twitch.

There is also a genetic influence on the predominance and distribution of muscle type. The ratio of slow to fast is about 50% for most people. However, some individuals inherit a much larger proportion of one or the other and this may determine their prowess in different sporting endeavours. Those born with a higher proportion of Type I slow-twitch fibres are more likely to become endurance athletes, while those born with more Type II fast-twitch fibres will do better as sprinters. Specialist training can change the balance somewhat, but a born marathon runner will never make a champion sprinter.

Exercising Your Muscles

This book does not specify which particular type of exercise could or should be taken; the options are too great. The important message is, to quote the Nike slogan, 'Just do it'. Exercise is far more likely to be sustained if it is enjoyable, so should be chosen with care.

There are three broad categories of exercise – isotonic, isometric and isokinetic:

1. *Isotonic (or dynamic) exercise* is that which uses the regular, purposeful movement of joints and large muscle groups, particularly their Type I fibres. This type of exercise will be the main concern of this book, because it yields the most health-giving benefit, including the treatment of chronic diseases.

2. *Isometric exercise*, on the other hand, involves static contraction of muscles with little or no joint movement, predominantly involving Type II fibres. Isometric exercise uses much strength but little movement. More mature readers will remember the once well-known Charles Atlas muscle-building techniques. These were pure isometrics, involving one muscle group straining against another without movement – a form of exertion designed to build up muscle bulk and strength. The muscle fibres used are the Type II, or fast-twitch, fibres. They do not use oxygen and they tire quickly. In a clinical context, isometric exercise is frequently used by physiotherapists in the treatment of joint injuries and after orthopaedic surgery.

3. *Isokinetic (same speed) exercise* gives maximal resistance to the muscles throughout the range of

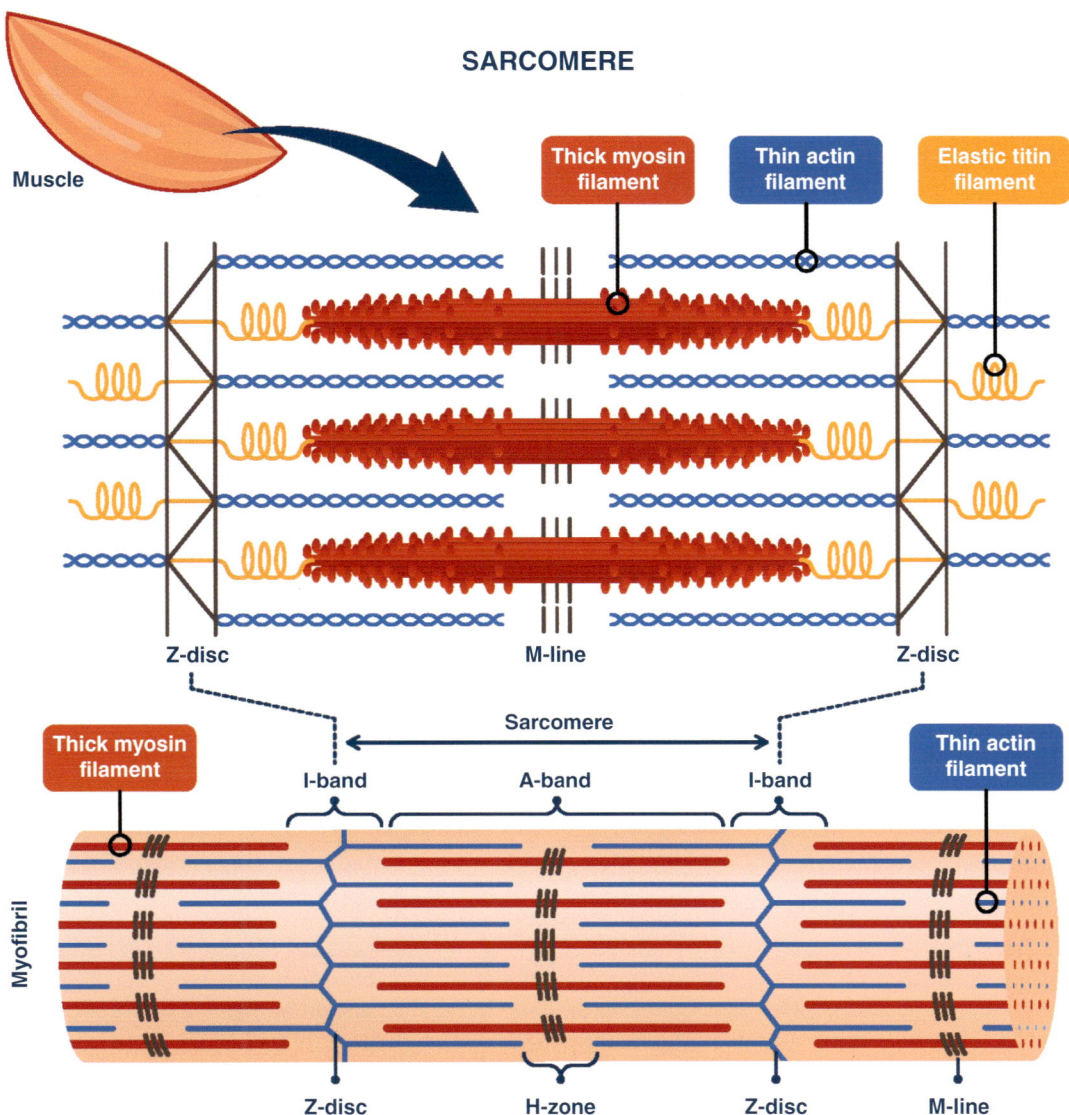

SARCOMERE

Muscle

Thick myosin filament

Thin actin filament

Elastic titin filament

Z-disc M-line Z-disc

Sarcomere

Thick myosin filament

I-band A-band I-band

Thin actin filament

Myofibril

Z-disc H-zone Z-disc M-line

Fig. 2.2. Diagrammatic view of sarcomere.

Table 2.1. Differences in muscle fibre characteristics.

	Type I	Type IIa	Type IIb
Speed of contraction	Slow	Fast	Very fast
Force produced	Low	Medium	High
Resistance to fatigue	High	Medium	Low
Colour	Red	Pink	White

motion. A simple way to illustrate this is the plunger in a cafetiere. The plunger can be pressed down either gently with a single finger or more forcibly with the flat of the hand. In both cases the cafetiere adjusts to the pressure and the full movement is at approximately the same speed. Most commonly, isokinetic training involves expensive equipment such as the Cybex machine, but it can produce a combination of both isotonic and isometric training with few disadvantages.

Table 2.2 shows the advantages of the three methods of training. The number 1 indicates good, 2 indicates medium and 3 indicates poor for each criterion.

Other ways of describing types of exercise include the aerobic (using oxygen) and anaerobic (not needing oxygen) energy systems. Most activities involve a combination of these factors and classification is typically determined by the dominant characteristics of the particular exercise.

Aerobic exercise includes such sports as running, cycling, swimming and aerobic dance. These involve significant movement and relatively little strength and can be continued for long periods; they are sometimes also referred to as 'cardiovascular' workouts.

They are dependent on a good supply of oxygen, which fuels the energy produced by the breakdown of carbohydrate into glucose and stored in the muscle as glycogen. Such exercise, performed at the appropriate level, can be continued as long as there is a sufficient supply of glycogen. If the duration and intensity of the exercise is sufficient to deplete the glycogen faster than it can be replenished, muscle fatigue sets in and the exercise must be greatly reduced or stopped. This is the experience of the marathon runner who 'hits the wall'. The effort of aerobic exercise is mainly performed by Type I, or slow-twitch, muscle fibres.

Most so-called anaerobic exercises do involve some movement but make much more use of strength. Examples are weightlifting and sprinting. They are predominantly exercises of short duration. The situation is complicated by a further subdivision of the anaerobic system into the ATP-PC and lactic acid systems. This is outside the scope of this book and more information can be found in standard exercise physiology texts.

Muscle strengthening is also very important in the treatment of frailty and balance problems in old age – both of which will be discussed later.

Nearly all exercise involves a mixture of aerobic and anaerobic effort, though one or the other usually predominates. Most gym fitness-training programmes use a mixture and the recommendations of the Department of Health include 'strengthening activities that work all the major muscles [legs, hips, back, abdomen, chest, shoulders and arms] on at least two days a week' (see Chapter 6, this volume).

In the gym a number of exercise types are usually available. Some examples are shown below, but often a combination of these will be recommended, depending on the needs of the individual:

- *Cardiovascular* – this includes mainly aerobic exercise such as cycling on a static bike or rowing machine, walking or running on a treadmill, skipping, aerobic dance and any other exercise designed to raise the heart rate and induce shortness of breath. Circuit training, which involves progressing from one station to another, is a popular form of cardiovascular activity, but can equally incorporate strengthening activities.
- *Bums and tums* – aimed mainly at young to middle-aged women concerned about their body image, this consists of a mixture of aerobic and isometric exercise concentrating on the abdomen, buttocks and thighs. Crunches, squats and jogging may be included.
- *Pilates* – an exercise system involving a mixture of mental concentration, economy of movement, building up core strength and breathing control. This may use free-standing exercise or weights and pulleys.

Table 2.2. Different aspects of three categories of exercise.

Criterion	Isokinetic	Isotonic	Isometric
Rate of strength gain	1	1	1
Strength gain throughout range of motion	Excellent	Good	Poor
Time per training session	2	3	1
Expense	3	2	1
Ease of performance	2	3	1
Adaptability to specific movement	1	2	3
Prospect of soreness	Little	Much	Little
Prospect of muscle injury	Slight	Moderate	Slight
Skill improvement	Some	Some	None

1, good; 2, medium; 3, poor.

- *Body balance* – uses a mixture of yoga, tai chi and Pilates to improve core strength, relax the mind and enhance flexibility.
- *Spinning* – group cycling under the direction of an instructor who changes the load and speed through the session; mainly aerobic.
- *Aquarobics* – exercise in the swimming pool that uses the resistance of the water to exercise different muscle groups and may be particularly suitable for those with lower-limb problems, which can be helped by the support provided by the flotation environment and who would be unable to exercise without support.
- *Calisthenics* – a variety of body movements, often rhythmical, generally without using equipment or apparatus, thus in essence bodyweight training. The exercises are intended to increase body strength, body fitness and flexibility through movements such as pulling or pushing oneself up, bending, jumping or swinging, using only one's body weight for resistance.
- *Zumba* – a form of aerobic dance with varying rhythms and intensity, which can be adapted to all age groups.
- *Boxercise* – an exercise based on the training concepts that boxers use to keep fit. Classes can take a variety of formats but a typical one may involve shadowboxing, skipping, hitting pads, kicking punchbags, press-ups, shuttle-runs and sit-ups.
- *Crossfit* – a strength and conditioning workout that is made up of functional movement performed at a high intensity.
- *Yoga* – an ancient form of exercise that concentrates on strength, flexibility and breathing to improve both physical and mental well-being.
- *Weight training* – the use of either free weights or weight machines to improve strength and/or muscle bulk.
- *Plyometrics* – also known as jump training. It involves exerting maximal force in short intervals of time, typically by jumping from a box and immediately springing upwards. The idea is to move from muscle extension to contraction in a rapid, explosive manner. Athletes such as sprinters and high jumpers most often use it.

The possible combinations of exercise are infinite and the effects of one form compared with another depend on the balance of dynamic, isometric and flexibility exercises. They are all beneficial and can be undertaken either in the outdoors or in the gym. Sustainability is always an issue with gym membership, so it is important to ensure that an enjoyable activity is selected from those on offer. There is no greater disincentive than engaging in a programme, but not wanting to be there. There is no evidence that one sort of exercise class is any better or worse than any other – whatever individual adherents may say.

For those who wish to create their own circuits, it is preferable to alternate the stations between 'cardiovascular' and 'MSE – muscular strength and endurance'. This can be undertaken at home using a staircase, a pair of dumbbells or 'TheraBands' – thick elastic bands for providing resistance. There is much to be said for competitive sports or outdoor exercise. Team sports are more sociable and are inherently more interesting because of their complexity. They have the disadvantage of having to find a number of like-minded individuals to join in and often demand membership of a specific sports club. There is strong evidence to show that those who participate in a number of team sports when young are more likely to continue some form of physical activity when older (Brodie *et al.*, 1991; Roberts and Brodie, 1992). Running, swimming and cycling can be performed in groups or individually and have the great convenience that they can be fitted in with whatever else is going on in life. Each individual should be encouraged to choose what exercise(s) suits them best and which they enjoy sufficiently to want to continue in the long term. As long as more people are moving and becoming out of breath, then the health of the nation can only improve.

Warming Up and Cooling Down

For any exercise, the usual advice is to warm up before starting – for anything from a few minutes to half an hour. This is received wisdom for exercise professionals and for anyone taking part in a supervised exercise class, the warm-up is an integral part of the session. The purpose is to loosen up and warm the joints, muscles and tendons, making them more flexible and ready for exercise, and thus less vulnerable to injury. Although it sounds a sensible thing to do, there is little evidence to support a lengthy warm-up. With limited time for exercising, most amateur sports people may prefer to minimize their warm-up and devote adequate time to a quality exercise session. Starting slowly is a perfectly adequate substitute for a long, ritual warm-up.

Another commonly promoted preliminary to taking exercise is stretching. Again the idea is to prepare the muscles and tendons for the more violent changes about to be brought on by exercise. There are two forms of stretch – static and dynamic. Both are beloved by exercise professionals, but they too have very little evidence to support them (Herbert and Gabriel, 2002). Indeed, it has been shown that static calf muscle stretches actually increase the risk of injury among runners, perhaps by reducing the strength in the stretched muscles (Simic *et al.*, 2013). Although there is some evidence that performance may be slightly improved by dynamic stretching, it is potentially tiring and questionably worthwhile.

Cooling down, however, is more valuable and really can prevent problems. At the end of a session, the exerciser is likely to be hot and sweaty with dilated blood vessels. Standing still at this stage results in a drop in heart rate, but the blood vessels tend to remain dilated to promote heat loss. The blood pressure (BP) tends to decrease, which may cause the subject to feel faint or even collapse. Unless the fall is near water or around something to cause injury, it is not dangerous. It is simply the body's attempt to achieve homeostasis by giving the heart less work to do. This is preventable by judicious cooling down, ideally by keeping on the move until the blood vessels have contracted enough to prevent the fall in BP.

Summary

The muscles are the engines of movement for the body and are responsible for the greatest proportion of energy production. There are two distinct varieties of skeletal (striated) muscle – slow-twitch and fast-twitch, with some subdivisions. Slow-twitch fibres contract slowly and can maintain their shortening for long periods. They are the endurance-giving fibres and are particularly used during such activities as distance running and cycling. Fast-twitch fibres contract rapidly but tire quickly and are those most used by sprinters and weightlifters. Repeated contractions give speed to action.

References

Brodie, D.A., Roberts, K. and Lamb, K. (1991) *City Sport Challenge.* Health Promotion Research Trust, Cambridge.

Herbert, R.D. and Gabriel, M. (2002) Effects of stretching before and after exercise on muscle soreness and risk of injury: systematic review. *BMJ* 325, 468.

Roberts, K. and Brodie, D.A. (1992) *Inner-City Sport: Who Plays, and What Are the Benefits?* Giordano Bruno Culemborg, Utrecht, The Netherlands.

Simic, L., Aarabon, N. and Markovic, G. (2013) Does pre-exercise static stretching inhibit maximal muscular performance? A meta-analytic review. *Scandinavian Journal of Medicine and Science in Sports* 23, 131–148.

3 Oxygen as the Fuel of Aerobic Exercise

Oxygen Uptake or Oxygen Consumption

This chapter concerns the role of oxygen in fuelling exercise. A grasp of this topic is essential to understanding how physical fitness is measured and how exercise dose is both measured and prescribed.

For a muscle to work it needs energy and energy requires fuel. The biochemical processes that fuel muscle contraction are immensely complicated – much too complicated to review here – except for the contribution of oxygen (O_2). Oxygen is an essential component of the metabolic conversion of various energy sources (sugars, fats, etc.) into action – in other words, muscle contraction. The supply of oxygen to the muscle and the muscle's use of it are the factors that decide how much work can be performed during aerobic exercise.

Oxygen makes up about 20% of the air breathed and it is absorbed from the lungs on to the haemoglobin molecules in the blood's red cells as they pass through the very small blood vessels (capillaries) supplying the air sacs (alveoli) in the lungs. Haemoglobin arrives in the lungs in the form of deoxyhaemoglobin and has a bluish hue. The oxygen picked up in the lungs converts it to oxyhaemoglobin, which is a much brighter red. The blood is pumped round the body to the various organs that need oxygen to maintain life – the brain, heart, kidneys, gut, liver, muscles of the respiration system, etc. There the oxygen is extracted into the cells. On average, oxygen uptake at rest is about 3.5 ml of oxygen per minute per kilogram of body weight, meaning that, for a 70 kg (11 stone) resting man, the rate of oxygen consumption is about 250 ml per minute. This is also known as 1 MET. The term MET – it stands for metabolic equivalent – is an extremely important measure of exercise intensity.

During exercise, muscles need more oxygen, and this is provided by breathing faster and by the heart pumping more blood to them. There is a straight-line relationship between muscular work and oxygen uptake, abbreviated as VO_2 ($\dot{V}O_2$ should correctly have a dot above the V, as shown, but as this is rarely used these days, it has also been abandoned throughout this text). This continues until the point at which no more oxygen can be absorbed and pumped round the body – known as the maximum oxygen uptake, or VO_{2max} (see Fig. 3.1). This is measured as millilitres of oxygen used per minute for each kilogram of body weight – ml/min/kg. Sometimes, oxygen uptake is expressed as litres per minute (l/min). Including body weight becomes more relevant when the person is carrying the weight of the body, such as in running. In sports such as cycling and rowing, it may be less relevant. This is aerobic exercise and at the point of maximum uptake, further exercise can only continue using anaerobic (not using oxygen) metabolism. This is fuelled by stored energy sources in the muscles, which quickly become depleted. Anaerobic exercise, therefore, can only be continued for a very short period.

As exercise workload increases, so does oxygen uptake to the point of exhaustion. For the unfit, this point is reached at a lower oxygen uptake and therefore a lower workload than for the fit individual. The fitter you are, the higher the rate at which you can take up and use oxygen and therefore the higher workload you can achieve – as illustrated in Fig. 3.2 showing the relationship between exertion and oxygen uptake.

The concept of VO_{2max} is very important. It is the most precise measure of physical fitness we have since it describes the maximum work rate of which a person is capable. In healthy young people it is usually between 35 and 55 ml/min/kg body weight (10–15 METs). Ultra-fit athletes may reach levels of 70–80 ml/min/kg, or 20–23 METs. Heart patients tend to have much lower levels, in the range of 10–30 ml/min/kg. With increasing age, after the late teens or early twenties, there is a decline in VO_{2max} of roughly 0.5–1.0 ml/min/kg each year. However, the variation in individual VO_{2max} is far greater than the age variation.

© H.J.N. Bethell and D. Brodie 2023. *Exercise: A Scientific and Clinical Overview* (H.J.N. Bethell and D. Brodie)
DOI: 10.1079/9781800621855.0003

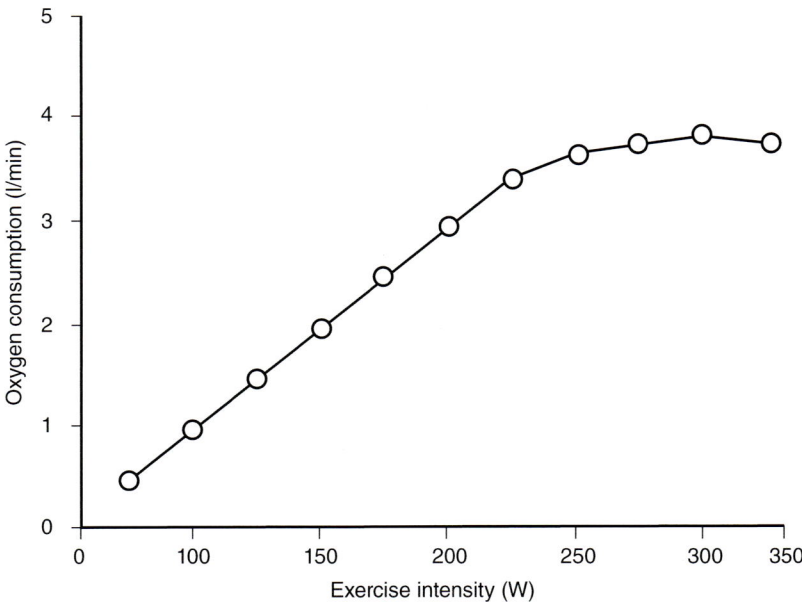

Fig. 3.1. Relationship between exercise intensity and oxygen uptake.

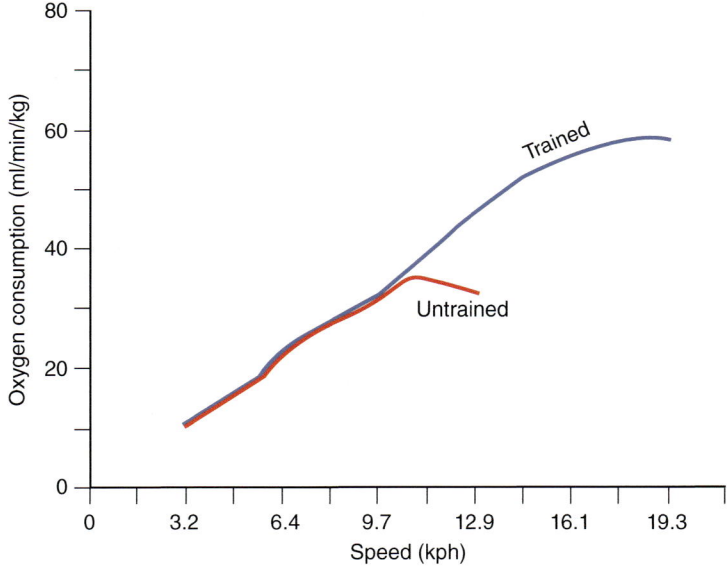

Fig. 3.2. Relationship between exercise intensity (running speed) and oxygen uptake – for the fit (trained) and unfit (untrained) subject.

Exercise to VO_{2max} can best be attained by using the large muscle groups of the legs. Because of their smaller bulk, maximum arm exercise will achieve only about two-thirds of maximum leg exercise. Also, once maximum oxygen uptake has been reached with leg exercise, bringing other muscles, like the arm muscles, into action will not increase oxygen uptake further. The limiting factor is not muscular effort, but the ability of the lungs and heart to supply oxygen to the muscles.

Oxygen Transport During Exercise

With progression from the resting state to exercise, the increase in oxygen uptake and transport is achieved by several changes, as follows.

Ventilation

Increased ventilation (breathing faster and deeper) brings more oxygen into contact with the capillary blood in the air sacs in the lungs. For people without lung disease, the saturation of oxygen in the blood does not fall with exercise, indicating that breathing and the lungs are not the limiting factor for exercise or for VO_{2max}.

Cardiac output – the amount of blood pumped out by the heart

At rest the normal heart rate is about 70 beats per minute (bpm). With each heartbeat about 70–80 ml of blood is pumped into the circulation – this is the stroke volume (SV). So the volume pumped out each minute is about 70×75, which comes to roughly 5.5 l/min – this is the resting cardiac output (CO).

With increasing exercise, the CO rises steadily with oxygen uptake to the point of VO_{2max} where it levels off at about 20–25 l/min. This four- to five-fold increase in CO is mediated by a more than doubling of the heart rate to 180–200 bpm and a less than doubling of SV to about 130 ml – i.e. the heart beats more rapidly and pumps out more blood with each stroke. There is an approximate straight-line relationship between increasing heart rate and increasing oxygen uptake.

The fit individual can perform a heavier workload than the unfit at any given heart rate. Getting fit by exercise training rarely changes the maximum heart rate (HR_{max}). The greater exercise level achieved by the fit individual is mediated by an increase in SV combined with more efficient oxygen use by the muscles (see Chapter 5, this volume).

In adults, HR_{max} reduces gradually with age and is very approximately 220 minus age. So a 20-year-old exercising maximally should reach a heart rate of about 200 bpm, while for a 70-year-old the rate would be around 150 bpm.

Extraction of blood by the muscles

The arteries supplying the muscles carry a full load of oxygen – the haemoglobin molecules are fully saturated with oxygen. The amount of oxygen extracted from the blood by the muscles depends on how hard the muscles are working. At rest the muscles extract about 5.5 ml of oxygen for every 100 ml of blood flow, rising to about 17 ml of oxygen during maximal exercise. This is achieved partly by an increased rate of oxygen uptake by each muscle fibre and partly by an increased blood flow to the muscles. Working muscles may use up to 18 times as much oxygen as at rest.

One set of muscles involved in exercise, the heart muscle or myocardium, differs from striated, voluntary muscle. Unlike the voluntary muscles, heart muscle extracts as much oxygen from its blood supply as it can at all times – both when 'resting' and when working at full capacity. Therefore the only way in which heart muscle can get more oxygen is by an increase in blood flow. This becomes important for people with narrowing of their coronary arteries (see 'Coronary Heart Disease (CHD)', Chapter 15, this volume).

Combined effect on oxygen uptake

For a young person of average fitness, the increase of VO_2 from rest to maximum exercise is about 12-fold – mediated by a fourfold rise in CO (heart rate up by 2.7 times and SV up by 1.4 times) and a threefold rise in arteriovenous oxygen difference.

VO_{2max} varies with age, sex and habitual physical activity. With increasing age, both HR_{max} and SV decline, as do muscle bulk and strength. The fall in VO_{2max} each year is between 0.5 and 1 ml/min/kg body weight. Although increasing age brings decreasing fitness, the variation between individuals is much greater than the variation with age – mainly because of the effect of habitual activity. Women, who have smaller frames and smaller hearts than men but more fat, have a VO_{2max} that is about 20% lower than in men. The influence of habitual activity on fitness will be discussed in Chapter 6 (this volume).

Summary

Oxygen is a major component of energy production in many exercises. Oxygen consumption rises in proportion to exercise intensity until alternative energy systems take over. This point of maximum oxygen uptake is a key measure in physical fitness. It is associated with ventilation, cardiac output and extraction of blood by the muscles. It is affected by a number of factors including training, age and gender.

4 Exercise Dose

There are two good reasons for considering exercise as a 'dose' and therefore wanting to measure it:

1. Exercise has widespread health benefits and can therefore be equated to medication. Sir Liam Donaldson, England's Chief Medical Officer in 2010 stated, 'If a medication existed which had a similar effect to physical activity, it would be regarded as a "wonder drug" or a "miracle cure".' The question remains about how big a dose is needed to help weight control, for instance, or to reduce the risk of diabetes or to lengthen life? What is the dose response – i.e. the ratio between the dose of exercise and the extent of any benefits? What would be the dose required to produce the same life-prolonging effect as, for example, taking a cholesterol-lowering drug like simvastatin at 40 mg per day? The answers are never straightforward. For instance, the intensity with which the exercise is performed changes its effect on health. An hour's brisk walking may equate to the same exercise dose as walking about slowly all day, but the effects will be very different.

2. Exercise is on one side of the equation that decides weight change. A comparison of the calorie content of ingested food with the calorie output of exercise helps to explain changes in weight and what is needed to reverse undesirable weight gain. For this purpose, the intensity of the exercise should be less important than the total dose.

There are several ways of expressing the amount of exercise undertaken and all are related to the oxygen cost of the activity.

Rate of Exertion

This is the measure of exercise intensity which tells us the rate of oxygen consumption. It can be expressed as an absolute rate – i.e. litres of oxygen per minute (l/min) – or, as was shown in Chapter 3 (this volume), relative to the exerciser's weight as millilitres of oxygen per minute per kilogram of body weight (ml/min/kg). The weight-related figure can be divided by 3.5 to give the rate of exertion in METs (metabolic equivalents). An example would be the rate of oxygen consumption required by a 70 kg man walking on a treadmill at, say, 4 miles/h (mph) – this takes approximately 17 ml/min/kg or 4.9 METs and equates to about 1.2 litres of oxygen per minute. The heavier the individual, the more effort is needed to move from one place to another. Thus for a 100 kg man the equivalent figures would still be 17 ml/min/kg or 4.9 METs, but this would equate to about 1.7 litres of oxygen per minute. This explains why fat people get more out of breath with exercise than thin people.

Total Energy Expended

This is represented by the total oxygen consumed by a particular period of exercise and is the actual dose of exercise taken. In the example given above, if the 70 kg man walks at 4 mph for 10 minutes, he will have consumed 12 litres of oxygen, while the heavier man will have consumed 17 litres. These figures can be converted into calories, or the metric equivalent, joules.

Unfortunately, common usage has made the calorie a more complicated unit than it need be. A calorie is the amount of energy (in the form of heat) needed to increase the temperature of 1 ml of water by 1°C. Since this is such a small amount of energy, nearly everybody works in kilocalories (kcals or Calories – note the capital C), i.e. calories multiplied by 1000. Confusingly, many people call the kcal a calorie! So for figures measured in calories, particularly in relation to food, the writer usually means kcals! It would be a lot simpler to change to the metric equivalent, joules, but calories are deeply ingrained in our language and culture, so that is unlikely to happen. One little calorie is equivalent to about 4.2 joules and one big Calorie or kcal is equivalent to about 4.2 kilojoules (kJ).

In human physiology, each litre of oxygen used is converted into about 5 Calories of energy or about 21 kJ. In the cases of the walking men above, in 10 minutes the thinner man has used 12 (litres) × 5 (Calories) = 60 Calories, or 12 × 21 = 252 kJ. The fatter man has used 85 Calories or 357 kJ. This system may be useful to assess the dose of exercise in relation to how much food it takes to fuel a certain amount of effort. It is a sad fact that it takes a disappointingly small quantity of food to fuel enormous efforts! One Mars bar will provide enough energy for 40 minutes of brisk walking at 4 mph for the thin man. An often-quoted index of high-calorie food is its equivalence in teaspoonfuls of sugar. A teaspoonful is just slightly over 5 ml, which converts to about 4 g of sugar, which is worth about 15 Calories.

Total exercise dose can also be calculated as MET minutes or MET hours (Bushman, 2012). As explained above, a MET, or metabolic equivalent, is the rate at which energy is used by the body at rest. It is expressed in relation to body weight and is taken as 3.5 ml of oxygen per minute per kilogram of body weight. A 70 kg man walking at 4 mph will be exercising at about 5 METs. If he maintains this pace for an hour, he will have expended 5 × 60 = 300 MET minutes. It is an interesting exercise to calculate the total number of MET minutes of exercise expended in a week – though it may demand a degree of obsessiveness to do so. It will require adding up the MET minutes of all the exercise undertaken overall. The actual energy cost of each exercise can only be an approximation and evidence from research into exercise recall suggests this will be an overestimate!

It is then possible to convert the exercise dose from MET minutes into Calories using this formula:

Total MET minutes × 3.5 ×
 body weight in kilograms ÷
 200 = number of Calories used

For example, the 70 kg man walking briskly for an hour will have used:

$$5 \times 60 \times 3.5 \times 70 \div 200 = 367.5 \text{ Calories}$$

For health benefits for most adults, the national guidelines suggest using exercise to burn about 900 Calories per week, roughly 150 minutes of brisk walking. Weight loss usually requires an expenditure of at least 1800 Calories per week, which is equivalent to about 5 hours of walking. This level of effort also brings appreciably greater benefits for other aspects of health.

Unfortunately it is not easy to measure exercise intensity or dose, however we choose to do it or to express it. It is difficult to specify an exact amount of energy for any given exercise. This is because very few exercises are sufficiently independent of the effort we put into them, or of our skill in their performance. Those that are more predictable include walking, cycling and running – on the flat without a wind, ideally indoors on a treadmill or cycle ergometer. For most other exercise we can only give approximations of energy expenditure. For instance, it is possible to give rough estimates of the energy costs of playing tennis or of various gym activities, but they will be very dependent on the amount of effort and skill put into the activity by the performer.

The use of modern accelerometer devices (Fitbit, Garmin, etc.) should allow more accurate estimates of the amount of exercise taken. They rely on heart-rate responses and often GPS (Global Positioning System) coordinates, so would need to be calibrated to the individual to produce anything like accurate measures of energy expenditure.

There are endless tables indicating the intensity of different sorts of exercise – usually expressed either as METs required or oxygen cost. None is particularly accurate because the answer depends so much on how hard the exerciser is working. However, they do give some idea of the exercise intensity of different activities. Table 4.1 below is an example. An approximation of the number of Calories used per hour for a 70 kg individual has been added.

Table 4.1 can give only a very rough estimate of the energy cost of these activities. The values approximate to the cost for the average-sized individual making an average effort. More detailed estimates can be found elsewhere (Ainsworth *et al.*, 2000). There are also online calculators for giving the energy cost of walking, running, cycling, skipping and rowing, taking into account the individual's weight, speed and duration of exercise (Mackenzie, 2002).

The exercise that the majority of people do most is walking – and excellent exercise it is too. Brisk walking is all that is needed to satisfy the recommendations of most health gurus, so Table 4.2 below gives exercise intensities of walking at different speeds.

Table 4.1. Approximate energy values for a range of physical activities.

Physical activity	MET value	VO$_2$ (ml/min/kg)	Calories per hour
Light-intensity activities	<3		
Sleeping	0.9	3.1	63
Watching television	1.0	3.5	70
Writing, desk work, typing	1.5	5.2	106
Strolling, 1.7 mph (2.7 kilometres per hour (kph), level ground)	2.3	8.1	162
Walking, 2.5 mph (4 kph)	2.9	10.1	205
Moderate-intensity activities	3 to 6		
Stationary cycling, 50 W, very light	3.0	10.5	212
Walking, 3 mph (4.8 kph)	3.3	11.5	233
Playing golf	3.5	12.2	247
Calisthenics, home exercise, light or moderate effort	3.5	12.2	247
Walking, 3.4 mph (5.5 kph)	3.6	12.6	254
Cycling, <10 mph (16 kph)	4.0	14.0	282
Doubles tennis	5.0	17.5	353
Heavy gardening	5.5	19.2	388
Stationary cycling, 100 W, light	5.5	19.2	388
Sexual activity	5.8	20.3	409
Vigorous-intensity activities	>6		
Jogging	7.0+	24.5+	494
Singles tennis, squash, racketball	7.0–12.0	24.5–42.0	494–847
Calisthenics (e.g. push-ups, sit-ups, pull-ups, star jumps), vigorous effort	8.0	28.0	565
Running on the spot	8.0	28.0	565
Rope skipping	10.0	35.0	706

Table 4.2. Energy expenditure for walking at different speeds.

Speed (mph)	Minutes per mile	MET value	VO$_2$ (ml/min/kg)	Calories per hour
2.0	30	2.5	8.9	176
2.5	24	2.9	10.2	205
3.0	20	3.3	11.5	233
3.5	17	3.7	12.9	261
3.75	16	4.4	15.3	310
4.0	15	4.9	17.1	346

The figures given are for walking on the flat with neither a following nor a head wind. The MET values are the same for everyone irrespective of weight. The final column is the Calories consumed per hour for a 70 kg (11 stone) individual. Lighter people will expend fewer Calories and heavier people will expend more. This implies that one advantage of being overweight is that the heavier the subject, the easier it *should* be to expend Calories to lose weight. Of course, it is never as simple as that because an overweight person is less likely to maintain a brisk pace for long.

The relationship between walking speed and oxygen need is a straight line at lower speeds, but above 3 mph it becomes harder to increase speed – and each increment in speed becomes more costly in terms of oxygen demand. For most people, brisk walking means travelling at between 3 and 4 mph.

Jogging/running is the most straightforward form of more vigorous exercise and is a highly efficient way of increasing fitness. It takes little time, needs minimal equipment and expenditure, and does not require an opponent. It can become a most satisfying social occasion as many running groups will testify. The exercise intensities for running at different speeds are given in Table 4.3 below. Again, the figures presume the unlikely scenario of no hills and no wind, and the Calorie

Table 4.3. Approximate energy values for running at different speeds.

Speed (mph)	Minutes per mile	MET value	VO$_2$ (ml/min/kg)	Calories per hour
3.5	17 min	6.4	22.3	451
4.0	15 min	7.1	24.9	501
4.5	13 min 20 s	7.9	27.6	558
5.0	12 min	8.7	30.3	614
5.5	10 min 54 s	9.4	33.0	663
6.0	10 min	10.2	35.7	720
6.5	9 min 13 s	11.0	38.3	776
7.0	8 min 34 s	11.7	41.0	826
7.5	8 min	12.5	43.7	882
8.0	7 min 30 s	13.3	46.4	939
8.5	7 min 40 s	14.0	49.1	988
9.0	6 min 40 s	14.8	51.7	1045
9.5	6 min 19 s	15.5	54.4	1094
10.0	6 min	16.3	57.1	1150

Table 4.4. Approximate energy values for cycling at different speeds.

Speed (mph)	MET value	VO$_2$ (ml/min/kg)	Calories per hour
10	5	17.5	470
12	7	24.5	514
14	9	31.5	661
16	11.5	40.2	845
18	14	49.0	1200

expenditure is that of an individual weighing 70 kg (11 stone).

Running at low speeds is less efficient than walking. At 4 mph, walking uses less energy than running.

Cycling is another exercise for which it is possible to calculate energy expenditure. Table 4.4 presents the very approximate figures for the MET value, oxygen cost and Calorie expenditure for cycling on the flat without wind for a 70 kg (11 stone) individual. Real-life conditions mean that the energy costs are usually much higher.

Summary

The measurement of exercise dose allows comparison of the effects of exercise with other health-giving measures such as nutrition and medication. Exercise dose is best expressed as oxygen uptake. The rate of oxygen uptake is used to define intensity of exercise and the total oxygen uptake over a period of exertion defines total exercise dose or volume. The rate of uptake can be expressed as litres of oxygen per minute, and this can be individualized by relating it to body weight – millilitres per minute per kilogram of body weight. The basal rate of oxygen use is approximately 3.5 ml/min/kg, and this is known as a metabolic equivalent (MET). METs multiplied by the duration of the activity (MET hours or MET minutes) reflect total exercise dose and can be converted to calories or joules.

References

Ainsworth, B.E., Haskell, W.L., Whitt, M.C., Irwin, M.L., Swartz, A.M., *et al.* (2000) Compendium of physical activities: an update of activity codes and MET intensities. *Medicine and Science in Sports and Exercise* 32(9 Suppl.), S498–S516.

Bushman, B.A. (2012) How can I use METs to quantify the amount of aerobic exercise? *ACSM's Health & Fitness Journal* 16(2), 5–7.

Mackenzie, B. (2002) Energy Expenditure. Available at: https://www.brianmac.co.uk/energyexp.htm (accessed 11 January 2023).

5 Physical Fitness: The Best Measure of Exercise Capacity

There are several ways to describe a person's level of physical fitness, including maximum oxygen uptake (VO_{2max}), exercise capacity and aerobic capacity. As seen previously, VO_{2max} is the standard measure of physical fitness. The level for a young to middle-aged adult averages between 30 and 50 ml/min/kg – about 8.5–14 METs.

The increase in VO_{2max} that can be attained by physical training is inversely proportional to the starting VO_{2max}. The less active the individual has been, the less fit he or she has become, the more will be gained from training. An inactive, unfit person can improve by a greater percentage than an out-of-training athlete, though they will not attain such a high level. The increase may exceed 30% in young, unfit individuals who begin to train intensively. Older subjects show a smaller response to training than younger ones.

Figure 5.1 shows the effects of fitness level on heart rate, and therefore on oxygen uptake, as exercise intensity increases. The fitter the individual, the more exercise can be performed, i.e. the more oxygen that can be absorbed and used, for any given heart rate. It is HR_{max}, the maximum heart rate, that limits the ability to exercise maximally. Subsequently, the higher the level of fitness, the greater will be an individual's maximal effort capacity. For most people, for most of the time, it is 'submaximal exercise' that is more important. Few people exercise maximally, but everyone exercises submaximally (i.e. at a defined level which is lower than the peak that can be reached). In this case, at any exercise level, a fit person will expend a lower proportion of what is maximally achievable. The consequence is that a standard effort becomes easier as fitness improves.

The increased aerobic capacity produced by training is brought about by a mixture of 'central' and 'peripheral' effects. Central effects include:

1. *Improved cardiac performance* – after training, the heart is able to contract more efficiently, pumping out a larger volume of blood with each beat. The SV increases. At rest, the body's need for oxygen and therefore the CO is the same for the fit as for the unfit person. A fit individual will pump out more blood with each beat (the SV) than the unfit. This results in a lower resting heart rate, perhaps as low as 50 bpm in a very fit person. In extremely fit people such as international cyclists, resting heart rates in the order of 40 bpm are not uncommon.

During submaximal exercise, again the need for circulating blood and oxygen delivery is the same in trained and untrained people. So at any given level of exercise the CO is the same for the fit as for the unfit. However, once again, the SV is higher and the heart rate is lower for the fit. Submaximal exercise is subsequently easier for the fit than for the unfit and achieved with a lower heart rate.

Maximal oxygen uptake, however, is increased by physical training. The HR_{max} does not increase, but CO is greater because SV is greater. More blood and oxygen can be pumped to the working muscles, which can therefore do more work. That is why the fit long-distance runner can run at a much higher, consistent pace than the unfit.

2. *Reduced sympathetic tone* – the resistance to flow in the peripheral blood vessels is partly determined by the tone of the 'sympathetic' nervous system. This includes the network of nerves that supply the tiny muscles which can contract and narrow small arteries. Physical training reduces this tone and opens up peripheral arteries, allowing blood to flow more freely through them and reducing BP at rest and during exercise. The heart has to work less hard to pump blood around the circulatory system.

3. *Changes in blood* – the trained individual has a greater total blood volume and more oxygen-bearing red cells. 'Blood doping' relies on this effect to improve the performance of athletes. Blood doping is a technique used by athletes to cheat the system. Blood is taken and stored long before a competition and is then transfused back just prior to the event.

DOI: 10.1079/9781800621855.0005

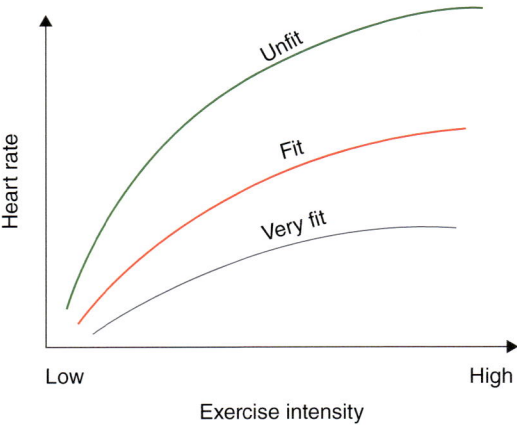

Fig. 5.1. Relationship between exercise intensity and heart rate at different levels of fitness.

This gives the athlete the enhanced advantage of a greater blood volume and red cell mass than could be achieved by simple training alone. A similar effect can also be achieved by training at high altitude or by sleeping in a tent with lower oxygen concentration than is found in the atmosphere.

Peripheral effects of physical training include:

1. *Increased muscle performance* – trained muscles exhibit a number of changes. They become larger, they develop more mitochondria (the enzyme packages within muscle cells that are concerned with energy production) and they have a better ability to extract oxygen and glucose from the blood.

2. *Increased muscle blood flow* – the larger muscles have a greater network of capillaries feeding them and the distribution of blood flow favours working muscles over inactive muscles.

3. *Increased arteriovenous oxygen difference* – better muscle performance and more efficient blood flow causes an increase in the overall extraction of oxygen from the blood. This results in the venous blood carrying blood back to the heart having less oxygen left in it. This is most marked at maximal effort.

Combined central and peripheral effects depend upon age:

1. In *young people*, the training-induced increase in maximal aerobic capacity is brought about equally by central and peripheral effects. The exact magnitude of the central training effect is related to the size of the muscles being used. Training of leg muscles has a greater effect than training of arm muscles.

Training of one set of muscles will result in increased exercise capacity when a different set of muscles is used, but the improvement is only about half that achieved by exercise with the trained muscles. Elegant experiments have shown that individuals trained in one-legged cycling on an ergometer do show an improved performance with the untrained leg, but this is still much less than for the trained leg (Klausen *et al.*, 1982).

2. *Older people* react rather differently – the central effects of training are less pronounced, and the peripheral effects are more important.

Measuring Physical Fitness

The basis for most measurements of physical fitness is observation of the level of key physiological indices during a standard amount of exercise. As fitness improves, then these indices will also improve when the specified amount of exercise is repeated.

As has been described in Chapter 3 (this volume), the best measure of physical fitness or aerobic capacity is the maximal oxygen uptake or VO_{2max}. However, most methods of measuring physical fitness or aerobic capacity estimate VO_{2max} rather than measuring it directly.

VO_{2max} can be measured directly, but it is a time-consuming business and needs specialized and expensive equipment. It is usually performed in a laboratory or clinical setting on a calibrated cycle ergometer or on a treadmill. The candidate performs the exercise while breathing through a tube connected to an oxygen analyser, which measures the rate at which oxygen is being extracted from the inhaled air. The individual is subjected to a steadily increasing workload until he or she can continue no longer. Real-time display of oxygen uptake shows a linear increase with increasing workload until the maximal oxygen uptake is reached. At this point the graph levels off at what is known as the 'anaerobic threshold' – the exerciser is capable of a bit more effort, but very soon has to stop from exhaustion. Increasing oxygen uptake is facilitated by increasing heart rate, which follows a similar trajectory, increasing to its maximum at peak exercise (Fig. 5.2).

Maximum oxygen uptake – VO_{2max} – is usually between 1.5 and 3.5 litres per minute. This is converted into millilitres per minute per kilogram of body weight by multiplying by 1000 and dividing by the weight of the individual. It can be further converted into metabolic equivalents (METs) by

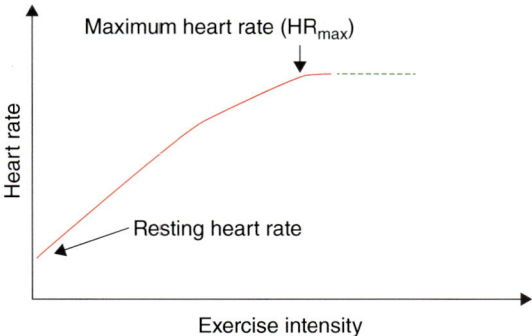

Fig. 5.2. Relationship between exercise intensity and heart rate.

dividing by 3.5, since a MET is 3.5 ml/min/kg (see Chapter 3, this volume). So for a 70 kg (11 stone) person with an oxygen uptake at maximum effort of 2 litres per minute:

$$VO_{2max} = 2000 \text{ ml/min}$$

and

2000 ÷ 70 gives the oxygen consumption in millilitres per minute per kilogram of body weight = 28.6 ml/min/kg

$$MET_{max} = 28.6 ÷ 3.5 = 8.16 \text{ METs}$$

Most measurements of fitness, however, estimate oxygen uptake by relying on the known oxygen cost of the exercise being undertaken.

The motorized treadmill is the most popular exercise machine for use in the laboratory or clinic. A variety of different protocols can be used, the most popular being the famous Bruce protocol, devised by the Seattle-based cardiologist Robert Bruce. The treadmill is started at 1.7 mph with a 10° slope and is increased every 3 minutes through seven stages to the maximum of 6.0 mph and a 22° slope. The time spent on the treadmill before exhaustion can be used to predict VO_{2max}. Even the standard Bruce protocol has a number of modifications. Some start at a higher speed and progress to ten stages, and others, more suitable for sedentary or elderly subjects, progress more slowly.

Cycle ergometers are much more portable than treadmills and are the most popular instruments for use in 'field' studies. Estimation of exercise intensity requires the work achieved on the cycle to be measured with as much precision as is possible. The resistance to pedalling and speed of pedalling decide the workload. With mechanically braked cycles the resistance depends upon a weight applied to the braking system, and if workload is to be calculated the subject must cycle at a constant speed, using a metronome. For electronically braked machines the workload is set at the required level and resistance then varies with pedal speed, so a constant pedalling rate is not required. Workload is usually measured in watts (W – i.e. joules per second). Peak wattage for a champion cyclist such as sprinter Mark Cavendish is about 1600 W and Chris Boardman could maintain 400 W for over an hour when he held the world one-hour record.

Again, a variety of protocols may be used. One such protocol starts the individual at 25, 50 or 75 W and increases the workload by 25 W every 3–5 minutes – long enough to reach 'steady-state' exercise. The cyclist continues to exhaustion and the oxygen uptake at this point is calculated from a knowledge of the oxygen cost of cycling.

Measuring Personal Fitness

There are a number of benefits from being able to measure your personal fitness:

- It can give an indication of personal fitness in comparison with others of the same sex and age. People should be concerned if they find themselves to be average or less than average. This is because most people are far less fit than they should be. Individuals should not be content with anything less than 'above average'.
- Measuring personal fitness should stimulate individuals to take up or increase exercise, especially if their levels are less than satisfactory.
- It gives a benchmark to measure future improvements and the effectiveness of whatever exercise is being undertaken.

The simplest approximate indicator of physical fitness is resting heart rate. For men any level above 70 and for women above 80 bpm may indicate reduced fitness. These levels work for large groups in identifying increased risk of cardiovascular disease (CVD) and cancers (Nanchen, 2017), but are too imprecise for the individual. Certain drugs such as beta blockers will artificially decrease the heart rate, thus providing a false indication of fitness using resting heart rate alone.

There are several ways in which you can estimate your own VO_{2max} accurately enough to be useful.

The Cooper test

One of earliest of these, and still highly regarded, is the Cooper test, devised by Dr Kenneth Cooper from the USA in the 1960s (Cooper, 1968). It is suitable for anyone with the ability to walk unaided and is simple to administer.

The Cooper test measures how far a person can travel on foot in 12 minutes. This may appear simple, yet it gives a remarkably accurate indicator of VO_{2max}. When covering the distance, it is important to be aware of personal limitations. Younger people and fitter older people can comfortably run for 12 minutes. For some, this is too demanding. If this is so, an alternative is to try a 'walk-jog', by alternating fast walking with jogging. Older people and those who have not run for many years are best doing it at the fastest walk they can manage. Sadly, 12 minutes of continuous exercise is longer than many people have experienced on a regular basis. It is important that the activity is undertaken at an even pace, so ensure that it is not started too fast.

There are several ways of undertaking the test with accuracy:

1. Using a smartphone, download a Cooper test app and just follow the instructions. The phone will measure the distance covered in 12 minutes, work out the VO_{2max} and record the results. The app will also explain how the results compare with others of the same age and gender. Misleadingly, it gives the same comparisons for everyone over the age of 60, so does not do justice to older people (see below for a broader age spread of normal values).
2. Use a GPS watch to measure the distance covered in 12 minutes.
3. Use a measured athletics track or undertake the measurements on any reasonable-sized playing field, and note the laps and the distance around the track covered in 12 minutes.

Tables 5.1 and 5.2, which are adapted from Dr Cooper's findings, set out the results from the distance covered in the 12 minutes and provide the normative results for 10-year age groups of men and women, respectively. They give both VO_{2max} and how to compare results with anyone of the same age and sex. Since Dr Cooper's figures stop at the age of 'over 60', age predictions for 70–79-year-olds and 80–89-year-olds have been added. These predictions apply only to those who are able to complete 12 minutes of walking/running, which may not be the case for many older people. For

Table 5.1. Results of the 12-minute run fitness test for men.

Age (years)	Average distance covered (m)	Average VO_{2max} (ml/min/kg)
20–29	2200–2399	40.1
30–39	1900–2299	35.6
40–49	1700–2099	31.2
50–59	1600–1999	28.9
60–69	1400–1700	23.4
70–79	1300–1600	21.1
80–89	1100–1400	18.0

Table 5.2. Results of the 12-minute run fitness test for women.

Age (years)	Average distance covered (m)	Average VO_{2max} (ml/min/kg)
20–29	1800–2199	33.4
30–39	1700–1999	30.1
40–49	1500–1899	26.7
50–59	1400–1699	23.4
60–69	1300–1600	21.1
70–79	1200–1500	18.9
80–89	1100–1400	17.8

them, the 6-minute walk test (see Tables 5.3 and 5.4 below) is a much better measure of their fitness and how it compares to the population at large.

To calculate your estimated VO_{2max} (in ml/kg/min) from the distance travelled in 12 minutes, use either of these formulas:

- In miles: $VO_{2max} = (35.97 \times miles) - 11.29$
- In kilometres: $VO_{2max} = (22.351 \times km) - 11.29$

The Rockport walk test

The Cooper test requires maximal energy expenditure and many middle-aged or older people find it daunting – or even frightening. An alternative is the Rockport test which depends upon heart-rate response to less extreme efforts. However, it cannot be used for people who take heart-rate-slowing medication like beta blockers. Some people have heart responses well below the normal response, known as chronotropic incompetence, and the test is unsuitable for them too.

This is a 1-mile walk test, which is suitable for those who do not wish to go at full speed. It uses weight (in kilograms), age (in years), gender (males = 1, females = 0), time taken to complete 1 mile (in minutes) and heart rate at completion of the test

Table 5.3. Results of the 6-minute walk fitness test for men.

Age (years)	Average distance covered (m)	Average VO$_{2max}$ (ml/min/kg)
65	596	18.6
70	568	18.0
75	534	17.2
80	487	16.3
85	427	15.5
90	403	14.2

Table 5.4. Results of the 6-minute walk fitness test for women.

Age (years)	Average distance covered (m)	Average VO$_{2max}$ (ml/min/kg)
65	535	17.3
70	510	16.7
75	482	16.0
80	443	15.1
85	406	14.3
90	358	13.1

(in beats per minute) to calculate VO$_{2max}$ using the following formula:

$$132.853 - 0.0769 \times (\text{Weight, kg}) - 0.3877 \times (\text{Age, years}) \\ + 6.315 \times (\text{Gender, 1 for males, 0 for females}) \\ - 3.2649 \times (\text{Time, min}) - 0.1565 \times (\text{Heart rate, bpm})$$

It is not necessary to work this all out. There are websites to do the numbers – once the age, weight, time taken and heart rate at the end are entered. Go to http://knightsofknee.com/calculators/Fitness TestCalc.htm (accessed 11 January 2023).

The 6-minute walk test

For older, less fit people and those with heart or lung diseases, a 6-minute walk is often used and has also been shown to give an acceptable prediction of VO$_{2max}$. The procedure is much the same as the Cooper test but for 6 rather than 12 minutes and walking as fast as possible. Table 5.3 (for men) and Table 5.4 (for women) present the normative results at different ages over 65. The estimate of fitness given by this method is considerably lower than that given by the Cooper 12-minute test. This is probably because the samples of individuals used to calculate the figures were rather different. This implies that the Cooper 12-minute test sample population was considerably fitter than the majority of

older people. Experience suggests that the 6-minute walk test results are more in keeping with the current UK population of elderly people.

There are numerous formulas for converting distance covered in the 6-minute test into VO$_{2max}$, but none is very accurate. Some involve body mass index (BMI) and can be very complicated to calculate. The best is this:

$$\text{VO}_{2max} = (\text{ml/min/kg}) = 0.023 \times 6\text{-minute} \\ \text{walk distance}(\text{m}) + 4.95$$

This works well for those whose maximum distance walked in 6 minutes is 600 metres or less, but underestimates VO$_{2max}$ for those who can go further. For such people, the full 12-min Cooper test is more accurate.

The 20-metre progressive shuttle test

This test, often called the bleep test, involves running between two lines spaced 20 metres apart, with the speed increasing approximately every minute. It was first described by Luc Léger (Léger et al., 1984) and is used to estimate the subject's aerobic capacity. If undertaken properly, the test is very demanding and is unsuitable for certain individuals as it can lead to exhaustion. The English rugby squad used it prior to winning the World Cup and described it as 'progressive paralysis'. One way to administer the test is to purchase a CD, which provides all the instructions. The test is used widely in many health-related fitness-test batteries but has been found to be unsuitable for some groups, including 11–14-year-old boys (Welsman and Armstrong, 2019).

Variations in Average Fitness Levels

The figures provided for average fitness levels at different ages must be considered cautiously. The average fitness level and the variation in fitness differ considerably from one test group to another. There have been many studies to try to determine the average fitness of the population as a whole, with variations from very unfit to very fit. The results of such surveys have produced wide discrepancies, largely because of the way in which the subjects have been selected and the nature of the testing systems used. In some cases the figures are derived from people who have volunteered to be tested; in other cases the sample is drawn from a particular set, such as those seeking routine health checks. In a relatively few cases the individuals being tested have been chosen randomly (Fentem *et al.*, 1994). Even for the most representative group tested, the average level of fitness will exceed reality because there will be a proportion of the subjects who have physical problems that prevent them completing the test. Their results are therefore discounted, thus raising the average of the group. Population measurements apply only to those who can complete the test. The proportion of people who are unable to do so increases with age, which means that the overestimate of population fitness levels is much greater for older age groups.

The difficulty in giving the normal range of physical fitness in the general population is illustrated by the two best and most representative investigations carried out in England over the past 30 years:

- The Allied Dunbar National Fitness Survey (ADNFS) in 1990 tested a sample of 1741 adults aged 16–74 chosen at random in 30 locations around the UK. They used a treadmill in a central mobile laboratory. For men, the average VO_{2max} fell from 55.5 ml/min/kg in the 16–34 age group to 32.0 ml/min/kg in the 65–74 age group (Fentem *et al.*, 1994).
- The Health Survey for England (HSE) in 2008 also tested a random sample – 1969 people – using a step test in the individuals' homes. For men, the average VO_{2max} fell from 40.9 ml/min/kg in the 16–34 age group to 29.9 ml/min/kg in

the 65–74 group (Health and Social Care Information Centre, 2009).

It would be expected that both studies should produce comparable results, but in practice the earlier study suggested that in 1990 the population of England was significantly fitter than it was in 2008. There are several explanations for such a disparity: perhaps the samples were in some way biased differently; the testing methods were not comparable; it was easier to get the subjects to exercise harder in a laboratory than in their own homes where emergency help was less available; or maybe we really are getting steadily less fit, the victims of our increasingly sedentary lifestyles.

All this explains why any table of normal fitness levels may be flawed. It can be helpful to know where an individual is placed in the range of possible fitness levels, so the tables below (Tables 5.5 and 5.6) have been constructed for this purpose. The tables have been compiled from a number of sources to give the best approximations for each age and sex (Fentem *et al.*, 1994; The Physical Fitness Specialist Certification Manual, 1997; Rikli and Jones, 1999; Fleg *et al.*, 2005; Health and Social Care Information Centre, 2009; Kokkinos *et al.*, 2014). They are only a guide but should permit interested parties to establish their position in the various fitness categories.

It is worth noting that after the mid-twenties, physical fitness declines throughout life – by about 0.5% per annum in early adult life but getting

Table 5.5. Range of VO_{2max} (in ml/min/kg) for men.

Age (years)	Poor	Below average	Average	Good	Very good
20–29	<35	35–38	38–45	45–50	>50
30–39	<31	31–35	35–41	41–49	>49
40–49	<30	30–33	33–39	39–48	>48
50–59	<26	26–31	31–36	36–45	>45
60–69	<21	21–29	29–33	33–41	>41
70–79	<15	15–25	25–29	29–36	>36

Table 5.6. Range of VO_{2max} (in ml/min/kg) for women.

Age (years)	Poor	Below average	Average	Good	Very good
20–29	<23	23–33	29–33	33–41	>41
30–39	<23	23–27	27–31	31–40	>40
40–49	<21	21–24	24–29	29–37	>37
50–59	<20	20–23	23–27	27–35	>35
60–69	<18	18–21.5	21–25	25–31	>31
70–79	<12	12–19	19–21	21–28	>28

steeper in middle age at about 1% each year and accelerating in old age to about 2% or more each year. This has been clearly demonstrated in a survey known as the FIT study of nearly 70,000 US citizens (Blaha *et al.*, 2016).

Undertaking moderate exercise does not change this rate of decline, but it does, of course, still give a higher fitness level at any age than being less active (Fleg *et al.*, 2005). More vigorous training in older athletes does decrease the rate of decline – to about 0.5% each year even in old age (Pollock *et al.*, 1987; Rogers *et al.*, 1990).

At any age, women are significantly less fit than men, mostly because they have a different body composition with a greater fat content. When the figures are adjusted so that the comparison is for fat-free mass, there is little difference between the sexes.

Summary

Physical fitness is influenced by improved cardiac performance, by reduced sympathetic tone, by changes in blood, by increased muscle performance and blood flow, and by increased arteriovenous oxygen difference. Physical fitness is measured by observing key physiological indices during standard exercise. Personal fitness can be measured by using simple tests such as the Cooper test, the Rockport walk test, the 6-minute walk test and the 20-metre progressive shuttle test.

References

Blaha, M.J., Hung, R.K., Dardarl, Z., Feldman, D.I., Whelton, S.P., *et al.* (2016) Age-dependent value of exercise capacity and derivation of fitness-associated biologic age. *Heart* 102, 431–437.

Cooper, K.H. (1968) A means of assessing maximal oxygen uptake. *Journal of the American Medical Association* 203, 201–204.

Fentem, P.H., Collins, M.F., Tuxworth, W., Walker, A., Hoinville, E., *et al.* (1994) *Allied Dunbar National Fitness Survey. Technical Report.* Allied Dunbar, Health Education Authority and Sports Council, London.

Fleg, J.L., Morrell, C.H., Bos, A.G., Brant, L.J., Talbot, L.A., *et al.* (2005) Accelerated longitudinal decline of aerobic capacity in healthy older adults. *Circulation* 112, 674–682.

Health and Social Care Information Centre (2009) *Health Survey for England – 2008: Physical Activity and Fitness.* Health and Social Care Information Centre, Leeds, UK.

Klausen, K., Secher, N.H., Clausen, J.P., Hartling, O. and Trap-Jensen, J. (1982) Central and regional circulatory adaptations to one-leg training. *Journal of Applied Physiology* 52, 976–983.

Kokkinos, P., Faselis, C., Myers, J., Sui, X., Zhang, J. and Blair, S.N. (2014) Age-specific exercise capacity threshold for mortality risk assessment in male veterans. *Circulation* 130, 653–658.

Léger, L., Lambert, J., Goulet, A., Rowan, C. and Dinelle, Y. (1984) Aerobic capacity of 6 to 17-year-old Quebecois – 20 meter shuttle run test with 1 minute stages. *Canadian Journal of Applied Sport Sciences/Journal Canadien des Sciences Appliquées au Sport* 9(2), 64–69.

Nanchen D. (2017) Resting heart rate: what is normal? *Heart* 104, 1076–1085.

The Physical Fitness Specialist Certification Manual (1997) The Cooper Institute for Aerobics Research, Dallas, Texas. Printed in Heyward, V.H. (1997) *Advance Fitness Assessment & Exercise Prescription*, 3rd edn. Human Kinetics Publishers, Champaign, Illinois, p. 48.

Pollock, M.L., Foster, C., Knapp, D., Rod, J.L. and Schmidt, D.H. (1987) Effect of age and training on aerobic capacity and body composition of master athletes. *Journal of Applied Physiology* 62, 725–731.

Rikli, R.E. and Jones, J.J. (1999) Functional fitness normative scores for community-residing older adults, ages 60–94. *Journal of Ageing and Physical Activity* 7, 162–181.

Rogers, M.A., Hagberg, J.M., Martin, W.H. 3rd, Ehsani, A.A. and Holloszy, J.O. (1990) Decline in VO_{2max} with aging in master athletes and sedentary men. *Journal of Applied Physiology* 68, 2195–2199.

Welsman, J. and Armstrong, N. (2019) The 20 m shuttle run is not a valid test of cardiorespiratory fitness in boys aged 11–14 years. *BMJ Open Sport & Exercise Medicine* 5(1), e000627. https://doi.org/10.1136/bmjsem-2019-000627

6 The Components of Overall Exercise Volume

This chapter is a summary of the elements that will contribute to most endurance (aerobic) exercise. The basic components of any exercise training programme involve the Frequency, Intensity, Time and Type of exercise, often abbreviated to the FITT principles. The success of any training programme will depend on the combination of these components. These will be considered in turn, and throughout this chapter the recommendations are aimed at the general population. Someone who is highly committed to exercise, such as an international athlete, will be capable of working at a much higher overall exercise volume.

Frequency

Figure 6.1 shows the relationship between exercise frequency and increase in fitness as measured by VO_{2max}.

Exercising once a week has little effect on improving fitness but may be just sufficient to maintain a given level of fitness. Twice weekly has a moderate effect, and three or four times weekly a far greater effect. Beyond that, in most people, there is a levelling off of the benefit of more frequent training. This does not suggest that there is *no* benefit from exercising more than, say, four times per week, but the increased benefit is substantially less. In addition, the more frequent the exercise sessions, the greater the risk of sprains and strains to joints and muscles. Thus the benefits of having a rest and recovery day in between exercise sessions are substantial, particularly in the older population.

In the special case of orthopaedic or cardiac complications, gains in fitness are less and progress slower. However, benefits can continue to increase when training daily. An example of this might be an elderly person recovering from certain types of hip replacement. The operation and early-stage recovery often involve lying in bed for some time and could have resulted in significant muscle wastage. As load bearing and movement will be very progressive, the increase in fitness will be slow, but will benefit most from daily exercise.

Intensity

Figure 6.2 shows the relationship between intensity of exercise, measured as the percentage of HR_{max} reached, and increase in fitness as measured by VO_{2max}.

Figure 6.2 shows that increasing effort results in increasing rewards, but there is a point beyond which the rate of increasing benefit becomes progressively less. This point is reached at approximately 70 to 85% of HR_{max}.

This figure of 70–85% of HR_{max} is therefore considered to be the optimal training threshold for improvements in aerobic fitness. As stated in Chapter 3 (this volume), peak or maximum heart rate is about 220 minus your age. This translates into 70% of HR_{max} being about 170 minus age and 85% of HR_{max} being about 195 minus age. These figures do not apply to those on heart-rate-slowing medication such as beta blockers and some calcium blocking agents.

For people with heart disease, exercising to very high heart rates brings an increased danger of complications, particularly disturbances of rhythm. For more specific guidance in such cases, it is prudent to follow the advice of a cardiac clinician or staff in a cardiac rehabilitation centre.

It is not always convenient to record heart rates while exercising. As a guide, when exercising at between 70 and 85% of HR_{max}, it is just about possible to talk to someone and be comfortably short of breath, but not gasping. As another rough guide, if it is possible to sing while exercising, the intensity is probably too low.

© H.J.N. Bethell and D. Brodie 2023. *Exercise: A Scientific and Clinical Overview*
(H.J.N. Bethell and D. Brodie)
DOI: 10.1079/9781800621855.0006

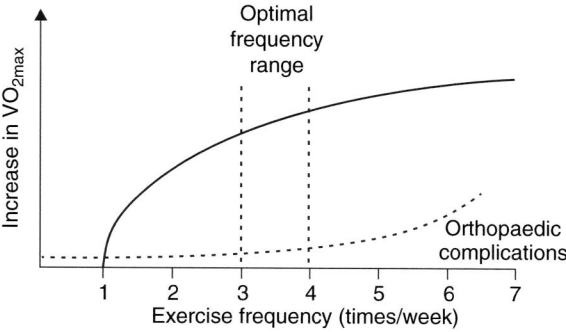

Fig. 6.1. Relationship between increase in fitness (VO_{2max}) and frequency of exercise sessions. (From Bethell, 1976.)

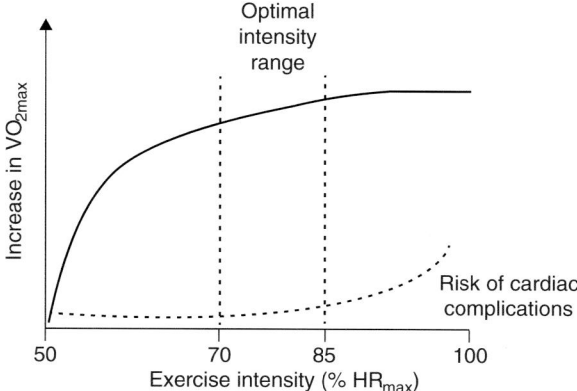

Fig. 6.2. Relationship between increase in fitness (VO_{2max}) and intensity of exercise sessions as measured by heart-rate response. (From Bethell, 1976.)

An alternative approach to establish the intensity of exercise is to rely on how hard it feels to exercise. This is termed a *rating of perceived exertion (RPE)*. The benefit of using the rating of perceived exertion is that it can be applied while exercising. When relying on heart rate, it is often necessary to stop to take the measurement. As soon as a person stops to measure the heart rate, it will slow down and give a false reading of exercise intensity. Pulse-rate monitors can overcome this, but many people prefer to rely simply on how hard the exercise *feels* to them. This is best achieved using the RPE scale devised by a Danish physiologist, Gunnar Borg, and named after him. There are two versions of the Borg scale (Tables 6.1 and 6.2) with one being linked more closely to exercise heart rate. The simpler one is expressed as a score from 0 to 10, with the numbers relating to a physical description of how hard the exerciser is finding the activity. Predicted HR_{max} usually reaches the 70–85% level at between

Table 6.1. The Borg scale of rating of perceived exertion – Version 1.

Score	Rating of perceived exertion
0	None
0.5	Very, very light
1	Very light
2	Light
3	Moderate
4	Somewhat heavy
5	Heavy
6	–
7	Very heavy
8	–
9	Very, very heavy
10	–

numbers 4 and 6 on the scale (Table 6.1). In the second version the numerical scale is set at one-tenth the expected heart rate for a young adult (Table 6.2).

Table 6.2. The Borg scale of rating of perceived exertion – Version 2.

Score	Rating of perceived exertion
6	–
7	Very, very light
8	–
9	Very light
10	–
11	Fairly light
12	–
13	Somewhat hard
14	–
15	Hard
16	–
17	Very hard
18	–
19	Very, very hard
20	–

Time

Figure 6.3 shows the relationship between duration of exercise sessions and increase in fitness as measured by VO_{2max}.

There is a steady increase in physical fitness for increase in duration of exercise up to about 30–40 minutes, but after that there is a flattening of the curve, with less and less benefit the greater the time spent training. Again, the more time spent training, the greater the risk of musculoskeletal injury.

Type of Exercise

The final 'T' in the FITT principle of Frequency, Intensity, Time and Type is the most variable. Different types of exercise are referenced throughout this book, but the Type of exercise is very much a matter of personal choice. The options are endless and lists of types of exercise that could be described as moderate, vigorous, best for aerobic fitness or for muscular strength are presented in the next section.

This book emphasizes the huge benefits to be gained by taking and increasing current levels of physical activity. Specific recommendations concerning the type of exercise to be undertaken are difficult, because everyone has different preferences, different needs, different experiences and different conditions imposed on their lifestyle. It is not uncommon to find high-class rowers who hate running. Similarly there are club runners who will avoid the weight room at all costs.

The key message is just do what will be enjoyable. There is substantial evidence, both from research and from experience, to demonstrate that an activity will do the most good if it is enjoyed and it results in being short of breath. If each person chooses an activity which satisfies these two criteria, then the outcome is most likely to be of greatest benefit. There is little evidence that any chosen type of exercise is better or worse than any other.

Overall Exercise Volume

The total amount of dynamic aerobic activity can be expressed as 'exercise volume', which is the product of average METs multiplied by the time involved in minutes. It has been suggested that the target for maintaining good health should be between 500 and 1000 MET minutes per week. As an example of walking at 3.5 mph, this uses about 6.4 METs. This good health target would take between 1 hour 18 minutes (500 MET minutes) and 2 hours 36 minutes (1000 MET minutes) of walking per week. If stepping out faster at, say, 4 mph (7.1 METs), the target is reached between 1 hour 10 minutes and 2 hours 20 minutes of walking per week.

The effectiveness of exercise is proportional to its intensity and total dose. From the above, it would be correct to presume that optimal exercising should be about 30 to 40 minutes of exercise three or four times per week to a level that makes you reasonably out of breath. This is also sufficient exercise to have a highly significant effect on both the prevention and treatment of a number of diseases.

It is insufficient exercise for those who wish to compete to a high level in their sport. Committed runners, cyclists, squash players, footballers, competitive tennis players and any other high-level performers need to be far fitter than would be allowed by this relatively modest regimen. As stated earlier, there is always the risk of injury for their sport as the total exercise volume increases. This is especially the case in older competitive sportspeople.

The current UK National Health Service (NHS) guidelines recommend a mix of aerobic exercise and muscle strengthening (Department of Health and Social Care, 2019).

To stay healthy, adults aged 19–64 should try to be active almost every day and should do:

- at least 150 minutes (2 hours and 30 minutes) of moderate-intensity aerobic activity such as cycling or fast walking every week, *and*

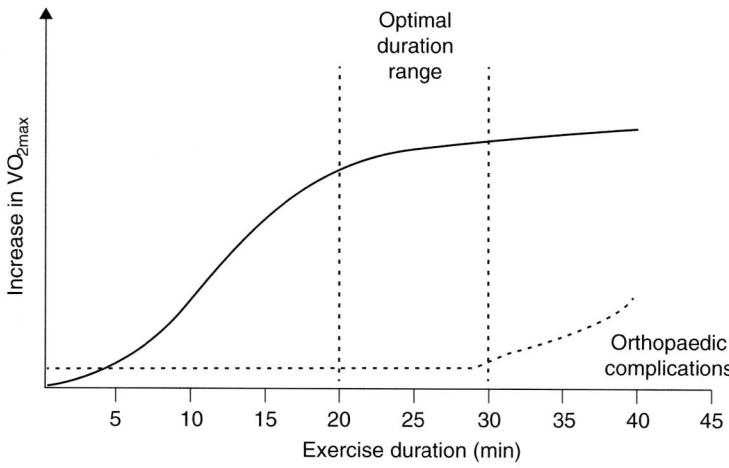

Fig. 6.3. Relationship between increase in fitness (VO_{2max}) and duration of exercise sessions. (From Bethell, 1976.)

- muscle-strengthening activities on two or more days a week that work all major muscle groups (legs, hips, back, abdomen, chest, shoulders and arms);

OR

- 75 minutes (1 hour and 15 minutes) of vigorous-intensity aerobic activity such as running or a game of singles tennis every week, *and*
- muscle-strengthening activities on two or more days a week that work all major muscle groups (legs, hips, back, abdomen, chest, shoulders and arms);

OR

- an equivalent mix of moderate- and vigorous-intensity aerobic activity every week (e.g. two 30-minute runs plus 30 minutes of fast walking), *and*
- muscle-strengthening activities on two or more days a week that work all major muscle groups (legs, hips, back, abdomen, chest, shoulders and arms).

As an indication, 1 minute of vigorous-intensity activity is about the same as 2 minutes of moderate-intensity activity.

One simple way to achieve the recommended 150 minutes of weekly physical activity is to exercise for 30 minutes on five days a week.

Moderate activities

Examples of activities that require moderate effort for most people include:

- walking fast;
- water aerobics;

- riding a bicycle on level ground or with few hills;
- doubles tennis;
- pushing a lawnmower;
- hiking;
- skateboarding;
- rollerblading;
- volleyball;
- basketball;
- gardening; and
- housework.

The first example given above is walking fast and this activity has received considerable interest in recent years. The key is the word *fast*. It has been shown (Zaccardi *et al.*, 2019) that the speed at which people walk is in itself a good indicator of overall fitness. They state that 'Fast walkers can live up to 20 years longer.' Speed of walking even seems to impact on the outcome of Covid-19. Slow walkers were 2.5 times more likely to develop severe Covid-19 than faster walkers, even among those of a healthy weight (Yates *et al.*, 2021). Dr William Bird, the general practitioner (GP) behind the Health Walks initiative, makes the point that fast walking will develop calf and thigh muscles, increase the resting metabolic rate and target the unhealthy visceral fat.

Brisk walks can reduce the risk of heart disease by a quarter in women under 50. A study of 97,000 women, undertaken at Indiana University (Chomistek *et al.*, 2016), showed that the most active women had a 25% lower incidence of coronary heart disease (CHD) 20 years later. This study was confirmed by Studentski (2019), who showed that slowest walkers aged roughly 5 years faster than the quickest. Slow walkers were also at greater risk of memory loss and dementia (see Chapter 20, this volume) and the author concludes by stating that a slow walk is a problem sign decades before old age (Studentski, 2019).

Another study (Grazzi et al., 2020) showed that the faster the walking speed, the lower the risk of hospitalization for people with heart disease and also the shorter the length of stay in hospital. The study was based on a group of nearly 2000 people and the difference was quite remarkable. Fast walkers spent almost 1000 days in hospital over the 3 years of the study, yet the slow walkers spent over 4000 days in hospital.

Walking faster improves heart health in people of all ages, but its greatest effect is with those over 60 years of age. A study involving 420,000 individuals from the UK Biobank showed a significant link between higher walking pace and reduced risk of death from CVD (Dempsey et al., 2022). As discussed in Chapter 9 (this volume), it is important to be careful about assigning one aspect of physical activity to be the cause of premature death. None the less, the health message is still the same: brisk walking appears extremely beneficial.

The penultimate item included in the list of moderate activities is gardening. The benefits of gardening have been shown from studies on both its energy cost and the impact on mortality. Digging can use up to 300 Calories per hour and pushing a manual lawnmower, even more. An American study on 88,000 people over 9 years has shown that for people aged 40 to 85 years, those who did from 10 to 60 minutes of activity, including gardening, were 18% less likely to die (Soga et al., 2016).

The last item in the list above is housework. It has been shown from a study in Amsterdam (Lachman et al., 2018) that doing the housework in retirement is enough to cut the risk of heart disease and strokes by 14%. This is especially true for people who are unable to hit the NHS target of 150 minutes of moderate exercise a week using other activities in the list. Another study, based on 130,000 people in 17 countries (Lear et al., 2017), supported the notion that the more active the better and housework and gardening can be included in the list of activities, provided they raise the heart rate for a time period like 30 minutes.

Moderate-intensity activity will raise the heart rate and make individuals breathe faster and feel warmer. As stated above, an indication of working at a moderate intensity is being able to talk but not able to sing the words to a song.

Vigorous activities

There is substantial evidence that vigorous-intensity activities can bring health benefits well above that of moderate-intensity activities. Examples of activities that require vigorous effort for most people include:

- jogging or running;
- swimming fast;
- riding a bike fast or on hills;
- singles tennis;
- football;
- rugby;
- rope-skipping;
- hockey;
- aerobics;
- gymnastics; and
- martial arts.

A vigorous-intensity activity means that the exerciser will be breathing hard and fast, and the heart rate will have increased substantially.

When working at this level, the individual will not be able to speak more than a few words without pausing for a breath.

In general, 75 minutes of a vigorous-intensity activity can give similar health benefits to 150 minutes of moderate-intensity activity.

Muscle-strengthening activities

Muscle strength is necessary for daily activities, to build and maintain strong bones, to regulate blood sugar and BP and to help maintain a healthy weight.

Muscle-strengthening exercises are counted in repetitions and sets. A repetition is one complete movement of an activity, such as lifting a weight or completing a sit-up. A set is a group of repetitions.

For each activity, try to complete 8–12 repetitions in each set. A minimum is at least one set of each muscle-strengthening activities. Even greater benefits will be gained by undertaking two or three sets (Department of Health and Social Care, 2019).

The following are some examples of muscle-strengthening activities. They suggest types of exercise that are also included in the 'moderate' and 'vigorous' categories above:

- lifting weights;
- using resistance bands;
- heavy gardening (think fork and spade work or pushing the lawnmower);
- stair-climbing, particularly carrying the shopping or the vacuum cleaner;
- hill walking;
- cycling, particularly on hills;
- dancing, particularly if you have to lift your partner;
- press-ups;
- sit-ups; and
- squats.

In older people, maintaining strength is crucial to decrease the risk of falls and other health problems. The trend towards home delivery of groceries is a worrying trend in this regard because online shopping can result in limited opportunity to push trolleys and carry home heavy bags of food. A survey of 2000 people by the Chartered Society of Physiotherapy (Hughes, 2017) found that a quarter of those aged over 65 did no muscle-strengthening activities at all each week. Such activities do not require a visit to the gym. Carrying shopping, lifting homemade weights and simple body-weight exercises such as standing up out of a chair ten times will all be beneficial.

The Benefits of These Recommendations

These proposals are both realistic and highly beneficial. The recommended level of 150 minutes of aerobic exercise a week is considerably less than the optimal dose. Yet it is still sufficient to cause an appreciable increase in physical fitness, together with health and longevity benefits. Note, however, that the NHS guidelines do suggest there is substantial evidence that more vigorous-intensity activities can bring health benefits above that of moderate-intensity activities (Department of Health and Social Care, 2019).

Almost identical recommended exercise guidelines have been produced by a number of countries and continental groups. There is limited science to support these recommendations. They are inevitably a compromise between what is ideal and what is achievable.

The benefits of exercise clearly increase with increasing exercise volume. However, as more exercise is recommended, the chance of it being implemented is reduced. No one, to date, has demonstrated the crossover point at which the benefit of exercise at a population level is cancelled out by the reduction in uptake. In 2018, the second edition of the Physical Activity Guidelines for Americans was published (Piercy et al., 2018). The overall levels of recommended activity were not changed from previous guidelines, but the way in which the exercise was broken up was different. The report quotes that 'Even short-duration activity lasting less than 10 minutes is beneficial.' A recent study compared a small group of people who either walked for 10,000 steps per day at their own pace or walked briskly for three bouts of 10 minutes. The results suggested that the shorter, more intense exercise was more beneficial in terms of fitness (Copeland and Moseley, 2018).

As the population gets older, the benefits of exercise increase dramatically but people in this age group routinely exercise far less. One study has used US figures to calculate that average walking time for 20–29-year-olds is about 30 minutes per day, falling to about 9 minutes per day by the age of 70–79 (Sparling et al., 2015). Very reasonably, it is argued, it is futile to advise the elderly to triple their exercise – they just will not do it. The target for everyone should not be a fixed amount of exercise but an increase within the bounds of possible attainment. This is supported by reference to the UK Chief Medical Officer's statement (Department of Health and Social Care, 2019): 'the majority of UK older adults have low levels of activity so it is important to emphasise that they can achieve some benefits from increasing their activity even if it is below the recommendation'. Indeed, the greatest relative benefit is achieved by increasing from doing nothing to doing something, even if that something is not very much (Fig. 6.4).

Even the somewhat modest levels of exercise recommended by the NHS are a long way from being achieved by the vast majority of UK citizens. This unfortunate statement will be explored more fully in the next chapter.

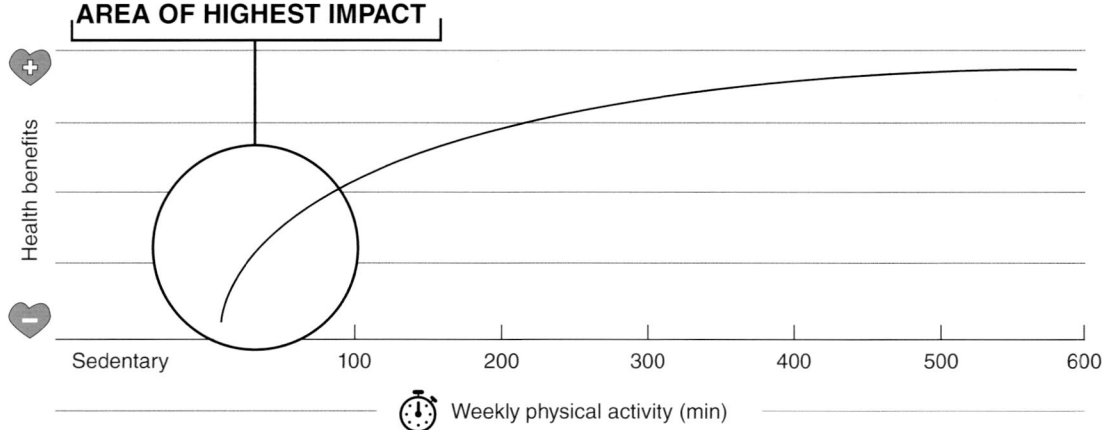

Fig. 6.4. Dose-response curve of physical activity and health benefits. (From https://gpcpd.heiw.wales/clinical/ motivate-2-move/chapter-1-the-uk-physical-activity-guidelines/key-principles-of-physical-activity/ (accessed 12 January 2023); adapted from Department of Health, Physical Activity, Health Improvement and Prevention, 2004.)

Summary

Total exercise volume is decided by the type of exercise and its duration, intensity and frequency. These are also related non-linearly to the effect of exercise on physical fitness. For most developed societies the recommended amount of exercise to promote good health is 150 minutes of moderate exercise or 75 minutes of intense exercise per week. This is equivalent to between 500 and 1000 MET minutes per week. Muscle-strengthening activities on two or more days per week are also recommended.

References

Bethell, H.J.N. (1976) *Exercise-Based Cardiac Rehabilitation*. Publishing Initiatives, Beckenham, UK.

Chomistek, A.K., Henschel, B., Eliassen, E.H., Mukamel, K.J. and Rimm, E.B. (2016) Frequency, type, and volume of leisure-time physical activity and risk of coronary heart disease in young women. *Circulation* 134, 290–299.

Copeland, R. and Mosley, M. (2018) *The Truth About Getting Fit* (BBC One documentary, televised 31 January 2018).

Dempsey, P.C., Musicha, C., Rowlands, A.V., Davies, M., Khunti, K., *et al.* (2022) Investigation of a UK biobank cohort reveals causal associations of self-reported walking pace with telomere length. *Communications Biology* 5, 381.

Department of Health and Social Care (2019) *UK Chief Medical Officers' Physical Activity Guidelines*. Department of Health and Social Care, London.

Department of Health, Physical Activity, Health Improvement and Prevention (2004) *At Least Five a Week: Evidence on the Impact of Physical Activity and Its Relationship to Health. A Report from the Chief Medical Officer*. HMSO, London.

Grazzi, G., Mazzoni, G., Myers, J., Caruso, L., Sassone, B., *et al.* (2020) Impact of improvement in walking speed on hospitalization and mortality in females with cardiovascular disease. *Journal of Clinical Medicine* 9(6), 1755. https://doi.org/10.3390/jcm9061755

Hughes, D. (2017) Carrying the shopping can improve strength in over-65s, say experts. *BBC News*, 29 September 2017. Available at: https://www.bbc.co.uk/news/health-41430301 (accessed 25 January 2023).

Lachman, S., Boekholdt, S.M., Luben, R.N., Sharp, S.J., Brage, S., *et al.* (2018) Impact of physical activity on the risk of cardiovascular disease in middle-aged and older adults: EPIC Norfolk prospective population study. *European Journal of Preventive Cardiology* 25(2), 200–208.

Lear, S.A., Hu, W., Rangarajan, S., Gasevic, D., Leong, D., *et al.* (2017) The effect of physical activity on mortality and cardiovascular disease in 130,000 people from 17 high-income, middle-income and low-income countries: the PURE study. *Lancet* 390, 2642–2654.

Piercy, K.L., Troiana, R.P., Ballard, R.M., Carlson, S.A., Fulton, J.E., *et al.* (2018) The Physical Activity Guidelines for Americans. *JAMA* 320, 2020–2028. https://doi.org/10.1001/jama.2018.14854

Soga, M., Gaston, K.J. and Yamaura, Y. (2016) Gardening is beneficial for health: a meta-analysis. *Preventive Medicine Reports* 5, 92–99.

Sparling, P.B., Howard, B.J., Dunstan, D.W. and Owen, N. (2015) Recommendations for physical activity in older adults. *BMJ* 350, h100.

Studenski, S. (2019) Gait speed reveals clues to lifelong health. *JAMA Network Open* 2(10), e1913112. https://doi.org/10.1001/jamanetworkopen.2019.13112

Yates, T., Razieh, C., Zaccardi, F., Rowlands, A.V., Seidu, S., *et al.* (2021) Obesity, walking pace and risk of severe COVID-19 and mortality: analysis of UK Biobank. *International Journal of Obesity* 45, 1155–1159.

Zaccardi, F., Davies, M.J., Khunti, K. and Yates, T. (2019) Comparative relevance of physical fitness and adiposity on life expectancy. A UK Biobank observational study. *Mayo Clinic Proceedings* 94, 985–994. https://doi.org/10.1016/j.mayocp.2018.10.029

7 Population Activity Levels

There are a number of answers to the question 'How much exercise do people take?' depending upon who is making the estimate and how they have measured it. Some of the regular surveys that assess physical activity in the population include the Health Surveys for England – HSE 2008 (Health and Social Care Information Centre, 2009), HSE 2012 (Health and Social Care Information Centre, 2013) and HSE 2016 (Health and Social Care Information Centre, 2017); the Active Lives Survey (Sport England, 2022); the National Travel Survey (Department of Transport, 2021); and the General Household Survey (Office for National Statistics, 2015).

The HSE surveys compare current population activity with the Department of Health recommendations. These have changed subtly over the years and the current guidelines (i.e. *UK Chief Medical Officers' Physical Activity Guidelines 2019*; Department of Health and Social Care, 2019) are described in Chapter 6 (this volume). The HSE uses validated questionnaires completed by wide sections of the population to assess the level of compliance with these guidelines. Different types of activity are summarized into a frequency–duration scale which takes into account the time spent participating in physical activities and the number of active days in the last week. By this measure the proportion of adults meeting the recommendation has increased steadily since 1997 for men and 1998 for women. In 1997, 32% of men met the recommendation, increasing to 43% in 2012. Among women, 21% met the recommendation in 1998, increasing to 32% in 2012 (HSE 2012). A similar increase in self-reported physical activity has been reported from the USA (Fig. 7.1).

After 2012 the recommendations changed to include shorter bursts of activity, so the figures for the past few years cannot be compared with the earlier figures. The most recent assessment of their level of physical activity (HSE 2016) indicates that 66% of men and 58% of women comply with the Department of Health guidelines. Caution needs to be applied, because these results depend upon the accuracy of the self-assessment of the individuals completing the questionnaires. They are likely to be substantial overestimates, as shown below.

The HSE 2008 found that, based on the participants' self-reported data, 39% of men and 29% of women in the whole survey met the exercise recommendations of the Chief Medical Officer. Increasing age and increasing BMI were associated with decreasing levels of activity. At the age range of 16–24 years, 52% of men and 35% of women met the recommendations. For those aged between 45 and 54 the compliance rate had fallen to 41% of men and 31% of women. Thereafter the fall was more precipitous, to 9% of men and 6% of women meeting the recommendations among the over-75s. Figure 7.2 illustrates the very similar findings in the Scottish population.

Like other HSE surveys, the HSE 2008 report gives a huge amount of additional data, including the effect of obesity and social status on activity as well as the different activities included in different age and sex groupings.

In 2011 the Department of Health modified its recommendations. It stated that adults should aim to be active daily. Over a week, activity should add up to at least 150 minutes (2½ hours) of moderate-intensity activity in bouts of 10 minutes or more – one way to approach this is to do 30 minutes on at least five days per week. Alternatively, comparable benefits can be achieved through 75 minutes of vigorous-intensity activity spread across the week or a combination of moderate- and vigorous-intensity activity (Department of Health and Social Care, 2019). The recommendations also added muscle-strengthening activities on two or more days per week that work all major muscle groups (legs, hips, back, abdomen, chest, shoulders and arms).

Using the new guidelines, the HSE 2012 estimated that 34% of men and 24% of women aged 16 and over met their recommendations. In both sexes, the proportion that met the guidelines generally

© H.J.N. Bethell and D. Brodie 2023. *Exercise: A Scientific and Clinical Overview*
(H.J.N. Bethell and D. Brodie)
DOI: 10.1079/9781800621855.0007

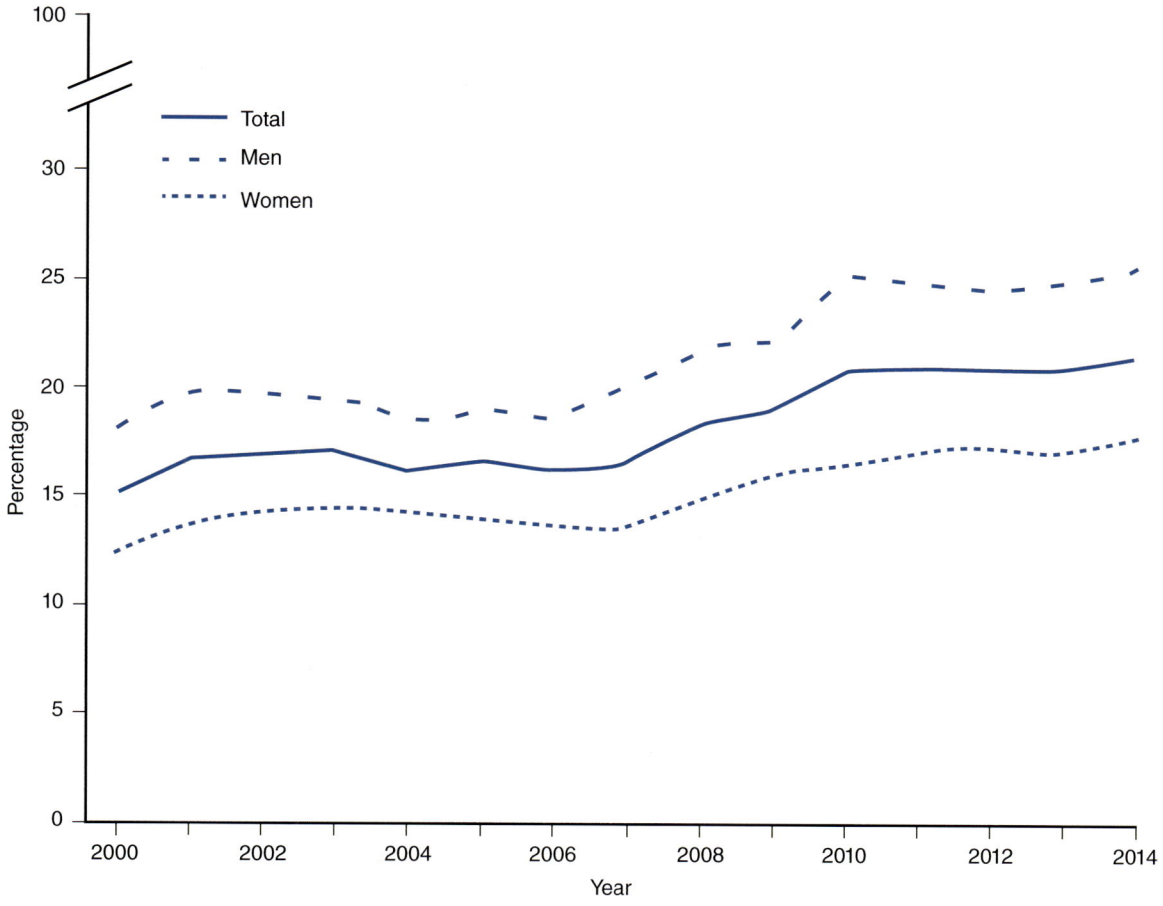

Fig. 7.1. Percentage of US adults meeting government exercise guidelines between the years 2000 and 2014. (From Centers for Disease Control and Prevention, 2016.)

decreased with age, reduced household income and increased BMI. Compared with 2008, there was an increase in those meeting the recommendation for aerobic activity. Considering just the aerobic exercise component, the numbers reaching the targets in HSE 2012 were 67% of men and 55% of women, and by HSE 2016 this had reduced to 65% for men and increased to 58% for women.

The details of the HSE 2008 report are important because that year the survey added a separate assessment of activity levels – it actually *measured* what people did. The comparison with what they *said* they did is startling. Questionnaire estimates of activity levels rely entirely on self-reporting, and it is well recognized that these are usually overestimates, usually in the region of 50%. The human tendency is to exaggerate – both those reporting participation and, perhaps even more to others, the amount of positive activity that is undertaken. This has been termed 'social desirability bias'. The unreliability of self-reported activity is particularly highlighted by the added information gleaned by the HSE 2008. The survey used accelerometers to record information on the frequency, intensity and duration of physical activity in 1-minute 'epochs', showing accurately the actual daily activity of their subjects over a period of 1 week. Based on the results of the accelerometer study, 6% of men and 4% of women achieved the government's recommended physical activity level, just 15% of the level of compliance indicated by individuals' own questionnaire responses. Men and women aged 16–34 were most likely to reach the recommended physical activity level (11 and 8%, respectively), while the proportion of both men and women meeting the recommendations fell in the older age

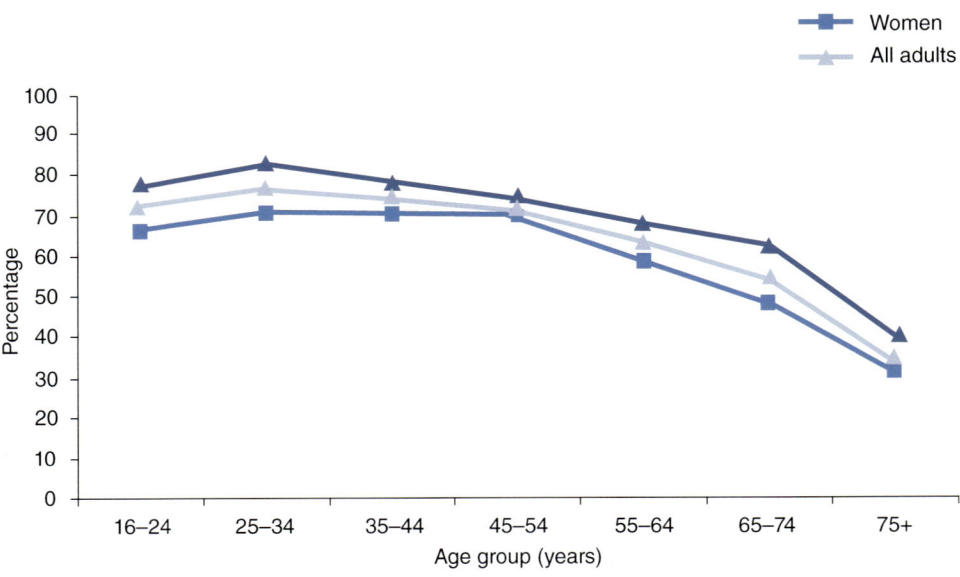

Fig. 7.2. Adult adherence to moderately vigorous physical activity guidelines, 2019, by age and sex. (From Scottish Government, 2020.)

groups. On average, men spent 31 minutes in moderate or vigorous physical activity in total per day and women an average of 24 minutes. However, most of this was sporadic activity, and only about a third of it was accrued in the bouts of 10 minutes or longer that count towards the government recommendations.

When the effects of physical fitness are compared with stated activity levels, it is physical fitness that is a far better predictor of future heart disease and mortality, particularly in younger subjects (Talbot *et al.*, 2002). Fitness level is a much better reflection than self-reported activity of how much exercise people actually undertake.

Summary

People vary greatly in the amount of exercise taken. The number of women meeting national recommendations has increased over time but is still only about 32% of the population. In men, the figure is slightly higher at 43%. However, it is recognized that these figures are often based on self-reports and usually overestimate the true figure. Exercise compliance is age-dependent, peaking at the 25–34 years age group.

References

Centers for Disease Control and Prevention (2016) Percentage of US adults who met the 2008 federal physical activity guidelines for aerobic and strengthening activity, by sex – National Health Interview Survey, 2000–2014. *MMWR Morbidity and Mortality Weekly Report* 65, 485. https://doi.org/10.15585/mmwr.mm6518a9

Department of Health and Social Care (2019) *UK Chief Medical Officers' Physical Activity Guidelines.* Department of Health and Social Care, London.

Department of Transport (2021) The National Travel Survey: 2021. Available at: https://www.gov.uk/government/collections/national-travel-survey-statistics (accessed 12 January 2023).

Health and Social Care Information Centre (2009) Health Survey for England – 2008: Physical activity and fitness. Available at: https://digital.nhs.uk/data-and-information/publications/statistical/health-survey-for-england/health-survey-for-england-2008-physical-activity-and-fitness (accessed 25 January 2023).

Health and Social Care Information Centre (2013) Health Survey for England – 2012: Chapter 2, Physical activity in adults. Available at: https://digital.nhs.uk/data-and-information/publications/statistical/health-survey-for-england/health-survey-for-england-2012 (accessed 12 January 2023).

Health and Social Care Information Centre (2017) Health Survey for England, 2016: Physical activity in adults. Available at: http://healthsurvey.hscic.gov.uk/support-guidance/public-health/health-survey-for-england-2016/physical-activity-in-adults.aspx (accessed 12 January 2023).

Office for National Statistics (2015) General Household Survey. Available at: https://data.gov.uk/dataset/138ca035-a90c-4e37-80f5-4c73eeb6ae04/general-household-survey (accessed 12 January 2023).

Scottish Government (2020) *The Scottish Health Survey, 2019 Edition, Volume 1: Main Report*. Scottish Government, Edinburgh.

Sport England (2022) Active Lives Survey. Available at: https://activelives.sportengland.org/ (accessed 12 January 2023).

Talbot, A., Morrell, C., Metter, E. and Fleg, J. (2002) Comparison of cardiorespiratory fitness versus leisure time physical activity as predictors of coronary events in men aged ≤65 years and >65 years. *American Journal of Cardiology* 89, 1187–1192.

8 How Fit is the General Population?

The answer to the question posed by the title of this chapter is: a lot less than it should be and a lot, *lot* less than people think.

The first attempt to assess physical fitness of the UK population was undertaken in 1990 – the ADNFS (Fentem *et al.*, 1994). This was conducted in a representative sample of English adults aged 16–96 years between February and November 1990. A total of 4316 participants (76% response rate) were interviewed about a range of sociodemographic characteristics and lifestyle factors, such as diet, physical activity (type, frequency and duration), smoking, alcohol, sleep, stress and social support. A subsample of 2767 participants also underwent a physical appraisal, which included objective assessment of body dimension, composition, flexibility, and cardiorespiratory and muscular fitness. The findings were shocking. More than seven out of ten men and eight out of ten women fell below their age-appropriate activity level for achieving a health benefit. Overall, about one in six had achieved no activity at all for 20 minutes or more in the past month. The level of inactivity increased with age: 10% of 16–20-year-olds took no exercise, increasing to 40% of 65–74-year-olds. When tested on a treadmill, the proportion of men unable to sustain walking up a gradient of 5% at 3 mph rose from 4% in the 16–24-year-olds to 81% in the 65–74 years age group. For women, the equivalent proportions were 34 and 92%. The figures for muscle strength were no more encouraging. Fifty per cent of women over 55 were unable to walk upstairs without assistance. Interestingly, although fitness tended to decline with age, many older individuals were as fit as, or fitter than, some of the much younger subjects. Astonishingly, 80% of both men and women of all ages incorrectly believed that they did enough exercise to keep fit. This provides yet more evidence of the human's capacity for self-deception.

The HSE 2008 is the best of the more recent sources of information on the measured cardiovascular fitness of a representative sample of the UK population (Health and Social Care Information Centre, 2019). Adults aged 16–74 underwent a step test. This involved stepping up and down a single step of a predetermined height at a standard rate for a maximum of 8 minutes. The pace of stepping increased throughout the test. Heart-rate measurements were taken during and after the test, then combined with the resting heart rate to provide an estimate of the individual's maximal oxygen uptake (VO_{2max}). The information in the HSE 2008 was analysed to allow comparisons to be made between the HSE 2008 and the ADNFS, which involved converting the results of the step test from the HSE to indicate the percentage of adults who could sustain walking at 3 mph on the flat and on a 5% incline. Key findings from HSE 2008 were:

- Men had higher cardiovascular fitness levels than women, with an average level of VO_{2max} of 36.3 ml/min/kg for men and 32.0 ml/min/kg for women. In both sexes, the mean VO_{2max} decreased with age.
- Cardiovascular fitness was lower on average among those who were obese (32.3 ml/min/kg among men and 28.1 ml/min/kg among women) than among those who were neither overweight nor obese (38.8 and 33.9 ml/min/kg, respectively).
- Virtually all participants were deemed able to walk at 3 mph on the flat but 84% of men and 97% of women would require moderate exertion for this activity. However, 32% of men and 60% of women were not fit enough to sustain walking at 3 mph up a 5% incline. Lack of fitness increased with age.
- Physical fitness was compared to self-reported physical activity. Average VO_{2max} decreased, and the proportion classified as unfit increased, as self-reported physical activity level decreased.

© H.J.N. Bethell and D. Brodie 2023. *Exercise: A Scientific and Clinical Overview*
(H.J.N. Bethell and D. Brodie)
DOI: 10.1079/9781800621855.0008

There have been a number of other studies of physical fitness in the 'population', but the HSE figures are probably the most meaningful in the real world because they deliberately included as broad a cross-section of society as possible. Longitudinal studies, which examine the same people over a number of years, give more accurate estimates of the effects of age than cross-sectional samples, which examine all the subjects at one point in time.

One consistent message given throughout this book is the importance of cardiorespiratory fitness (CRF) as an indicator of general health and as a risk factor for a number of different chronic and non-communicable diseases. CRF is also a significant prognostic factor for lifespan and healthspan. A convincing argument has been provided that CRF is a measure which can be as useful as BMI, resting heart rate, BP and many routinely performed observations and tests in the risk assessment, management and follow-up of these conditions. It is certainly a better predictor of future health than self-reported physical activity (Arena and Lavie, 2019). CRF is a vital measurement, which should be included in routine health checks, risk assessments, treatment recommendations and follow-up evaluations of patient progress. It could also be a very important developmental test for children and adolescents.

In the UK and in most other countries routine measurement of CRF is not carried out, so there are insufficient data to validate the usefulness of CRF from epidemiological studies. For CRF to become a useful clinical observation there need to be tables of normative reference values. Population studies of fitness by age and gender have been carried out in Germany (Koch et al., 2009; Rapp et al., 2018),

in the Brazilian Fleury study (Rossi Neto et al., 2019), in the US FRIEND study (Kaminsky et al., 2015, 2017), in the Norwegian HUNT study (Edvardsen et al., 2013; Loe et al., 2013) and in the UK (Ingle et al., 2020). Unfortunately some of the potentially useful clinical data are hidden behind a paywall, but Ingle et al. (2020) and Rossi Neto et al. (2019) summarize the comparison between the results of the different surveys. The differences are wide and the results of most seem to indicate unfeasibly high levels of fitness, particularly in older age groups. For instance, taking the mean VO_{2max} of men aged 70 to 75, the results vary from 28 ml/min/kg, which is equivalent to running at 4.5 mph, which does sound possible, to 37 ml/kg/min, equivalent to running at 6 mph which does not.

One cause of the variation is the difference in methods of measurement. Cycle ergometry gives consistently lower figures than treadmill testing. The other cause is variations in the composition of the populations sampled. It is very difficult to get a truly representative sample, partly because the less physically active will be less willing to volunteer for such studies and partly because an appreciable number will be unable to complete the test. The older the sample the more likely this is, which also leads to artificially high results in older people. Indeed in one study, the oldest group tested were found to be fitter than the younger cohort.

Although HSE annual surveys indicate that more people are complying with the government's exhortations to reach their exercise targets, there is evidence that this is not always translating into increased levels of fitness. For instance, the number of British military reservists failing their fitness assessments increased from 20% in 2015 to 29% in 2018.

Summary

There have been a number of attempts to measure population levels of physical fitness and thus produce normative tables. Unfortunately, different surveys have produced widely differing results, mainly because of differences between the populations surveyed and the methods used for fitness measurements. All studies, however, have found very low levels of fitness in populations as a whole and this is related to generally inadequate levels of physical activity.

References

Arena, R. and Lavie, C.J. (2019) Cardiorespiratory fitness and physical activity: two important but distinct clinical measures with different degrees of precision – a commentary. *Progress in Cardiovascular Diseases* 62(1), 74–75. https://doi.org/10.1016/j.pcad.2018.11.011

Edvardsen, E., Hansen, B.H., Holme, I.M., Dyrstad, S.M. and Anderssen, S.A. (2013) Reference values for cardiorespiratory response and fitness on the treadmill in a 20- to 85-year-old population. *Chest* 144(1), 241–248. https://doi.org/10.1378/chest.12-1458

Fentem, P.H., Collins, M.F., Tuxworth, W., Walker, A., Hoinville, E., *et al.* (1994) *Allied Dunbar National Fitness Survey. Technical Report.* Allied Dunbar, Health Education Authority and Sports Council, London.

Health and Social Care Information Centre (2019) Health Survey for England – 2008: Physical activity and fitness. Available at: https://digital.nhs.uk/data-and-information/publications/statistical/health-survey-for-england/health-survey-for-england-2008-physical-activity-and-fitness (accessed 13 January 2023).

Ingle, L., Rigby, A., Brodie, D.A. and Sandercock, G. (2020) Normative reference values for estimated cardiorespiratory fitness in apparently healthy British men and women. *PLoS One* 15(10), e0240099. https://doi.org/10.1371/journal.pone.0240099

Kaminsky, L.A., Arena, R. and Myers, J. (2015) Reference standards for cardiorespiratory fitness measured with cardiopulmonary exercise testing: data from the Fitness Registry and the Importance of Exercise National Database. *Mayo Clinic Proceedings* 90(11), 1515–1523. https://doi.org/10.1016/j.mayocp.2015.07.026

Kaminsky, L.A., Imboden, M.T., Arena, R. and Myers, J. (2017) Reference standards for cardiorespiratory fitness measured with cardiopulmonary exercise testing using cycle ergometry: data from the Fitness Registry and the Importance of Exercise National Database (FRIEND) Registry. *Mayo Clinical Proceedings* 92(2), 228–233. https://doi.org/10.1016/j.mayocp.2016.10.003

Koch, B., Schäper, C., Ittermann, T., Spielhagen, T., Dörr, M., *et al.* (2009) Reference values for cardiopulmonary exercise testing in healthy volunteers: the SHIP study. *European Respiratory Journal* 33(2), 389–397. https://doi.org/10.1183/09031936.00074208

Loe, H., Rognmo, Ø., Saltin, B. and Wisløff, U. (2013) Aerobic capacity reference data in 3816 healthy men and women 20–90 years. *PLoS One* 8(5), e64319. https://doi.org/10.1371/journal.pone.0064319. Erratum in: *PLoS One* 2013, 8(11). https://doi.org/10.1371/annotation/e3115a8e-ca9d-4d33-87ef-f355f07db28e

Rapp, D., Scharhag, J., Wagenpfeil, S. and Scholl, J. (2018) Reference values for peak oxygen uptake: cross-sectional analysis of cycle ergometry-based cardiopulmonary exercise tests of 10 090 adult German volunteers from the Prevention First Registry. *BMJ Open* 8(3), e018697. https://doi.org/10.1136/bmjopen-2017-018697

Rossi Neto, J.M., Tebexreni, A.S., Alves, A.N.F., Smanio, P.E.P., de Abreu, F.B., *et al.* (2019) Cardiorespiratory fitness data from 18,189 participants who underwent treadmill cardiopulmonary exercise testing in a Brazilian population. *PLoS One* 14(1), e0209897. https://doi.org/10.1371/journal.pone.0209897

9 Evidence: Interpreting the Science

The main thrust of this book is the effect of exercise (or lack of it) on health and disease. It explores the extent to which exercise can both prevent a number of diseases and also contribute to their treatment. The text contains numerous references, citations and apparent facts, but it is important to understand the quality and limitations of these statements. This chapter should help the reader to assess evidence and, in doing so, be able to interpret the science better. A starting point is to consider evidence as applied to facts and beliefs in a medical or clinical setting. In the context of exercise and health, an important principle is that of cause and effect.

When it comes to exercise as a factor in health and disease, an important source of evidence is found in epidemiology:

Epidemiology is the study and analysis of the distribution (who, when, and where), patterns and determinants of health and disease conditions in defined populations. It is the cornerstone of public health, and shapes policy decisions and evidence-based practice by identifying risk factors for disease and targets for preventive healthcare.

(Wikipedia, 2023)

In simple terms, epidemiology is the observation of associations between disease and certain behaviours, environmental conditions and physical states. For example, when Professors Richard Doll and Tim Peto from Oxford University identified cigarettes as the main cause of lung cancer, they used epidemiological evidence – the observation that people who smoked cigarettes had a far higher incidence of lung cancer than those who did not. A substantial amount of the evidence related to the effects of exercise is epidemiologically based. A specific example is the finding that people who take a large amount of exercise are less likely to develop type 2 diabetes.

Both these examples demonstrate only associations, not proof of cause. Association is not the same as causation – though it may be! The following is a light-hearted example: during the period in the 20th century when the incidence of coronary disease was increasing rapidly, so was the use of the radio. Clearly, few people believe that coronary disease is *caused* by radio waves. In the case of smoking and lung cancer, however, there is no other reasonable explanation and there are good biological reasons to believe that smoking might cause lung disease. In the case of exercise and diabetes, it is not possible to be quite so certain. There may be other 'confounders'. Confounders are other factors with which both exercise and diabetes are associated, such as sugar consumption. If exercisers consume less sugar than non-exercisers, that might be the explanation for the association. There are many differences between exercisers and non-exercisers, and it would be impossible to find groups of each whose other characteristics were identical. This means that many of the associations described below are just that – associations with a very strong presumption of a causal link.

Stronger evidence of causation is provided by the clinical trial. The purest form is the randomized, double-blind, controlled trial (RCT). This is best understood in the example of a drug trial. A group of individuals with a particular condition is selected to clarify the effect of the drug and they are divided randomly into two groups. One group receives the treatment and the other (the control group) receives a placebo. A placebo is simply an inert pill that looks the same as the real treatment. Neither the person giving the treatment and assessing its effect, nor the patient receiving it, knows who is getting the real treatment and who is getting the placebo. At the end of a predefined period the code is broken and the difference between the two groups analysed. If a trial of a cancer treatment is being tested, this might be the cure rate, and if the cure rate is significantly higher in the treatment group than in the control group it can be inferred that the drug is effective.

There are lots of possible pitfalls even in this very straightforward scenario. The patients might not have complied properly with the treatment. This is most likely for the treatment group if the drug has

© H.J.N. Bethell and D. Brodie 2023. *Exercise: A Scientific and Clinical Overview* (H.J.N. Bethell and D. Brodie)
DOI: 10.1079/9781800621855.0009

unpleasant side effects. The randomization process might not be perfect. Despite the randomization, there may be unexpected differences between the two groups. The statistical analysis has its own problems. In clinical trials, statistical significance is reached if the chance of the difference found between the two groups is less than 1 in 20 (in statistical shorthand, $P < 0.05$). With a clearly effective treatment this can be derived from a trial with small numbers of patients. The less obvious the effect, the more patients will be needed in the trial to demonstrate it. The more patients needed in the trial to show an effective outcome, the less effective the drug must be. If the number needed is very great, a statistically significant effect might be clinically insignificant. This means that although statistical significance is eventually reached, the clinical outcome is questionable. The counter side to this is that small trials are more likely to produce erroneous results. The bigger the trial, the more reliable the test will be. Even apparently well-conducted RCTs can yield results with problems of interpretation. When such trials are carried out by pharmaceutical firms on their own products, they are far more likely to have a positive outcome than independently funded and conducted trials.

Even well-conducted clinical trials of drugs can present problems. However, these are far fewer than the difficulties associated with carrying out randomized, controlled trials of exercise. For a start, trials of exercise cannot be double-blind. Treatment group members know they are in the treatment group, and it is quite hard to prevent the observers from knowing too. Compliance can be a nightmare and there may be cross-contamination. This means that members of the control group may start exercising, even if they have been asked not to. On the occasion that a randomized, controlled, but not blinded, trial of exercise was conducted for patients following heart attacks, one of the non-exercise controls bought himself a static cycle on his way home from his initial exercise test!

A further difficulty in most epidemiological studies and in many trials of exercise is that the estimated amount of physical activity depends on the evidence of the individual. Unfortunately this is highly unreliable, as was seen in Chapter 7 (this volume), since most people greatly overestimate how much exercise they take. An alternative measure is the physical fitness of the person involved. This is independent of the exaggerations told by the subject, both to the researcher and to themselves, so

should be a much more reliable measure. In the majority of cases, it most certainly is. However, fitness level is not wholly determined by the amount of exercise undertaken. There is also a genetic component, and this reduces the accuracy of fitness level as a reflection of exercise-taking.

There is one more level of evidence, which in some instances can provide the strongest information. This is the systematic review and meta-analysis. These are most useful when the numbers required to show an effect in an RCT are larger than can be reasonably recruited in a single trial. It is also an essential technique for unravelling the facts when different studies of the same topic come up with different answers. A systematic review answers a defined research question by collecting and summarizing all the evidence collected through observation that fits prespecified eligibility criteria. A meta-analysis uses statistical methods to summarize the results of these studies. In other words, a meta-analysis is a summation of the results of all the trials carried out using the particular intervention under investigation. The total number of subjects is much larger than in single trials and the results should therefore be that much more convincing. Again, there are problems. Different trials are different in many aspects and combining them sometimes involves mixing 'oranges and pears'. The choice of trials for inclusion is crucial if a particular question is to be answered – there must be as many similarities as possible. Unfortunately, there is the ever-present bias of the tendency to publish trials with a positive outcome but not those with a negative outcome.

Medicine is very far from being a perfect science. It is said that half of what doctors believe to be true today will, in time, be shown to be wrong. The problem is that no one knows which half. Interpreting evidence is a huge problem, but it is at the core of 'evidence-based medicine'. This book does not attempt to give a full systematic review of all the evidence for each statement on the effects of exercise, but it will include some of the more important or convincing research. In particular, the text will be referring frequently to 'Cochrane Reviews'. The Cochrane Collaboration is an independent non-profit group that conducts systematic reviews and meta-analyses of RCTs of healthcare interventions across all aspects of medical treatments. If the reader needs or wishes to check on the evidence for any particular treatment, it is recommended to Google 'Cochrane' and enter their website for the most comprehensive assessment of evidence-based interventions or drugs available in the world. Helpfully, the Cochrane Reviews include a layman's summary of the evidence and what it means.

Presentation of Evidence

It is very easy to be misled by the way in which evidence is presented. Those with a predetermined view, including those funding the study, tend to present their results in the way that is most likely to persuade the reader that the treatment is effective. Also, negative studies are much less likely to be published than those with positive findings. This is particularly likely to bias the published results of drug trials (Lundh *et al.*, 2017).

Fortunately, exercise studies are seldom sponsored by commercial organizations, but nevertheless the authors of such studies do sometimes have an interest in the outcomes. It is instructive to be aware of this possible bias.

One further point on the presentation of evidence. The benefit of a particular intervention is usually expressed in terms of change in risk and may be presented as a change in relative risk or a change in absolute risk. A change in relative risk usually makes the treatment seem much more attractive than a change in absolute risk:

- *Absolute risk* of a disease is the risk of developing the disease over a period of time and may be expressed as a fraction. An example would be, say, one in 20. Expressed as a percentage, this case would be 5% – or as a decimal, a 0.05 risk.
- *Relative risk* is used to compare the risk in two different groups of people. For example, the groups could be smokers and non-smokers. All sorts of groups are compared to others in medical research to see if belonging to a particular group increases or decreases the risk of developing certain diseases. For instance, research has shown that smokers have a higher risk of developing heart disease compared to (relative to) non-smokers. A reasonable assumption is that the absolute risk of developing heart disease is four in 100 (4%) in non-smokers, and that the relative risk of the disease is increased by 50% in smokers. The 50% relates to the four. This means that the absolute increase in the risk is 50% of four, which is two. So, the absolute risk of smokers developing this disease is six in 100. If the two groups are compared, the increase in risk brought about by smoking is two in 100 – for every 100 smokers. In summary, two more

individuals will develop heart disease compared with non-smokers.

When comparing the results of treatments, the choice of whether the outcomes are expressed as absolute or relative improvements can have a major effect on how effective the treatment appears. The less common the condition, the truer this is. An appropriate example is to examine the risk of a heart attack and how this can be reduced by taking a particular drug. The risk of a heart attack over the next 10 years in a group of women aged between 40 and 50 may be, say, one in 100, i.e. 1%. If taking the drug in question reduces the risk to one in 200 (0.5%), it may be reported that the risk of a heart attack, the relative risk, was halved in this group. However, the absolute risk is a reduction from two deaths to one death for every 200 women – an absolute reduction of one in 200. In other words, 200 women would have to take the drug for 10 years to prevent one new heart attack. This clearly seems rather less impressive than halving the risk. Sometimes the effectiveness of a treatment is then expressed as 'number needed to treat'. This is the number of people who need to take the treatment for just one person to benefit – in this case 200.

Mortality

Mortality rates are often used as outcome measures to compare the efficacy of different drugs and other treatments. The ultimate mortality for any treatment regimen is 100% because everyone will die in the end. This means that 'mortality' when used in this context has to be qualified. There are two ways of doing this:

1. Mortality is expressed as the death rate over the period of study and compared between the groups being studied.
2. The death rate of the group being studied is compared with the known death rate of the whole population of the same age and gender. This is usually expressed as deaths per 1000 persons per year.

Interpreting the Evidence

In conclusion, facts unsupported by evidence should be questioned. Even when the evidence seems to support the facts, individuals must be alert to the possibilities of error. Very little evidence is totally unarguable. However, it is a great deal better than any other way of reaching the truth. This applies equally to exercise as to any other treatment.

Summary

This book presents numerous references, citations and apparent facts. Evidence is found from many sources, often from epidemiology. It is important to recognize the distinction between association and causation. The ideal clinical trial is randomized, controlled and double-blind. However in clinical trials of exercise this is very difficult, and this limitation is recognized. A systematic review and meta-analysis can provide strong evidence for the benefits of exercise. Evidence can be presented as absolute risk or relative risk, with qualified mortality often used as an outcome measure for drug and other treatments.

References

Lundh, A., Lexchin, J., Mintzes, B., Schroll, J.B. and Bero, L. (2017) Industry sponsorship and research outcomes. *Cochrane Database of Systematic Reviews* 2(2), MR000033. https://doi.org/10.1002/14651858.MR000033.pub3

Wikipedia (2023) Epidemiology. Available at: https://en.wikipedia.org/wiki/Epidemiology (accessed 15 January 2023).

10 Obesity

The standard unit for measuring weight compared with height is body mass index (BMI), which is weight in kilograms divided by height in metres squared. So a 70 kg (about 11 stone) person who is 1.75 m (about 5 foot 9 inches) tall has a BMI of 70 divided by 1.75 squared, which is 70 divided by 3.0625, which is about 22.9 kg/m². The easiest way to avoid the maths is to find a BMI website and feed in the height and weight in either kilograms and centimetres or pounds and feet.

The ideal BMI is generally accepted as between 18.5 and 25 kg/m². Between 25 and 30 kg/m² is 'overweight', between 30 and 40 kg/m² is 'obese' and over 40 kg/m² is 'morbidly obese'. Obesity is also defined as Class 1 (BMI = 30–35 kg/m²), Class 2 (BMI = 35–40 kg/m²) and Class 3 (BMI > 40 kg/m²). For the purposes of longevity, a BMI between 20 and 25 kg/m² is optimal (Global BMI Mortality Collaboration, 2016). Weights higher than this carry an increasing risk of coronary disease and type 2 diabetes, of which much more later.

However, there is more to weight than BMI. It also matters where excess fat is stored. Obesity can be predominantly either central or peripheral. Those with central obesity store fat in the abdominal cavity and have paunches or beer bellies – the 'apple' shape. Those with peripheral obesity store it on their hips, bottoms and thighs – the 'pear' shape. It is much more dangerous to be an 'apple' than to be a 'pear'. So when it comes to assessing risk from obesity, mainly risk for CVD and premature death, waist measurement seems to give a better assessment than BMI. The upper limit of recommended waist size for men is 102 cm (40 inches) and for women 88 cm (35 inches). With higher measurements, the risks for CVD, diabetes and high BP all rise steeply. Alternative parameters include the waist-to-hip ratio (waist circumference divided by hip circumference). For men this should be below 1.0 and for women below 0.8. Another parameter is the waist-to-height ratio, which is supported by the National Institute for Health and Care Excellence (NICE) (Wise, 2022). They recommend that waist circumference should not be more than half of height – an easy measure for the individual to make. Such measures are used to refine the predictive power of simple BMI, which can be misleadingly high in very muscular people with normal body fat. A group based at the University of Wolverhampton found in a cohort of over 4700 people that waist-to-height ratio correlated much better than BMI with cardiometabolic scores determined from treadmill exercise (Nevill *et al.*, 2020).

Obesity is not a new condition. One of the oldest surviving human carvings, the Venus of Willendorf, created some 27,000 years ago, depicts a strikingly obese woman (Fig. 10.1).

Hippocrates, in about 500 BC, reported that obese people were at increased risk of sudden death. In 1727, a British physician named Thomas Short wrote, 'No age has seen more instances of corpulency than our own' (Bray, 1990).

Obesity is a huge and growing problem in most Western countries and the figures published about its extent are as gross as the problem itself. The weight of the average person in the UK has risen by more than 1.5 kg (3 lb) every decade since 1970 and Britain is currently the most overweight nation in Western Europe. Over the past 20 years, the proportion of adults in the UK who are obese has increased from 13.2% in 1993 to 26.0% in 2020 for men, and from 16.4 to 29.0% for women over the same period. Adding the number of overweight men and women increases these figures alarmingly. The proportions that were overweight or obese increased from 57.6 to 67.1% in men and from 48.6 to 60.0% in women from 1993 to 2020 (NHS Digital, 2020) (and see Fig. 10.2).

From 1999–2000 through 2017–March 2020, US obesity prevalence increased from 30.5 to 41.9%. During the same time, the prevalence of severe obesity increased from 4.7 to 9.2% (Stierman

© H.J.N. Bethell and D. Brodie 2023. *Exercise: A Scientific and Clinical Overview*
(H.J.N. Bethell and D. Brodie)
DOI: 10.1079/9781800621855.0010

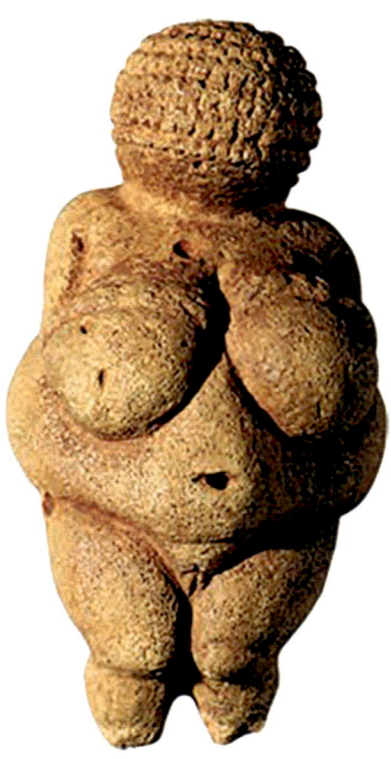

Fig. 10.1. The Venus of Willendorf.

et al., 2021). Globally in 2016, more than 1.9 billion adults, 18 years and older, were overweight. Of these over 650 million were obese (World Health Organization, 2021)

The seeds of obesity are sown in childhood. In the UK, among Year 6 pupils, who are aged 10 and 11, obesity prevalence increased from 21.0% in 2019/20 to 25.5% in 2020/21 (NHS Digital, 2021). In the USA, rates of obesity have also been rising steadily – from 13.9% in 1999 to 18.5% in 2016 among children and adolescents aged 2 to 19 years (Sanyaolu *et al.*, 2019). A systematic review showed that 16.8% of boys and 15.2% of girls were obese in 2008 and that the associated health problems included psychological difficulties such low self-esteem (Canoy and Bundred, 2011). That review included 14 systematic reviews and RCTs and is recommended reading for anyone wishing to explore obesity in children more thoroughly. The prevalence of severe obesity in the USA has risen from 1.0% in 1971–1974 to 6.1% in 2017–2018 (Fryar *et al.*, 2020) and the inexorable increase in childhood obesity is behind the very serious problem of rising levels of childhood type 2 diabetes (see Chapter 13, this volume). A worrying fact is that one in four obese teenagers is unaware that they are obese. Government initiatives to reduce

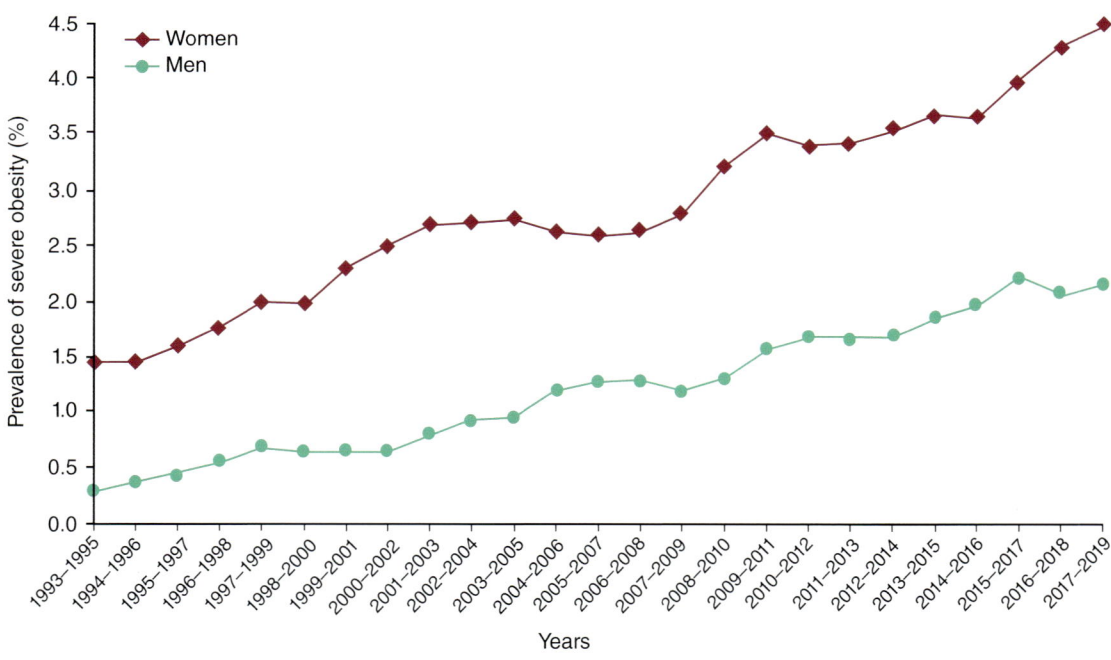

Fig. 10.2. Prevalence of severe obesity in UK adults between 1993 and 2019. (From Hancock, 2021. Used with kind permission of the UK Health Security Agency.)

childhood obesity have failed miserably and interventions in schools have also mostly been unsuccessful. This may not be unrelated to the selling off of school playing fields. Maternal lifestyle is also a very prominent contributor to the risk of obesity in the child, so targeting overweight and obese parents may be a better option. It has even been suggested that obesity in children should be made a childhood protection issue.

Causes of Obesity

This huge increase in obesity would seem to be explained by the rise in availability of high-calorie foods, particularly sweet, fizzy drinks and the widespread use by the food industry of high-fructose corn syrup. Surprisingly, however, a team of economists from the Institute of Fiscal Studies published a paper in 2016 showing that, judging by the sale of calorific foods, the average daily calorie intake of adults in the UK had actually fallen by 20% over the previous 30 years (Griffith *et al.*, 2016). They concluded that the rise in obesity was a result of 'a decline in the strenuousness of work and daily life'. Their figures are supported by the Department for Food, Environment and Rural Affairs (DEFRA), which has shown that overall our calorie intake peaked in the 1970s, declined until the 2000s and has flattened since (DEFRA, 2013). This view of the cause of our increasing obesity is not shared by all. The Obesity Health Alliance is firmly convinced that the causes are changes in diet, increased portion size, far more meals eaten outside the home and a shift to ready meals, junk food and snacks (Obesity Health Alliance, 2021). The whole problem is made more obtuse by the fact uncovered by the Office of National Statistics that the average Briton consumes 50% more calories than they estimate for themselves – so-called social desirability bias (Bailey, 2018). As one representative of the National Obesity Forum is quoted as saying, 'People lie and I am not surprised that they do when it comes to food. They wish not to be taken for slobs, even though they may be just that!' As has been seen, the same bias results in a similar degree of overestimation of exercise taken. People take about 50% less exercise than they claim. Moreover, the more overweight the individual, the greater the overestimate (Guo *et al.*, 2019).

For an individual's weight to increase, the number of calories absorbed and used (bioavailable calories) must exceed the number expended in physical activity. The bioavailability of calories in food items is not the same as the calorific value – this is exemplified by the high glycaemic load from sugary foods compared with the lower energy provided by protein and fats of similar calorific value (Ludwig *et al.*, 2021). There is a variety of reasons for weight gain leading to obesity including both over-eating and under-exercising, and it is not easy for some people to control this energy balance. The genetic influence contributes up to 80% of the difference between the slim and the fat and is mediated by the hypothalamus and hippocampus, which control appetite, hunger and satiety (Miras, 2020). It is also likely that satiety is influenced by habitual food intake – both type and quantity – which becomes ingrained during childhood and adolescence.

There is a great number of variables contributing to excessive weight gain. The loss of necessity for physical activity, the ready availability of calorie-rich foods and the increase in dining out all contribute. The energy-balance equation is also made more complicated by the fact that exercise can increase appetite and eating is often taken as a reward for participating in competitive sport (Bennion *et al.*, 2020). Changing societal circumstances can also be involved. The Covid-19 pandemic has seen weight gains for both children and adults, most marked in those who were already obese (Robinson *et al.*, 2021; Woolford *et al.*, 2021).

The Costs of Obesity

Obesity is much more than a medical problem. In 2015 in the UK, the cost to the NHS directly attributable to obesity was £6.1 billion and the cost to the wider economy was £27 billion (National Audit Office, 2020). In the USA the medical costs of obese people have been calculated to be US$2505 per annum greater than for those of normal weight – an uplift of 100% – with a 'dose response' effect. The costs increased from 68% excess for Class 1 obesity to 234% for Class 3. The overall cost to the USA was considered to be US$260 billion (Cawley *et al.*, 2021). There are also hidden costs such as the reduction in productivity associated with obesity (Rozjabek *et al.*, 2020).

The Medical Ill Effects of Obesity

Obesity is not a disease, but it is a powerful risk factor for a number of dangerous and debilitating illnesses, including such age-related conditions as lower-limb osteoarthritis, type 2 diabetes, dementia, hypertension, heart attacks, atrial fibrillation, strokes, oesophageal reflux, fatty liver and several varieties of cancer (uterus, breast, bowel, gullet, ovary, liver and pancreas). The charity Cancer Research UK (2021) states 'overweight and obesity is the second biggest cause of cancer in the UK – more than 1 in 20 cancer cases are caused by excess weight.' Around 12% of postmenopausal breast cancers are blamed on obesity.

In men it is a similar story, with 4.4% of all cancers being due to obesity. There is a direct relationship between obesity and cancer with every 10 cm (3.9 inches) of waist circumference raising the risk of dying from prostate cancer by 7% and every 5 kg/m^2 of extra BMI increasing the risk by 10% (Perez-Cornago et al., 2022).

The risk of dying from Covid-19 is doubled for obese patients (Tan et al., 2020). On a national scale, coronavirus death rates were up to ten times greater in countries with high levels of obesity compared with those with low levels of obesity (World Obesity Federation, 2021). Both quality of life and productivity are considerably reduced for the obese. Obesity also contributes significantly to disability in later life, making old people less able to carry out normal activities of daily living (ADL) and more likely to become frail and dependent (Somoes et al., 2006). The risk of needing hospital admission is also increased for the obese. In a cohort of nearly half a million men and women, a 2 kg/m^2 higher BMI (above 20 kg/m^2) was associated with a 6.2% higher admission rate and an 8.6% higher annual cost in men and with a 5.7% higher admission rate and an 8.4% higher annual cost in women (O'Halloran et al., 2020). Obese older people have a significantly greater risk of needing care and help with daily life than those of normal weight (Landré et al., 2020). They have a reduction of about a quarter in disease-free life (see Chapter 26, this volume) in old age. Again there is a relationship between degree of obesity and loss of disease-free years, ranging from 1.1 years for men who are overweight to 8.5 years for those with a BMI over 40 kg/m^2. The equivalent figures for women are 1.1 years and 7.3 years (Nyberg et al., 2018).

Mortality rate increases by 30% for every increment of 5 kg/m^2 above a BMI of 25 kg/m^2 (Prospective Studies Collaboration, 2009). Yet, while 45% of deaths of those with a BMI of 30 kg/m^2 or more are due to obesity-related diseases, obesity is seldom recorded as a contributory factor on death certificates (Ranjbar et al., 2020). A recent study of more than 10.5 million people over four continents has clarified the mortality risk of being overweight or obese. Compared with those of normal weight (BMI = 18.5–25 kg/m^2), having a BMI between 25 and 27.5 kg/m^2 increases the risk of death over the following 5 years by 7%. A BMI between 27.5 and 30 kg/m^2 increases risk by 20%; a BMI between 30 and 35 kg/m^2 increases risk by 45%; a BMI between 35 and 40 kg/m^2 increases risk by 94%; and a BMI over 40 kg/m^2 increases risk by a staggering 276% (Global BMI Mortality Collaboration, 2016). It has been estimated that the obesity epidemic shortens lives overall by as much as 9 years. Figure 10.3 illustrates the relationship between BMI and mortality.

The risks are much greater for men than for women at all levels of obesity. About one in seven premature deaths in Europe are due to being overweight or obese. Overweight people lose on average 1 year of life, and obese people lose about 3 years of life. However, being thin is not always healthy. BMIs below 22 kg/m^2 are also associated with increased mortality. It is presumed that thin people include those who are thin because they suffer ill health or practise unhealthy behaviour such as smoking (Aune et al., 2016).

Other important ill effects of obesity include aggravation of breathlessness; worsening of asthma; damage to joints, particularly knees and hips; abnormal blood lipids; depression; and sleep apnoea.

Exercise in the Prevention of Obesity

Staying a normal weight is much easier than losing weight. Those who take regular exercise from childhood and continue into adult life seldom become obese.

Weight can be compared with a bank balance. Calories replace money, but with an opposite desirable outcome! Calories can be considered as cash – if more is taken in than taken out, then weight increases. Obesity is caused neither by a slow metabolism nor by big bones. It is caused by energy intake being greater than output. Some figures have been produced to illustrate the effectiveness of exercise in burning off excess calories. It has even been suggested that food packaging should include the exercise required to work off the contents. The labels would not make comfortable reading. Walking at between 3.5 and 4 mph burns off about

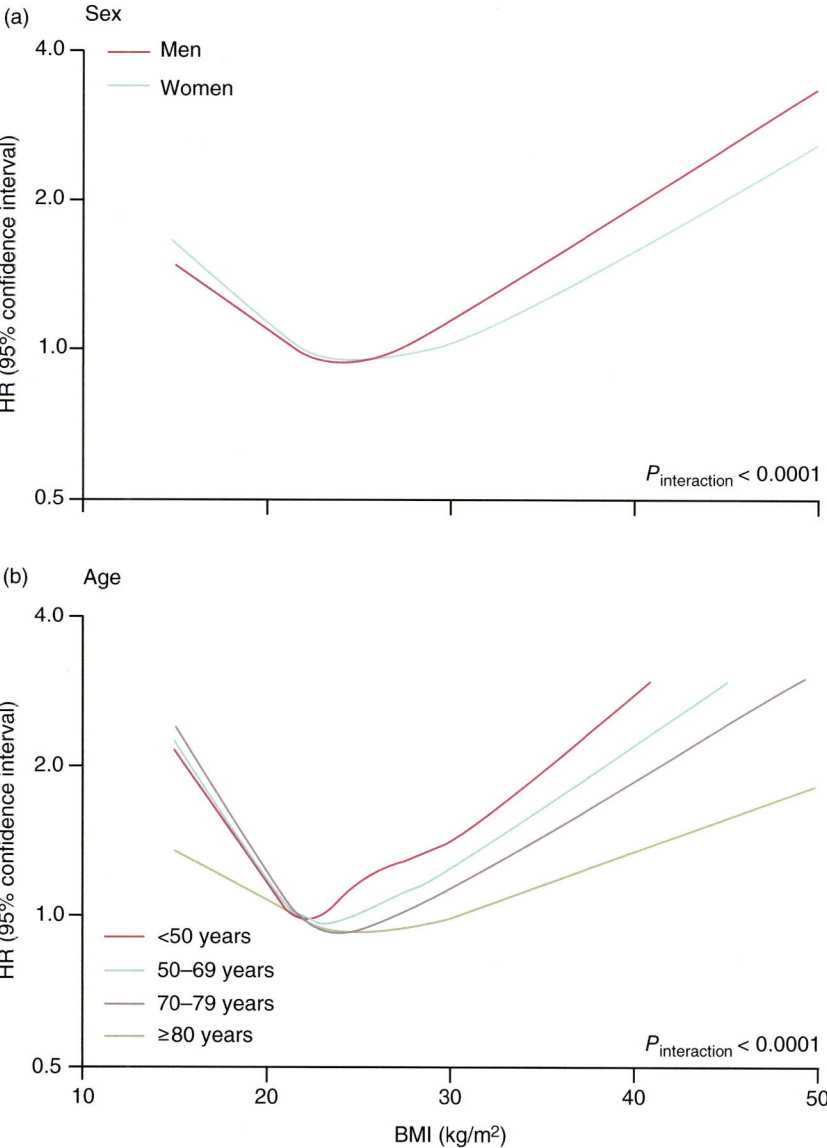

Fig. 10.3. Relationships between BMI and hazard ratio (HR) for all-cause mortality in UK adults according to sex (a) and age (b). (From Bharaskan *et al.*, 2018. Article available under the terms of the Creative Commons Attribution License (CC BY): https://creativecommons.org/licenses/by/4.0/.)

5 Calories per minute, so about 26 minutes of walking is needed to walk off a can of fizzy drink. A digestive biscuit might be metabolized by climbing 25 floors of stairs and a quarter of a pizza fuels running for 43 minutes.

Reaching a steady state with equal intake and output of calories is relatively easy for a regular exerciser. This demonstrates the advantage of starting young – exercising from childhood. It is not known just how much exercise is needed to prevent obesity, nor to prevent weight being regained by those who have slimmed down. The figure of 60–90 minutes of moderately intense exercise per day has been calculated (Wareham *et al.*, 2005). This is considerably more than the level recommended by the UK Department of Health for the maintenance of good health. For runners, 15 miles per week seems to be the required amount (Slenz *et al.*, 2004). However, the level of activity in day-to-day living is just as important as formal exercise for increasing energy output. There are numerous ways for increasing energy expenditure. These include walking upstairs instead of taking the lift, walking up escalators, opting for active transport such as walking or cycling for getting to and from work, getting off the bus a stop earlier than the destination, walking short journeys rather than taking the car, etc., etc. It is reported that the winners of a lottery in Beijing for a free car showed a 10 kg weight gain compared to the losers over the following 10 years (Anderson *et al.*, 2019). Regular participators in sports are much less likely to be obese than non-participants (Mielke *et al.*, 2020). Another important element in daily energy expenditure is fidgeting. People who fidget are thinner than those who do not, and the energy expenditure of fidgeting can be as much as 600 Calories per day. Being a fidget has a strong inherited component and it may be difficult to become a fidgeter – though special fidget chairs have shown some promise. Another suggestion is to exercise before breakfast. It is believed that the muscles will expend more energy, use more fat as the energy source and subsequently reduce more body fat.

Exercise in the Treatment of Obesity

Most adults in the developed world weigh too much and for them the problem is a difficult one. Removing unwanted weight is much harder than avoiding adding it in the first place. Anyone who has ever considered the need to go on a diet can testify that it is *extremely* difficult to lose weight. Eating fewer calories than is expended in exercise is really, really hard – but it *can* be done. Some people have the willpower to cut their food intake to the level where they lose weight, but by adulthood, dietary habits are hard-wired into us and most people who lose weight by diet alone subsequently put it all back on again. There are good reasons why dieting is so ineffective. When the body is deprived of nutrition, various contributions to energy expenditure, including involuntary movement, are reduced – probably via in-built homeostatic adjustments to save energy.

Some people can increase their exercise level to the point where they lose weight, but this does need a lot more effort than is recommended by government or than most people are prepared to incorporate into their daily life. Typical exercise regimens, which may take 150 minutes per week, are occupying only 2% of total waking hours. Increasing effort during these sessions makes a tiny contribution to overall energy expenditure and is easily neutralized by the resulting increase in appetite (Beaulieu *et al.*, 2020). Moderate-intensity exercise for an hour a day (Flack *et al.*, 2020) or running more than 15 miles per week are required to guarantee weight loss without cutting back on food. The popular belief that 10,000 pedometer steps daily are enough is wrong. This number is only about half of the number of paces required (Bailey *et al.*, 2019). Those with low fitness levels find it much harder to lose weight with exercise – it just takes them too long (The Endocrine Society, 2020). Finding out how difficult it is to exercise out of obesity is demoralizing and often results in giving up. People need to be realistic from the outset about how much exercise is needed. The mode of exercise has an influence on its effectiveness. Moderate-intensity exercise has been compared with high-intensity interval (HIIT) training and sprint-interval training (SIT) (Viana *et al.*, 2020). HIIT consists of short intervals of extreme exertion punctuated by rest periods. SIT is a more extreme form of HIIT. The primary difference between HIIT and SIT is that HIIT, despite what the name may suggest, reaches hard, but not *maximal* intensities, whereas SIT does require maximal and even supramaximal intensities. Studies have shown that all three regimens were associated with similar reductions in body-fat percentages, but interval training provided greater reductions in total fat mass. The time spent in moderate-intensity exercise averaged 38 minutes, HIIT averaged 28 minutes and SIT averaged 18 minutes. This suggests that the time saving of interval regimens might appeal to busy individuals. When it comes to the efficacy of different regimens, a combination of endurance training with strength training may be the most beneficial (Stankovic *et al.*, 2021).

The most successful weight-losing strategy is a combination of diet, exercise and, most important of all, maintenance of this changed lifestyle in perpetuity. Most people find it too difficult, perhaps because it means both taking an unaccustomed amount of exercise (which may increase the appetite) and being hungry. In a world where many people are surrounded by too much high-calorie food, such self-denial may seem close to masochism. In the specific case of mid-life bulge, some of the effect of exercise may be mediated by sleep. Exercise lowers the production of stress hormones and makes it easier to sleep and to avoid stress eating (Novak, 2022a). Anti-obesity medication is now being used in some countries for chronic weight management. One example, approved by both NICE in the UK and the Food and Drug Administration (FDA) in the USA, is the GLP-1 receptor agonist group of antidiabetic drugs which include semaglutide. The use of such drugs must coincide with lifestyle changes, such as exercise; otherwise the prospect of maintaining any weight loss is significantly reduced (Novak, 2022b).

The Cochrane Review on 'Exercise for overweight or obesity' (Shaw et al., 2006) analysed the results of 43 studies involving 3476 participants. Overall, they found exercise programmes without dietary changes produced a modest effect, with weight losses of between 2 and 7 kg. More vigorous exercise was more effective than less vigorous. However, the most effective treatment was a combination of diet and exercise, with diet alone being rather more effective than exercise alone.

Benefits of Weight Loss

Those who exercise to lose weight achieve other benefits. These include a reduction in risk factors for CVD, with lowering of BP and blood sugar and an improvement in blood lipids. These improvements are seen even in those who take up exercise but fail to lose weight. This fact is confirmed by studies that have shown that while both BMI and fitness are strong independent predictors of all-cause mortality, fit obese patients have a lower mortality than unfit people of normal weight (Verheggen et al., 2016). In middle-aged and more elderly people, it has been shown that exercise reduces the risk of stroke or a heart attack, regardless of BMI. A Dutch study tracked 5300 people aged 55 and over for 15 years. Those who were both inactive and overweight were a third more likely to suffer a cardiovascular event. Unfortunately, very few obese people take enough exercise to counteract the ill effects of obesity. One estimate calculated that just 2.2% of all men and 4.1% of all women in England could be classed as both obese and fit (Sui et al., 2007).

Diabetic control is improved by losing weight and in one study 86% of type 2 diabetics who lost 15 kg or more became normoglycaemic (Lean et al., 2018).

Another great benefit of using exercise as part of a weight-control programme is that it helps to maintain and increase muscle mass – starvation diets are no respecters of which part of the body shrinks. Fat is not the only part to be diminished, as can be seen in the pictures of the victims of famines or wartime privation. Exercise training increases muscle mass – and muscle is somewhat more dense than fat. Those who fail to lose weight during exercise programmes may have lost fat but replaced it with muscle. One meta-analysis involving 4815 subjects found that, in the absence of weight loss, exercise produces a 6.1% decrease in 'visceral adiposity' (i.e. paunch size) while diet showed virtually no change (1.1%) (Verheggen et al., 2016). A 24-year follow-up study of 116,564 women aged 30–55 found that the death rate in the inactive obese was two-and-a-half times greater than in the lean active group (Hu et al., 2004).

Weight loss may be particularly important for those in early or mid-life and lead to significant lowering of premature mortality (Xie et al., 2020). Lower mortality is also seen in obese men who have high levels of physical fitness (Tarp et al., 2021). Indeed, taken separately, increasing physical fitness protects against premature mortality to a greater extent than weight loss (Gaesser et al., 2015).

Maintenance of Weight Loss

Once weight has been lost by whatever combination of diet and exercise, there is a depressing tendency for the weight lost to be regained. More than 70% of people who succeed in losing weight will have returned to their usual weight within 2 years (Jakicic et al., 2008). Scientists at Lawrence Berkeley National Laboratory in California studied more than 20,000 people over 7 years. They found that recreational runners who stopped exercising subsequently put on significant amounts of weight. However, when they resumed the same level of running, they did not reverse the weight gain (Williams, 2008). A confounding factor is that these runners would have been older when they resumed their running and may have been more sedate in their approach to exercise. It takes about 275 minutes of moderate exercise per week to maintain weight loss, which is considerably more than the Department of Health recommendations for healthy living. However, exercise is more effective than diet in maintaining weight loss (Ostendorf *et al.*, 2018). Those who are successful in maintaining a lowered body weight eat more than unsuccessful dieters but expend significantly more energy in daily activity. Regular exercise also promotes maintenance of weight loss after bariatric surgery (Pouwels *et al.*, 2020).

Summary

The easiest way to lose weight and retain the loss is to combine eating less with exercising more. For maintenance, continuing the exercise habit is crucial. Anyone can theoretically lose weight, but for some it is much harder than for others. Success depends upon the balance between determination to do so, the desire to eat and the disdain for exercise. It is a balance between motivation and deprivation.

Weight-losing groups such as WW (Weight Watchers) and Slimming World can be helpful. Bariatric surgery is highly effective (Arterburn *et al.*, 2020). A new group of antidiabetic drugs – the GLP-1 receptor agonists, which include semaglutide and liraglutide – is soon to be launched as aids to weight loss (Yanovski and Yanovski, 2021).

There has been a move in the medical profession to label obesity as 'an ongoing chronic disease' and to reduce the 'shaming' of fat people. Rather, clinicians are encouraged to sympathize with fat people for the 'health inequalities, genetic influences and social factors' that have contributed to their problem. This philosophy is more common in the USA than in the UK. Not all agree with this approach. It is quite valid to question how anyone who believes they are a victim of uncontrollable outside forces can come to understand that they are able to change their own situation for the better. On the whole, people believe that they eat much less than they really do and exercise more than they think. The discrepancy between perception and reality grows with increases in BMI (Ekelund *et al.*, 2019). If the fat are to become thin, they need more reality and a huge amount of motivation. Understanding the difficulty of losing weight and the very serious consequences of not doing so may help.

Sadly, however, as we get fatter our perceptions change: the new norm is to be overweight or obese, with the likely subsequent consequence of an increasingly corpulent population.

Summary

There is no very good way of expressing body weight but one of the best and convenient is body mass index (BMI), which is weight divided by height squared. Normal BMI is between 18.5 and 25 kg/m^2, between 25 and 30 kg/m^2 is termed overweight, between 30 and 40 kg/m^2 is obese and over 40 kg/m^2 is morbidly obese. The ill effects of obesity include lower-limb osteoarthritis, type 2 diabetes, dementia, hypertension, heart attacks, atrial fibrillation, strokes, oesophageal reflux, fatty liver and several varieties of cancer (uterus, breast, bowel, gullet, ovary, liver and pancreas). The prevalence of obesity has increased steadily over the past four decades and is responsible for the huge increase in the diseases with which it is associated, particularly type 2 diabetes.

References

Anderson, M.L., Lu, F. and Yang, J. (2019) Physical activity and weight following car ownership in Beijing, China: quasi-experimental cross sectional study. *BMJ* 367, l6491. https://doi.org/10.1136/bmj.l6491

Arterburn, D.E., Telem, D.A., Kushner, R.F. and Courcoulas, A.P. (2020) Benefits and risks of bariatric surgery in adults: a review. *JAMA* 324(9), 879–887.

Aune, D., Sen, A., Prasad, M., Norat, T., Janszky, I., *et al.* (2016) BMI and all cause mortality: systematic review and non-linear dose-response meta-analysis of 230 cohort studies with 3.74 million deaths among 30.3 million participants. *BMJ* 353, i2156.

Bailey, B.W., Bartholomew, C.L., Summerhays, C., Deru, L., Compton, S., *et al.* (2019) The impact of step recommendations on body composition and physical activity patterns in college freshman women: a randomized trial. *Journal of Obesity* 2019, 4036825. https://doi.org/10.1155/2019/4036825

Bailey, R. (2018) Evaluating calorie intake. *Data Science Campus*, 15 February 2018. Available at: https://datasciencecampus.ons.gov.uk/eclipse/ (accessed 16 January 2023).

Beaulieu, K., Hopkins, M., Gibbons, C., Oustric, P., Caudwell, P., *et al.* (2020) Exercise training reduces reward for high-fat food in adults with overweight/obesity. *Medicine and Science in Sports and Exercise* 52(4), 900–908.

Bennion, N., Spruance, L.A. and Maddock, J.E. (2020) Do youth consume more calories than they expended in youth sports leagues? An observational study of physical activity, snacks and beverages. *American Journal of Health Behaviour* 44(2), 180–187.

Bharaskan, K., dos-Santos-Silva, I., Leon, D.A., Douglas, I.J. and Smeeth, L. (2018) Association of BMI with overall and cause-specific mortality: a population-based cohort study of 3.6 million adults in the UK. *Lancet Diabetes & Endocrinology* 6, 944–953.

Bray, G.A. (1990) Obesity: historical development of scientific and cultural ideas. *International Journal of Obesity* 14, 909–926.

Cancer Research UK (2021) Does Obesity Cause Cancer? Available at: https://www.cancerresearchuk.org/about-cancer/causes-of-cancer/obesity-weight-and-cancer/does-obesity-cause-cancer (accessed 30 January 2023).

Canoy, D. and Bundred, P. (2011) Obesity in children. *BMJ Clinical Evidence* 2011, 0325.

Cawley, J., Biener, A., Meyerhoefer, C., Ding, Y., Zvenyach, T., et al. (2021) Direct medical costs of obesity in the United States and the most populous states. *Journal of Managing Care and Speciality Pharmacy* 27(3), 354–366. https://doi.org/10.18553/jmcp.2021.20410

DEFRA (2013) Family Food Datasets: Detailed annual statistics on family food and drink purchases. Available at: https://www.gov.uk/government/statistical-data-sets/family-food-datasets (accessed 30 January 2023).

Ekelund, U., Tarp, J., Steene-Johannessen, J., Hansen, B.H., Jefferis, B., et al. (2019) Dose-response associations between accelerometry measured physical activity and sedentary time and all cause mortality: systematic review and harmonised meta-analysis. *BMJ* 366, l4570. https://doi.org/10.1136/bmj.l4570

Endocrine Society (2020) Poor fitness may impede long-term success in weight loss program. *Science Daily*, 31 March 2020. Available at: https://www.sciencedaily.com/releases/2020/03/200331130033.htm (accessed 16 January 2023).

Flack, K.D., Hays, H.M., Moreland, J. and Long, D.E. (2020) Exercise for weight loss: further evaluating energy compensation with exercise. *Medicine and Science in Sports and Exercise* 52(11), 2466–2475. https://doi.org/10.1249/MSS.0000000000002376

Fryar, C.D., Carroll, M.D. and Afful, J. (2020) Prevalence of overweight, obesity, and severe obesity among children and adolescents aged 2–19 years: United States, 1963–1965 through 2017–2018. *NCHS Health E-Stats*. Available at: https://www.cdc.gov/nchs/data/hestat/obesity-child-17-18/obesity-child.htm (accessed 30 January 2023).

Gaesser, G.A., Tucker, W.J., Jarrett, C.L. and Angadi, S.S. (2015) Fitness versus fatness: which influences health and mortality risk the most? *Current Sports Medicine Reports* 14(4), 327–332. https://doi.org/10.1249/JSR.0000000000000170

Global BMI Mortality Collaboration (2016) Body-mass index and all-cause mortality: individual-participant-data meta-analysis of 239 prospective studies in four continents. *Lancet* 388, 776–786.

Griffith, R., Lluberas, R. and Luhrmann, M. (2016) Gluttony and sloth? Calories, labor market activity and the rise of obesity. *Journal of the European Economic Association* 14, 1253–1286.

Guo, W., Key, T.J. and Reeves, G.K. (2019) Accelerometer compared with questionnaire measures of physical activity in relation to body size and composition: a large cross-sectional analysis of UK Biobank. *BMJ Open* 9, e024206. https://doi.org/10.1136/bmjopen-2018-024206

Hancock, C. (2021) Patterns and trends in excess weight among adults in England. *UK Health Security Agency Blog*, 4 March 2021. Available at: https://ukhsa.blog.gov.uk/2021/03/04/patterns-and-trends-in-excess-weight-among-adults-in-england/ (accessed 17 October 2022).

Hu, F.B., Willett, W.C., Li, T., Stampfer, M.J., Colditz, G.A. and Manson, J.E. (2004) Adiposity as compared with physical activity in predicting mortality among women. *New England Journal of Medicine* 351, 2694–2703.

Jakicic, J.M., Marcus, B.H., Lang, W. and Janney, C. (2008) Effect of exercise on 24-month weight loss maintenance in overweight women. *Archives of Internal Medicine* 198, 1550–1559.

Landré, B., Czernichow, S., Goldberg, M., Zins, M., Ankri, J. and Herr, M. (2020) Association between life-course obesity and frailty in older adults: findings in the GAZEL cohort. *Obesity* 28(2), 388–396. https://doi.org/10.1002/oby.22682

Lean, M.E.J., Leslie, W.S., Barnes, A.C., Brosnahan, N., Thom, G., et al. (2018) Primary care-led weight management for remission of type 2 diabetes (DiRECT): an open-label, cluster-randomised trial. *Lancet* 391, 541–551. https://doi.org/10.1016/S0140-6736(17)33102-1

Ludwig, D.S., Aronne, L.J., Astrup, A., de Cabo, R., Cantley, L.C., et al. (2021). The carbohydrate–insulin model: a physiological perspective on the obesity pandemic. *American Journal of Clinical Nutrition* 114, 1873–1885. https://doi.org/10.1093/ajcn/nqab270

Mielke, G.I., Bailey, T.G., Burton, N.W. and Brown, W.J. (2020) Participation in sports/recreational activities and incidence of hypertension, diabetes, and obesity in adults. *Scandinavian Journal of Medicine and Science in Sports* 30(12), 2390–2398. https://doi.org/10.1111/sms.13795

Miras, A. (2020) Royal Society of Medicine, Endocrinology and Diabetes section webinar series, entitled 'Respect and treat obesity like any other endocrine disease', EDN50, 22 September. Available at: https://www.medscape.co.uk/viewarticle/royal-society-medicine-respect-and-obesity-like-any-other-2020a1000yp6 (accessed 30 January 2023).

National Audit Office (2020) *Childhood Obesity. Report by the Comptroller and Auditor General*. National Audit Office, London.

Nevill, A.M., Stewart, A.D., Olds, T. and Duncan, M.J. (2020) A new waist-to-height ratio predicts abdominal adiposity in adults. *Research in Sports Medicine* 28(1), 15–26. https://doi.org/10.1080/15438627.2018.1502183

NHS Digital (2020) Statistics on Obesity, Physical Activity and Diet, England, 2020. Available at: https://digital.nhs.uk/data-and-information/publications/statistical/statistics-on-obesity-physical-activity-and-diet/england-2020 (accessed 30 January 2023).

NHS Digital (2021) National Child Measurement Programme, England 2020/21 School Year. Available at: https://digital.nhs.uk/data-and-information/publications/statistical/national-child-measurement-programme/2020-21-school-year (accessed 30 January 2023).

Novak, S. (2022a) Battle of the mid-life bulge. *New Scientist*, 12 March 2022, 39–41.

Novak, S (2022b) Obesity blockers. *New Scientist*, 7 May 2022, 46–49.

Nyberg, S.T., Batty, G.D., Pentti, J., Virtanen, M., Alfredsson, L., *et al.* (2018) Obesity and loss of disease-free years owing to major non-communicable diseases: a multicohort study. *Lancet Public Health* 3(10), e490–e497. https://doi.org/10.1016/S2468-2667(18)30139-7

Obesity Health Alliance (2021) *Turning the Tide: A 10-Year Health Weight Strategy*. Obesity Health Alliance. Available at: https://obesityhealthalliance.org.uk/turning-the-tide-strategy/ (accessed 16 January 2023).

O'Halloran, R., Mihaylova, B., Cairns, B.J. and Kent, S. (2020) BMI and cause-specific hospital admissions and costs: the UK Biobank cohort study. *Obesity* 28(7), 1332–1341. https://doi.org/10.1002/oby.22812

Ostendorf, D.M., Caldwell, A.E., Creasy, S.A., Pan, Z., Lyden, K., *et al.* (2018) Physical activity energy expenditure and total daily energy expenditure in successful weight loss maintainers. *Obesity* 27, 496–504.

Perez-Cornago, A., Dunneram, Y., Watts, E.L., Key, T.J. and Travis, R.C. (2022) Adiposity and risk of prostate cancer death: a prospective analysis in UK Biobank and meta-analysis of published studies. *BMC Medicine* 20, 143. https://doi.org/10.1186/s12916-022-02336-x

Pouwels, S., Sanches, E.E., Cagiltay, E., Severin, R. and Philips, S.A. (2020) Perioperative exercise therapy in bariatric surgery: improving patient outcomes. *Diabetes, Metabolic Syndrome and Obesity* 13, 1813–1823. https://doi.org/10.2147/DMSO.S215157. Erratum in: *Diabetes, Metabolic Syndrome and Obesity* 2022, 13, 2603. https://doi.org/10.2147/DMSO.S272430

Prospective Studies Collaboration (2009) Body-mass index and cause-specific mortality in 900,000 adults: collaborative analyses of 57 prospective studies. *Lancet* 373, 1083–1096.

Ranjbar, N., Turner, L. and Wanklyn, P. (2020) Obesity – the deadly disease no one dies of. Presented at the virtual *European and International Conference on Obesity (ECOICO), 1–4 September 2020*.

Robinson, E., Boyland, E., Chisholm, A., Harrold, J., Maloney, N.G., *et al.* (2021) Obesity, eating behavior and physical activity during COVID-19 lockdown: a study of UK adults. *Appetite* 156, 104853. https://doi.org/10.1016/j.appet.2020.104853

Rozjabek, H., Fastenau, J., LaPrade, A. and Sternbach, N. (2020) Adult obesity and health-related quality of life, patient activation, work productivity, and weight loss behaviors in the United States. *Diabetes, Metabolic Syndrome and Obesity* 13, 2049–2055.

Sanyaolu, A., Okorie, C., Qi, X., Locke, J. and Rehman, S. (2019) Childhood and adolescent obesity in the United States: a public health concern. *Global Pediatric Health* 6, 2333794X19891305. https://doi.org/10.1177/2333794X19891305

Shaw, K.A., Gennat, H.C., O'Rourke, P. and Del Mar, C. (2006) Exercise for overweight or obesity. *Cochrane Database of Systematic Reviews* 2006(4), CD003817. https://doi.og/10.1002/14651858.CD003817.pub3

Slenz, C.A., Duscha, B.D., Johnson, J.L., Ketchum, K., Aiken, L.B., *et al.* (2004) Effects of the amount of exercise on body weight, body composition and measures of central obesity: STRRIDE – a randomized controlled study. *Archives of Internal Medicine* 164, 31–39.

Somoes, E.J., Kobau, R., Kapp, J., Waterman, B., Mokdad, A. and Anderson, L. (2006) Associations of physical activity and body mass index with activities of daily living in older adults. *Journal of Community Health* 31, 453–467.

Stankovic, M., Djodjevic, S., Hadzovic, M., Djordjevic, D. and Katanic, B. (2021) The effects of physical activity on obesity among the population of different ages: a systematic review. *Journal of Anthropology of Sport and Physical Education* 5(3), 19–26. https://doi.org/10.26773/jaspe.210704

Stierman, B., Afful, J., Carroll, M.D., Chen, T.-C., Davy, O., *et al.* (2021) National Health and Nutrition Examination Survey 2012–March 2020 prepandemic data files – development of files and prevalence estimates for selected health outcomes. *National Health Statistics Reports* No. 158(14 June). https://doi.org/10.15620/cdc:106273

Sui, X., LaMonte, M.J., Laditka, J.N., Hardin, J.W., Chase, N., *et al.* (2007) Cardiorespiratory fitness and adiposity as mortality predictors in older adults. *JAMA* 298, 2507–2516.

Tan, M., He, F.J. and MacGregor, G.A. (2020) Obesity and covid-19: the role of the food industry. *BMJ* 369, m2237. https://doi.org/10.1136/bmj.m2237

Tarp, J., Grøntved, A., Sanchez-Lastra, M.A., Dalene, K.E., Ding, D. and Ekelund, U. (2021) Fitness, fatness, and mortality in men and women from the UK Biobank: prospective cohort study. *Journal of the American Heart Association* 10(6), e019605. https://doi.org/10.1161/JAHA.120.019605. Erratum in: *Journal of the American Heart Association* 2021, 10(8), e020837. https://doi.org/10.1161/JAHA.121.020837

Verheggen, R.J.H.M., Maessen, M.F.H., Green, D.J., Hermus, A.R.M.M., Hopman, M.T.E. and Thijssen, D.H.T. (2016) A systematic review and meta-analysis on the effects of exercise training versus hypocaloric diet: distinct effects on body weight and visceral adipose tissue. *Obesity Reviews* 17, 664–690. https://doi.org/10.1111/obr.12406

Viana, R.B., Naves, J.P.A., Coswig, V.S., de Lira, C.A.B., Steele, J., *et al.* (2020) Is interval training the magic bullet for fat loss? A systematic review and meta-analysis comparing moderate-intensity continuous training with high-intensity interval training (HIIT). *British Journal of Sports Medicine* 53, 655–664.

Wareham, N.J., van Sluijs, E.M.F. and Ekelund, U. (2005) Physical activity and obesity prevention: a review of the current evidence. *Proceedings of the Nutrition Society* 64, 229–247.

Williams, P.T. (2008) Asymmetric weight gain and loss from increasing and decreasing exercise. *Medicine and Science in Sports and Exercise* 40(2), 296–302. https://doi.org/10.1249/mss.0b013e31815b6475

Wise, J. (2022) Advise adults to keep waist size to less than half their height, says NICE. *BMJ* 377, o933. https://doi.org/10.1136/bmj.o933

Woolford, S.J., Sidell, M., Li, X., Else, V., Young, D.R., *et al.* (2021) Changes in body mass index among children and adolescents during the COVID-19 pandemic. *JAMA* 326(14), 1434–1436. https://doi.org/10.1001/jama.2021.15036

World Health Organization (2021) Obesity and Overweight. Available at: https://www.who.int/news-room/fact-sheets/detail/obesity-and-overweight (accessed 30 January 2023).

World Obesity Federation (2021) *Covid-19 and Obesity: The 2021 Atlas*. World Obesity Federation, London. Available at: https://www.worldobesity.org/resources/resource-library/covid-19-and-obesity-the-2021-atlas (accessed 16 January 2023).

Xie, W., Lundberg, D.J., Collins, J.M., Johnston, S.S., Waggoner, J.R., *et al.* (2020). Association of weight loss between early adulthood and midlife with all-cause mortality risk in the US. *JAMA Network Open* 3(8), e2013448. https://doi.org/10.1001/jamanetworkopen.2020.13448

Yanovski, S.Z. and Yanovski, J.A. (2021) Progress in pharmacotherapy for obesity. *JAMA* 326(2), 129–130. https://doi.org/10.1001/jama.2021.9486

11 High Blood Pressure (BP)

High BP is classified as a disease – but it is better seen as a risk factor for a number of other diseases, most notably for coronary disease and stroke. BP is expressed as a two-figure quantity – say, 120/80. The higher figure is the systolic pressure, which is the peak pressure reached when blood is pumped out from the heart to the main arteries. The arterial pressure then falls to the lower figure, which is the diastolic pressure, the lowest level reached before it is increased again by the next contraction of the heart. A level of 140/90 or less is usually taken as normal.

The unit of measurement used is millimetres of mercury, mmHg. This strangely antique unit came into being because BP was always measured with a mercury sphygmomanometer, which uses the height of a column of mercury as the measure of pressure. Modern sphygmomanometers no longer use mercury, so it would be more logical to use the Système International (SI) unit of pressure, the Pascal. However, the long-established mmHg is so ingrained into doctors' psyche that they have retained this archaic unit, rather as we continue to measure distance in the UK in miles rather than kilometres.

The distribution of BP in the population follows the usual distribution of most human characteristics – the bell-shaped curve (Fig. 11.1). As with height, for instance, there are a few people at the lower end of the range and a few at the upper end, but most are somewhere in between.

For the majority, high BP is not a disease – just a measurement within the upper range of a continuous scale. For a few people, high BP is due to some other condition, particularly kidney disease. Someone deemed by the medical profession to have high BP is labelled as having 'hypertension'. It is a very difficult condition to define – just where is the cut-off between acceptable upper level of BP and unacceptable hypertension? It could be the level above which the complications of raised BP start to become relevant. Unfortunately the ill effects develop insidiously and the higher the pressure the higher the risk. Wallis Simpson said that 'you can never be too thin or too rich' and to that one could add 'nor have too low a blood pressure'.

A better definition of hypertension would be the level above which lowering the BP reduces risk. Theoretically, this approach should be on firmer ground, but unfortunately even this soil is somewhat boggy. For decades it has been assumed that when a mildly raised pressure is treated with the appropriate medication to reach a more acceptable figure, risk is automatically reduced. However, there has been no evidence for reducing the systolic level below 140 mmHg until a recent study from the USA, the SPRINT study. This has indicated that reducing the systolic pressure down to 120 mmHg may have substantial advantages over the higher target of 140 mmHg (SPRINT Research Group, 2015; Vaduganathan et al., 2020). There is less certainty about appropriate BP levels in people over the age of 80. Enthusiastic lowering of BP in this group carries the risk of postural hypotension – low BP when standing (Masoli et al., 2020). This may cause faintness, dizziness and possibly dangerous falls in the elderly. It may also aggravate cognitive decline in older people (Pajewski et al., 2020).

Another confusion in the assessment of BP is that it is not a fixed figure; it is a fiction of the moment. It varies with time of day, pressure of work, timing of meals and contact with other people – particularly doctors. Most people are aware of 'white coat' hypertension, which is the condition in which BP is markedly higher when measured by a doctor. The most representative measurements of BP are those taken by the individual at home. There are plenty of reliable automatic home BP machines that will give a much more accurate picture of BP and its fluctuations than does the occasional snapshot BP taken in the surgery. The alternative is the 24-hour BP recorder, which is available to most GP surgeries.

DOI: 10.1079/9781800621855.0011

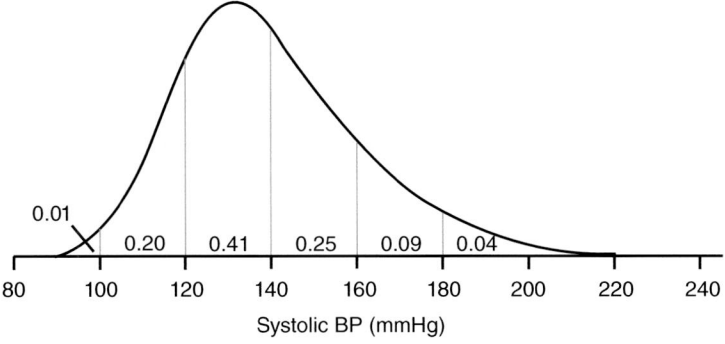

Fig. 11.1. Range of systolic BP in the population, following the Gaussian or bell-shaped distribution.

However it is measured, raised BP is common in Western societies and it continues to rise steadily with age. An American study found the prevalence of hypertension to be 9% for those aged 18–44, 40% for those aged 45–64 and 75% for those aged 65 and over (Gillespie and Hurvitz, 2013). Across the world more than 1 billion people are diagnosed as hypertensive and the condition is responsible for more than 10 million deaths annually (Zhou *et al.*, 2017).

The Medical Ill Effects of Raised BP

Persistently raised BP damages the walls of the arteries and this predisposes affected people to atheroma. There is a narrowing of the blood vessels by patchy plaques, which build up over many years, reducing the internal dimensions – or lumen – of the vessels and sometimes leading to complete blockage. The most damaging results include heart attacks, strokes and, less commonly, gangrene of the legs. Other ill effects of hypertension include kidney failure, heart failure, vascular dementia, visual loss, peripheral arterial disease and erectile dysfunction. Hypertension is the largest of all the risk factors for stroke, responsible for about 54% of cases. It is also an important risk factor for heart attacks, being implicated in about 47% of cases (Lawes *et al.*, 2008).

Exercise in the Prevention of Raised BP

Physical fitness has a direct effect on BP. A large Harvard alumni study showed that those who engaged in regular vigorous leisure activities had a 33% lower risk of developing hypertension than those who took little exercise (Paffenbarger *et al.*, 1983). There is a dose-response relationship between physical fitness and BP. A fitter person is likely to have a lower BP. In a study of 5249 middle-aged males in Copenhagen, every increase in VO_{2max} of 10 ml/min/kg was associated with a 2-mmHg reduction in both systolic and diastolic BP (Gyntelberg and Meyer, 1974). Researchers at University College London tracked 138 first-time runners who were training for the 2016 and 2017 London Marathons (Bhuva *et al.*, 2020). They compared the BPs and arterial stiffness 6 months before and 3 weeks after the race. They concluded that the 'heart age' of these novice runners dropped by almost 4 years in line with their reduced BP. A study that examined exactly which form of sport or exercise was most effective found that running, tennis, team sports, exercise classes and resistance training were best for keeping BP low (Mielki *et al.*, 2020). More specifically, regular muscle strengthening lowers the risk of developing hypertension by about 60% (Bennie *et al.*, 2020).

Exercise in the Treatment of Raised BP

Whatever a person's BP may be, they would probably be better off if, by their own efforts, they could bring it down. There are many aspects of lifestyle that contribute to increasing BP. The most important are eating too much salt, drinking too much alcohol, being obese and taking too little exercise. Before embarking on drug treatment for hypertension these should be corrected as far as is possible.

Exercise has well-documented benefits in lowering BP (Whelton *et al.*, 2002). Exercise as simple as walking reduces BP and the higher the BP, the greater the effect. A single bout of exercise reduces BP for several hours, while exercise training reduces BP both at rest and during exercise (Pescatello *et al.*,

2004). This training effect is reflected in a dose-related lowering of the risk of CVD and premature death at all degrees of hypertension. The more exercise that is taken, the lower the rate of both CVD and premature death. One report of a random study of 19,000 white men and women compared mortality with BP and activity level. At all levels of BP, physical activity was associated with a reduction in mortality in a dose-response pattern. In hypertensive individuals, light activity reduced mortality by 22% and moderate to high levels reduced mortality by 31% (Joseph *et al.*, 2019). Researchers at the University of California in San Francisco tracked the daily steps of 638 people using an Apple watch, while recording their BP weekly. They found that for every 1000 steps, BP reduced by 0.45 mmHg (Sardana *et al.*, 2021). In a further study in San Diego, 6000 women with an average age of 79 were studied. The researchers found that those women taking between 2100 and 4500 steps a day reduced their risk of dying from CVD by 38% (La Croix *et al.*, 2020). In Western Australia the effect of three different exercise regimens was tested in a number of older sedentary adults (Wheeler *et al.*, 2019). It was found that the best results for lowering BP were when participants did 30 minutes of walking on a treadmill in the morning followed by 6.5 hours of sitting, as long as they walked around for a few minutes every hour. People following this regimen reduced their systolic pressure by 5.1 mmHg, enough to significantly cut their chances of a heart attack or stroke.

It has been thought that only aerobic exercise was suitable for managing hypertension – but recent studies have shown that isometric exercise is perfectly safe in this condition (Hansford *et al.*, 2021) and may enhance the effect of aerobic exercise on its own. In a meta-analysis of 93 RCTs conducted among 5223 healthy adults, systolic BP was shown to be reduced after endurance, dynamic resistance and isometric resistance exercise regimens (Cornelissen and Smart, 2013).

The effect of exercise on BP is greatest in those who already have hypertension. It is likely that reducing BP with exercise and other lifestyle changes, such as losing weight and cutting back on salt and alcohol, are more effective at reducing risk than taking pills. Each lifestyle change has many other benefits. Often these can reduce BP sufficiently to allow the previously hypertensive patient to stop taking medication. The American Heart Association has summarized the benefits of exercise as well as other treatments in the management of high BP, concluding that 'moderate-intensity dynamic aerobic regimens are capable of significantly lowering BP among most individuals within a few months' (Brook *et al.*, 2013). In some cases, hypertension that is resistant to medication can respond to exercise training (Dimeo *et al.*, 2012).

After an extensive appraisal of the evidence, the American College of Cardiology concluded that for adult men and women regular aerobic physical activity decreases systolic and diastolic pressure significantly:

> The amount of physical activity recommended for lowering BP is congruent with the amount of physical activity recommended in 2008 by the federal government for overall health. Most health benefits occur with at least 150 minutes a week of moderate intensity physical activity such as brisk walking. *Additional benefits occur with more physical activity* [our emphasis].
>
> (Eckel *et al.*, 2014)

No trial has directly compared the effect of exercise with that of medication in reducing BP. However, comparative analysis of many trials of both approaches has indicated that exercise does have a very similar effect on BP as medication (Pescatello, 2019). The largest meta-analysis carried out compared the results of medication in 29,000 subjects with exercise in 10,000 subjects and concluded at an individual patient basis that medication was slightly more effective, but in groups the average response showed no difference (Naci *et al.*, 2019).

Summary

High blood pressure (BP) is a risk factor for a number of diseases, especially coronary disease and stroke. The population incidence follows a Gaussian curve, but var-ies throughout the day, with age and situation. Physical fitness has a beneficial effect on BP and appropriate exercise is a valid form of treatment for raised BP.

References

Bennie, J.A., Lee, D.C., Brellenthin, A.G. and De Cocker, K. (2020) Muscle-strengthening exercise and prevalent hypertension among 1.5 million adults: a little is better than none. *Journal of Hypertension* 38(8), 1466–1473. https://doi.org/10.1097/HJH.0000000000002415

Bhuva, A.N., D'Silva, A., Torlasco, C., Jones, S., Nadarajan, N., *et al.* (2020) Training for a first-time marathon reverses age-related aortic stiffening. *Journal of the American College of Cardiology* 75(1), 60–71. https://doi.org/10.1016/j.jacc.2019.10.045

Brook, R.D., Appel, L.J., Rubenfire, M., Ogedegbe, G., Bisognano, J.D., *et al.* (2013) Beyond medications and diet: alternative approaches to lowering blood pressure. A scientific statement from the American Heart Association. *Hypertension* 61, 1360–1383.

Cornelissen, V.A. and Smart, N.A. (2013) Exercise training for blood pressure: a systematic review and meta-analysis. *Journal of the American Heart Association* 2, e004473.

Dimeo, F., Pagonas, N., Seibert, F., Arndt, R., Zidek, W. and Westhoff, T.H. (2012) Aerobic exercise reduces blood pressure in resistant hypertension. *Hypertension* 60, 653–658.

Eckel, R.H., Jakicic, J.M., Ard, J.D., de Jesus, J.M., Houston Miller, N., *et al.* (2014) 2013 AHA/ACC guideline on lifestyle to reduce cardiovascular risk: a report of the American College of Cardiology/American Heart Association Task Force on Practice Guidelines. *Journal of the American College of Cardiology* 63(25 Pt B), 2960–2984.

Gillespie, C.D. and Hurvitz, K.A. (2013) Prevalence of hypertension and controlled hypertension – United States, 2007–2010. *MMWR Supplements* 62(3), 144–148.

Gyntelberg, F. and Meyer, J. (1974) Relationship between blood pressure and physical fitness, smoking and alcohol consumption in Copenhagen males aged 40–59. *Acta Medica Scandinavia* 195, 375–380.

Hansford, H.J., Parmenter, B.J., McLeod, K.A., Wewege, M.A., Smart, N.A., *et al.* (2021) The effectiveness and safety of isometric resistance training for adults with high blood pressure: a systematic review and meta-analysis. *Hypertension Research* 44, 1373–1384. https://doi.org/10.1038/s41440-021-00720-3

Joseph, G., Marott, J.L., Toorp-Pedersen, C., Biering-Sørensen, T., Nielsen, G., *et al.* (2019) Dose-response association between level of physical activity and mortality in normal, elevated and high blood pressure. *Hypertension* 74, 1307–1315.

La Croix, A.Z., Bellettiere, J., Di, C. and Lamonte, M.J. (2020) Every step counts in reducing cardiovascular disease among older women. Presented at *American Heart Association (AHA) EPI Lifestyle Scientific Sessions, Phoenix, Arizona, 3–6 March 2020* (abstract 30).

Lawes, C.M., Vander Hoorn, S. and Rodgers, A. (2008) Global burden of blood-pressure-related disease, 2001. *Lancet* 371, 1513–1518.

Masoli, J.A.H., Delgado, J., Pilling, L., Strain, D. and Melzer, D. (2020) Blood pressure in frail older adults: associations with cardiovascular outcomes and all-cause mortality. *Age and Ageing* 49(5), 807–813. https://doi.org/10.1093/ageing/afaa028

Mielki, G.I., Bailey, T.G., Burton, N.W. and Brown, W.J. (2020) Participation in sports/recreational activities and incidence of hypertension, diabetes and obesity in adults. *Scandinavian Journal of Medicine and Science in Sports* 30(12), 2390–2398.

Naci, H., Salcher-Konrad, M., Dias, S., Blum, M.R., Sahoo, S.A., *et al.* (2019) How does exercise treatment compare with antihypertensive medications? A network meta-analysis of 391 randomised controlled trials assessing exercise and medication effects on systolic blood pressure. *British Journal of Sports Medicine* 53, 859–869. https://doi.org/10.1136/bjsports-2018-099921

Paffenbarger, R.S. Jr, Wing, A.L., Hyde, R.T. and Jung, D.L. (1983) Physical activity and incidence of hypertension in college alumni. *American Journal of Epidemiology* 117(3), 245–257.

Pajewski, N.M., Berlowitz, D.R., Bress, A.P., Callahan, K.E., Cheung, A.K., *et al.* (2020) Intensive vs standard blood pressure control in adults 80 years or older: a secondary analysis of the Systolic Blood Pressure Intervention Trial. *Journal of the American Geriatric Society* 68(3), 496–504. https://doi.org/10.1111/jgs.16272

Pescatello, L.S. (2019) Exercise measures up to medication as hypertensive therapy: its value has long been underestimated. *British Journal of Sports Medicine* 53(14), 849–852. https://doi.org/10.1136/bjsports-2018-100359

Pescatello, L.S., Franklin, B.A., Fagard, R., Farquhar, W.B., Kelley, G.A. and Ray, C.A. (2004) American College of Sports Medicine position stand: exercise and hypertension. *Medicine and Science in Sports and Exercise* 36(3), 533–553.

Sardana, M., Lin, H., Zhang, Y., Liu, C., Trinquart, L., *et al.* (2021) Association of habitual physical activity with home blood pressure in the electronic Framingham Heart Study (eFHS): cross-sectional study. *Journal of Medical Internet Research* 23(6), e25591. https://doi.org/10.2196/25591

SPRINT Research Group (2015) A randomized trial of intensive versus standard blood-pressure control. *New England Journal of Medicine* 373, 2103–2116.

Vaduganathan, M., Claggett, B., Juraschek, S. and Solomon, S. (2020) Assessment of long-term benefit of intensive blood pressure control on residual life span: secondary analysis of the Systolic Blood Pressure Intervention Trial (SPRINT). *JAMA Cardiology* 5(5), 576–581.

Wheeler, M.J., Dunstan, D.W., Ellis, K.A., Cerin, E., Phillips, S., *et al.* (2019) Effect of morning exercise with or without breaks in prolonged sitting on blood pressure in older overweight/obese adults. *Hypertension* 73(4), 859–867. https://doi.org/10.1161/HYPERTE NSIONAHA.118.12373

Whelton, S.P., Chin, A., Xin, X. and He, J. (2002) Effect of aerobic exercise on blood pressure: a meta-analysis of randomized, controlled trials. *Annals of Internal Medicine* 136, 493–503.

Zhou, B., Bentham, J., Di Cesare, M., Bixby, H., Danaei, G., *et al.* (2017) Worldwide trends in blood pressure from 1975 to 2015: a pooled analysis of 1479 population-based measurement studies with 19.1 million participants. *Lancet* 389, 37–55. https://doi.org/10.1016/S0140-6736(16)31919-5. Erratum in: *Lancet* 2020, 396, 886. https://doi.org/10.1016/S0140-6736 (20)31972-3

12 Dyslipidaemia

Dyslipidaemia means undesirable changes in your blood fats. This is a complicated field and what follows is a simplification.

Blood Fats

Cholesterol

There are a number of different forms of fat in the bloodstream, the best known of which is cholesterol. Cholesterol is an important component of cell walls. Everyone needs it to function properly. Proteins called lipoproteins, which can very roughly be divided into two forms, carry the cholesterol in the blood. These are low-density lipoprotein cholesterol (LDL-C) and high-density lipoprotein cholesterol (HDL-C).

LDL-C can become established in the walls of the arteries in the plaques of atheroma ('hardening of the arteries') – the 'pinch points' that narrow the artery. This is the so-called 'bad' cholesterol. A high level of LDL-C is a risk factor for atheroma, leading to heart attacks and strokes.

There are various causes of high LDL-C, including genetic factors; being overweight; having an underactive thyroid gland; some forms of kidney disease; and eating a high-fat diet, particularly a diet with a lot of 'saturated' fat. There are three main categories of fats: saturated fats, unsaturated fats and trans fats. All are made up of carbon, hydrogen and oxygen molecules. Saturated fats are saturated with hydrogen molecules and contain only single bonds between carbon molecules. They tend to be solid at room temperature. Unsaturated fats have at least one double bond between carbon molecules and tend to be liquid at room temperature. Trans fats are vegetable oils which have been artificially hydrogenated to extend their shelf life. Consumption of trans fats increases LDL-C and lowers HDL-C and is associated with an increase in all forms of CVD. Examples include margarine and frying oils.

Saturated fat is largely derived from animals – being found in cream, butter, fatty joints of meat and, particularly, prepared meat products such as meat pies, pâtés and sausages. Fat is cheaper than lean meat, so food manufacturers use it liberally. Unsaturated fat is usually of plant origin and sources include peanut oil; vegetable oils, such as sunflower and corn oil; fatty fish, such as salmon and mackerel; and nuts and seeds, such as almonds, peanuts, cashews and sesame seeds.

HDL-C is the form that transports cholesterol to the liver where it is broken down and excreted in the bile. This is the so-called 'good' cholesterol. A high level of HDL-C is protective while a low level is a risk factor for atheroma. The main causes of a low HDL-C are cigarette smoking, obesity, diabetes and physical inactivity.

The 'normal' level of these fat fractions is somewhat arbitrary and there is a tendency for each new generation of cholesterol recommendations to set the limits for total cholesterol and LDL-C lower and lower. Levels are measured in millimoles per litre, mmol/l. Currently the recommended upper limit for total cholesterol is 5.0 mmol/l and for LDL-C it is 3.0 mmol/l. The bell-shaped curve of normal distribution would put most of the population in the too-high category. HDL-C makes up around one-quarter of the total cholesterol – the current recommendation is that it should be above 1.0 mmol/l. A better measure of risk for atheroma and CVD is the ratio between total cholesterol and HDL-C. This should be below 4.0 and preferably much lower. This is the measure of cholesterol level used in algorithms for calculating risk of CVD ('Q-Risk3'; https//qrisk.org (accessed 17 January 2023)).

The treatment of dyslipidaemia should involve changes in diet, but in practice most people find it nearly impossible to change the way they eat and maintain it. The modern treatment is the group of drugs known as the statins, which are very effective. Not only do they reduce LDL-C by up to 30% as

© H.J.N. Bethell and D. Brodie 2023. *Exercise: A Scientific and Clinical Overview* (H.J.N. Bethell and D. Brodie)
DOI: 10.1079/9781800621855.0012

well as reduce the LDL-C/HDL-C ratio, but they also reduce the risk of atheroma substantially. The risk is reduced so substantially that it is regarded as obligatory to prescribe them for all those deemed to be at high risk and particularly for those who already have evidence of arterial disease.

Triglycerides

Triglycerides are esters derived from glycerol and three fatty acids. They are the main constituents of body fat in humans and other vertebrates and are carried in the bloodstream. Raised levels are associated with genetic factors, unhealthy diet, obesity, diabetes, sedentary living and cigarette smoking. They carry an increased risk for atheroma – heart attacks, strokes and peripheral vascular disease (PVD).

The Medical Ill Effects of Dyslipidaemia

The main ill effect is the promotion of atheroma. A high total cholesterol, a high ratio of total cholesterol to HDL-C and raised triglyceride levels are all powerful risk factors for heart attacks, strokes and PVD (see Chapter 16, this volume). For this reason, the total cholesterol/HDL-C ratio is an important element of the Q-Risk assessment for predicting CVD. Dyslipidaemia is also a feature of the 'metabolic syndrome' (see Chapter 14, this volume), which is a combination of obesity, hypertension, diabetes and lipid abnormalities. The metabolic syndrome carries a high risk of CVD, particularly heart disease.

Effect of Exercise on Lipids

The effect that exercise has on the different fat fractions found in the blood is not straightforward and some of the studies are contradictory. There are age-related changes in total cholesterol and LDL-C, both of which increase gradually with time. Regular exercise and high levels of physical fitness delay this undesirable progression. A study of physical fitness in 11,400 people who had several treadmill tests over 36 years found those in the lower third for fitness developed abnormal lipids 10 to 15 years earlier than those in the fittest third (Park *et al.*, 2015).

The data on the response of lipid abnormalities to exercise alone are surprisingly and disappointingly sparse, and sometimes contradictory. A 2001 meta-analysis concluded that regular aerobic exercise does raise HDL-C levels (Leon and Sanchez, 2001), but that the effect on other lipid levels was less certain. It also seemed that exercise alone was less effective than the combination of diet and exercise (Varady and Jones, 2005). A meta-analysis of the effects of exercise training on HDL-C involving 25 studies found a modest increase in HDL-C, with a threshold for producing this effect being about 120 minutes of moderate exercise weekly. Exercise duration per session was the most important element of an exercise prescription. Exercise was more effective in subjects with initially high total cholesterol levels or low BMI (Kodama *et al.*, 2007). Confusingly, a further meta-analysis found that diet and exercise reduce total cholesterol, total cholesterol/HDL-C ratio and LDL-C but have little effect on HDL-C (Kelley *et al.*, 2012). The same group had previously reported that regular walking reduces both total cholesterol and the ratio of total cholesterol to HDL-C (Kelley *et al.*, 2004). For the most part, however, exercise alone has small effects on dyslipidaemia unless it is accompanied by weight loss (Gordon *et al.*, 2014). There does appear to be a level of disparity in these studies, but all are agreed that regular exercise does reduce the all-important total cholesterol/HDL-C ratio.

Triglyceride levels are reduced acutely by exercise for up to 24 hours. Physical training can increase this effect because fitter people can take more prolonged and more vigorous exercise (Thompson *et al.*, 2001).

The most effective management of dyslipidaemia is the combination of statins, diet and exercise. A cohort of 10,043 Americans with dyslipidaemia was studied. Among men treated with statins, the risk of dying over the next 10 years for the most fit was just 30% of the risk for the least fit (Kokkinos *et al.*, 2012).

Finally, it is appropriate to take heed of the conclusions of the American Heart Association and the American College of Cardiology. After a thorough appraisal of all the evidence, they concluded that it might require 12 MET hours of exercise per week to lower LDL-C (Eckel *et al.*, 2014). That is about 1 hour and 40 minutes of very brisk walking at 4 mph, every week.

Summary

Disturbances of the normal patterns of blood fats are known as dyslipidaemia and include raised blood cholesterol and triglyceride levels. The contributors to dyslipidaemia include inherited factors, diet, diseases of the thyroid and kidneys, and lack of exercise. Dyslipidaemia is one element of the 'metabolic' syndrome and is a powerful risk factor for atheroma, heart disease and strokes.

References

Eckel, R.H., Jakicic, J.M., Ard, J.D., de Jesus, J.M., Houston Miller, N., et al. (2014) 2013 AHA/ACC guideline on lifestyle management to reduce cardiovascular risk: a report of the American College of Cardiology/American Heart Association Task Force on Practice Guidelines. *Journal of the American College of Cardiology* 63(25 Pt B), 2960–2984.

Gordon, B., Chen, S. and Durstine, J.L. (2014) The effects of exercise training on the traditional lipid profile and beyond. *Current Sports Medicine Reports* 13(4), 253–259. https://doi.org/10.1249/JSR.0000000000 000073

Kelley, G.A., Kelley, K.S. and Tran, Z.V. (2004) Walking, lipids, and lipoproteins: a meta-analysis of randomized controlled trials. *Preventive Medicine* 38, 651–661.

Kelley, G.A., Kelley, K.S., Roberts, S. and Haskell, W. (2012) Combined effects of aerobic exercise and diet on lipids and lipoproteins in overweight and obese adults: a meta-analysis. *Journal of Obesity* 2012, 985902. https://doi.org/10.1155/2012/985902

Kodama, S., Tanaka, S., Saito, K., Shu, M., Sone, Y., et al. (2007) Effect of aerobic exercise training on serum levels of high-density lipoprotein cholesterol: a meta-analysis. *Archives of Internal Medicine* 167, 999–1008.

Kokkinos, P.F., Faselis, C., Myers, J., Panagiotakos, D. and Doumas, M. (2012) Interactive effects of fitness and statin treatment on mortality risk in veterans with dyslipidaemia: a cohort study. *Lancet* 381, 394–399.

Leon, A.S. and Sanchez, O.A. (2001) Response of blood lipids to exercise training alone or combined with dietary intervention. *Medicine and Science in Sports and Exercise* 33(6 Suppl.), S502–S515.

Park, Y.M., Sui, X., Liu, J., Zhou, H., Kokkinos, P.F., et al. (2015) The effect of cardiorespiratory fitness on age-related lipids and lipoproteins. *Journal of the American College of Cardiology* 65, 2091–2100.

Thompson, P.D., Crouse, S.F., Goodpaster, B., Kelley, D., Moyna, N. and Pescatello, L. (2001) The acute versus the chronic response to exercise. *Medicine and Science in Sports and Exercise* 33(6 Suppl.), S438–S445. https://doi.org/10.1097/00005768-200106001-00012

Varady, K.A. and Jones, P.J. (2005) Combination diet and exercise interventions for the treatment of dyslipidemia: an effective preliminary strategy to lower cholesterol levels? *Journal of Nutrition* 135, 1829–1835.

13 Diabetes

The main consideration for this chapter is type 2 diabetes mellitus (T2DM). Type 1 diabetes mellitus (T1DM) is something totally separate, although it is also a risk factor for CVD. T1DM is a condition whose onset is usually in young people whose pancreas fairly suddenly fails and stops producing insulin. T2DM develops later in life and the problem is not an absence but an insufficiency of insulin.

Insulin is essential for the control of sugar in the blood, ushering the sugar into the cells to help fuel activity and ensuring that the level of glucose in the blood is kept within narrow limits. People with T1DM can survive only by regularly injecting themselves with insulin for the rest of their days. T2DM develops later in life and is largely a result of an unhealthy lifestyle. There is a genetic element – the tendency to develop T2DM is inherited, but it rarely manifests in the absence of too much food and too little exercise. Some 80–85% of the risk of developing T2DM is down to obesity (Diabetes UK, 2020) and exercise has a major part to play, as shown in Chapter 10 (this volume). The pancreas in normal people responds to the flood of glucose into the bloodstream after each meal by increasing the output of insulin. The insulin helps the cells to absorb the glucose, keeping blood glucose level constant and fuelling cellular activity. Exercise assists this process by enhancing absorption of glucose into muscle cells.

People who carry too much weight, particularly those with central obesity, and take too little exercise develop a state called *insulin resistance*. In this condition, insulin becomes less effective at keeping blood glucose levels normal and a greater production of insulin is needed to maintain homeostasis (normal blood levels). So the pancreas has to work ever harder to produce enough insulin for normal metabolism and eventually becomes unable to satisfy the body's ability to keep its sugar level within normal limits. Consequently, the blood sugar rises producing hyperglycaemia, the hallmark of diabetes,

in this case T2DM. The laying down of fat where it is not wanted aggravates the problem. In the liver this further increases insulin resistance while in the pancreas it further reduces the production of insulin. Physical inactivity is a major factor in facilitating insulin resistance.

T2DM is a growing epidemic, with ever-rising rates of diagnosis as the population becomes older, fatter and less active. In the mid-1990s, about 2 to 3% of the UK population was known to be affected by diabetes. The figure now is about 6% and growing (Saeedi *et al.*, 2020), with about 100,000 people newly diagnosed with diabetes each year. There are about 4 million diabetic patients in the UK, with more than 21,000 deaths per annum. With the enormous increase in childhood obesity, T2DM in children, which used to be a rarity, is on the rise too. In England and Wales about 7000 people under the age of 25 are diabetic (Diabetes UK, 2020) and this is the tip of the iceberg of the threat for the future. A Bristol University study of 4000 participants from the 'Children of the 90s' showed subtle differences in the metabolism of young people who were more prone to developing diabetes later in life (Boyd *et al.*, 2013).

The annual cost to the NHS of managing diabetes is a staggering £11.7 billion, which is more than 12% of the total NHS budget.

Side Effects of Diabetes

The complications of diabetes are legion. It is a risk factor for atheroma of large vessels, which leads to heart attacks and strokes and may also result in gangrene of the legs. Small blood vessels are also affected leading to kidney disease and impairment of sight and ultimately to blindness. Damage to nerves causes numbness and neuralgic pain. Diabetic patients are particularly susceptible to infections. Since most type 2 diabetics are obese, they are at increased risk of a number of different cancers, but

DOI: 10.1079/9781800621855.0013

there is also a link between diabetes and cancer that is independent of their obesity. Untreated diabetes is a risk factor for dementia, which develops more rapidly in diabetic sufferers. Frailty of old age is an increasing end-stage for many.

T2DM is a most unpleasant disease and in most cases it is preventable. Indeed, too much food and too little exercise are such important causative factors that diabetes can be cured in a proportion of sufferers simply by eating less and exercising more (The Look Ahead Research Group, 2007). The fact that this is so seldom achieved indicates the difficulty in stimulating inactive, overweight individuals to change their lifestyles. Part of the problem may lie in the fact that so many diabetics seem to be unaware that they have the cure for their disease in their own hands. Education of diabetics with a clear focus on the dangers of poor control can be a powerful tool in the management of this condition (Gagliardino et al., 2012).

Exercise in the Prevention of Diabetes

There is growing awareness in the health profession that prevention of T2DM is both desirable and achievable with the main emphasis on weight loss. Weight loss equivalent to 13% of body weight reduces the risk of progression to T2DM by about 40% (Haase et al., 2021). Sedentary time is a risk factor and replacing as little as 30 minutes of sitting per week with physical activity reduces the risk of developing T2DM by between 6 and 31% (Li et al., 2021) The NHS has set up a nationwide Diabetes Prevention Programme (DPP). An analysis of the first 100,000 referrals to the programme found an uptake of 56% but a disappointing completion rate of 12% (Howarth et al., 2020). However, some promising results are being achieved. A number of studies have confirmed that diet and exercise reduce the chance of developing T2DM in susceptible people (i.e. obese people or those with insulin resistance) to as much as half the expected level (Knowler et al., 2002; Orozco et al., 2008; Tuomilehto et al., 2016). The response has a curvilinear distribution, with the steepest section of the curve at the lower levels of exercise but continuing effectiveness with increasing levels of activity up to 300 minutes of moderate-to-vigorous exercise per week. This is equivalent to 22 MET hours weekly (Mutie et al., 2020; Zhao et al., 2020). When considering specific exercise types, running, cycling, resistance training and yoga have all been found to reduce the risk of developing T2DM (Mielke et al., 2020). Exercise is also as effective as medication for preventing the progression from 'pre-diabetes' to clinical T2DM (Naci et al., 2019).

It is difficult to disentangle the effects of diet and exercise in a condition which is so dependent on body weight. It is possible, however, to be confident that any intervention that reduces body weight – which certainly includes exercise (see Chapter 10, this volume) – will also reduce the incidence of T2DM. Some studies of exercise as preventive treatment have shown that almost any level of activity is beneficial, though with smaller gains for increased effort at higher levels of exertion (Yerramalla et al., 2020). Curiously, leisure-time activity is more effective than occupational exertion (Mutie et al., 2020).

The latest Cochrane Review examined 12 RCTs of diet and exercise for over 5000 people at high risk of T2DM (Hemmingsen et al., 2017). The review concluded that the effects of diet or exercise alone were relatively small, but the combination did have a significant effect, reducing the risk from 26% in the control group to 15% in the combined group. Additional benefits of this approach to prevention are reduction in weight, waist circumference and BP.

Exercise in the Treatment of Diabetes

As with prevention, diet and exercise should be the centrepieces of any treatment for diabetes. It should aim to reduce weight and thereby lessen insulin resistance. If this is done quickly and effectively, many patients with diabetes can be cured (Christian et al., 2008). The loss of at least 15% of body weight should become the initial treatment goal (Lingvay et al., 2022). Studies of diet and exercise in the treatment of T2DM have indicated that up to nearly 50% can be cured of their disease in this way (McInnes et al., 2017). A highly successful RCT of lifestyle management of T2DM was reported from Scotland and Newcastle in 2018, with 298 obese diabetic patients receiving either intensive weight management or their usual care. The intervention group had their medication withdrawn and were given a carefully controlled diet completely different to their usual regimen. This lasted for a period of 12 weeks, followed by a 4-week food-reintroduction phase and a further weight-management phase lasting up to 2 years. The weight-management phase used diet and exercise programmes to try to prevent them regaining weight. After 1 year, 46% of the intervention group had remission of their diabetes compared with only 4% in the control group (Lean *et al.*, 2017). There was a reduction of an amazing 86% in the incidence of diabetes among those who lost 15 kg or more (Fig. 13.1).

For some, such an approach is too late to effect a cure – the pancreas is already exhausted and cannot keep up with the body's demands. Nevertheless, diet and exercise enhance the effects of other treatments and sometimes make them unnecessary. Most diabetics need tablets to reduce their blood sugar to reasonable levels and some require insulin. Diet and exercise, combined with weekly counselling, has been shown to reduce considerably the need for medication even in those not cured (Colberg *et al.*, 2016). Results were best for those who lost the most weight or who started the programme with less severe or with newly diagnosed diabetes. Those who do not achieve remission with diet and exercise still have much to gain from regular physical activity. Exercise can greatly improve diabetic control (Kurniawati *et al.*, 2019). Regular exercise improves glycaemic control, reduces glycated haemoglobin (HbA1c), improves blood lipids, lowers BP and increases physical fitness (Barbosa *et al.*, 2021). Better sexual function and quality of life are additional benefits (Martenstyn *et al.*, 2020). The response to exercise for diabetic control is, like the response for prevention, related to dose of exercise (Sigal *et al.*, 2007) and curvilinear (Gay *et al.*, 2016). Both aerobic and combined aerobic and resistance exercise have these effects but not resistance exercise on its own.

Diabetics who respond favourably to diet and exercise and maintain their improved control or remission for over 2 years or more have been shown to have an increase in pancreatic volume. This suggests that their response may be mediated partly through recovery of beta-cell function (Al-Mrabeh *et al.*, 2020).

Exercise in the Prevention of the Complications of Diabetes

Intensive lifestyle interventions have many other benefits for the type 2 diabetic. These include better glucose and lipid control, improved BP, less sleep apnoea, lower liver fat, less depression, less urinary incontinence, less severe kidney disease, less retinopathy (i.e. blindness and sight loss), reduced need of diabetes medications, maintenance of physical mobility, improved quality of life, less knee pain, improved sexual function, lowered inflammation and reduced overall health costs (Pi-Sunyer, 2014). The Whitehall study has shown an increase in life expectancy for diabetics who take regular exercise (Yerramalla *et al.*, 2020) and this has been confirmed in a study of the cycling habits of diabetics followed over 15 years. Cycling for 150 to 300 minutes per week was associated with 35% lower mortality than in non-cyclists (Redberg *et al.*, 2021). Walking has also been shown to reduce mortality in diabetics. A study from the National Center for Chronic Disease Prevention and Health Promotion in the USA examined the activity levels of nearly 3000 adults. Compared with inactive individuals, those who walked at least 2 hours per week had a 39% lower all-cause mortality rate and a 34% lower CVD mortality rate (Gregg *et al.*, 2003).

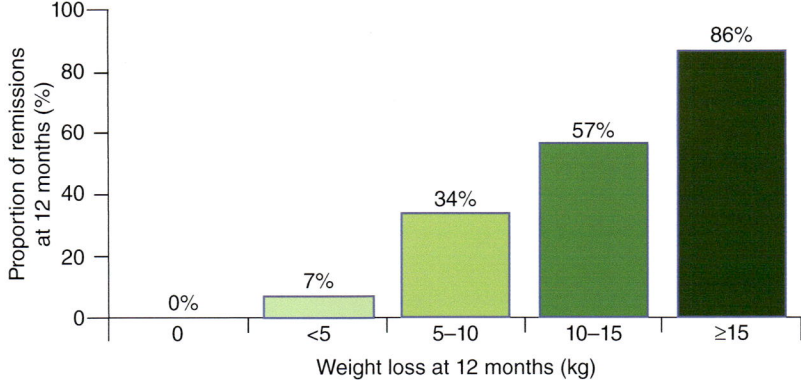

Fig. 13.1. Effect of weight loss on remission of type 2 diabetes. (From Sbraccia *et al.*, 2021. Article available under the terms of the Creative Commons Attribution 4.0 International License; https://creativecommons.org/licenses/by/4.0/.)

Summary

Type 2 diabetes mellitus most often develops later in life and is largely a result of an unhealthy lifestyle. It costs more than 12% of the NHS budget. Exercise has been shown in numerous reviews to reduce the risk of diabetes. Exercise is a valid treatment for diabetes and can assist in the prevention of the complications of diabetes. Cycling and walking have been shown to be especially beneficial.

References

Al-Mrabeh, A., Hollingsworth, K.G., Shaw, J.A.M., McConnachie, A., Sattar, N., *et al*. (2020) 2-year remission of type 2 diabetes and pancreas morphology: a post-hoc analysis of the DiRECT open-label, cluster-randomised trial. *Lancet Diabetes & Endocrinology* 8(12), 939–948. https://doi.org/10.1016/S2213-8587(20)30303-X

Barbosa, A., Brito, J., Figueiredo, P., Seabra, A. and Mendes, R. (2021) Football can tackle type 2 diabetes: a systematic review of the health effects of recreational football practice in individuals with prediabetes and type 2 diabetes. *Research in Sports and Medicine* 29(3), 303–321. https://doi.org/10.1080/15438627.2020.1777417

Boyd, A., Golding, J., Macleod, J., Lawlor, D.A., Fraser, A., *et al*. (2013) Cohort profile: the 'Children of the 90s' – the index offspring of the Avon Longitudinal Study of Parents and Children. *International Journal of Epidemiology* 42(1), 111–127. https://doi.org/10.1093/ije/dys064

Christian, J.G., Bessesen, D.H., Byers, T.E., Christian, K.K., Goldstein, M.G. and Bock, B.C. (2008) Clinic-based support to help overweight patients with type 2 diabetes increase physical activity and lose weight. *Archives of Internal Medicine* 168(2), 141–146.

Colberg, S.R., Sigal, R.J., Yardley, J.E., Riddell, M.C., Dunstan, D.W., *et al*. (2016) Physical activity/exercise and diabetes: a position statement of the American Diabetes Association. *Diabetes Care* 39(11), 2065–2079. https://doi.org/10.2337/dc16-1728

Diabetes UK (2020) Diabetes Statistics. Available at: https://www.diabetes.org.uk/professionals/position-statements-reports/statistics (accessed 30 January 2023).

Gagliardino, J.J., Aschner, P., Baik, S.H., Chan, J., Chantelot, J.M., *et al*. (2012) Patients' education, and its impact on care outcomes, resource consumption and working conditions: data from the International Diabetes Management Practices Study (IDMPS). *Diabetes & Metabolism* 38(2), 128–134. https://doi.org/10.1016/j.diabet.2011.09.002

Gay, J.L., Buchner, D.M. and Schmidt, M.D. (2016) Dose-response association of physical activity with HbA1c: intensity and bout length. *Preventive Medicine* 86, 58–63. https://doi.org/10.1016/j.ypmed.2016.01.008

Gregg, E.W., Gerzoff, R.B., Caspersen, C.J., Williamson, D.F. and Narayan, K.M. (2003) Relationship of walking to mortality among US adults with diabetes. *Archives of Internal Medicine* 163(12), 1440–1447. https://doi.org/10.1001/archinte.163.12.1440

Haase, C.L., Lopes, S., Olsen, A.H., Satylganova, A., Schnecke, V. and McEwan, P. (2021) Weight loss and risk reduction of obesity-related outcomes in 0.5 million people: evidence from a UK primary care database. *International Journal of Obesity* 45, 1249–1258. https://doi.org/10.1038/s41366-021-00788-4

Hemmingsen, B., Gimenez-Perez, G., Mauricio, D., Figuls, M.R.I., Metzendorf, M.-I. and Richter, B. (2017) Diet, physical activity or both for prevention or delay of type 2 diabetes mellitus and its associated complications in people at increased risk of developing type 2 diabetes. *Cochrane Database of Systematic Reviews* 12(12), CD003054. https://doi.org/10.1002/14651858.CD003054.pub4

Howarth, E., Bower, P.J., Kontopantelis, E., Soiland-Reyes, C., Meacock, R., *et al*. (2020) 'Going the distance': an independent cohort study of engagement and dropout among the first 100 000 referrals into a large-scale diabetes prevention program. *BMJ Open Diabetes Research & Care* 8, e001835. https://doi.org/10.1136/bmjdrc-2020-001835

Knowler, W.C., Barrett-Connor, E., Fowler, S.E., Hamman, R.F., Lachin, J.M., *et al*. (2002) Reduction in the incidence of type 2 diabetes with lifestyle intervention or metformin. *New England Journal of Medicine* 346(6), 393–403.

Kurniawati, Y., Baridah, H.A., Kusumawati, M.D. and Wabula, I. (2019) Effectiveness of physical exercise on the glycemic control of type 2 diabetes mellitus patients: a systematic review. *Jurnal Ners* 14(3si), 199–204. https://doi.org/10.20473/jn.v14i3(si).17059

Lean, M.E.J., Leslie, W.S., Barnes, A.C., Brosnahan, N., Thom, G., *et al*. (2017) Primary care-led weight management for remission of type 2 diabetes (DiRECT): an open-label, cluster-randomised trial. *Lancet* 391, 541–551.

Li, X., Zhou, T., Ma, H., Liang, Z., Fonseca, V.A. and Qi, L. (2021) Replacement of sedentary behavior by various daily-life physical activities and structured exercises: genetic risk and incident type 2 diabetes. *Diabetes Care* 44(10), 2403–2410. https://doi.org/10.2337/dc21-0455

Lingvay, I., Sumithran, P., Cohen, R.V. and le Roux, C.W. (2022) Obesity management as a primary treatment goal for type 2 diabetes: time to reframe the conversation. *Lancet* 399, 394–405. https://doi.org/10.1016/S0140-6736(21)01919-X

Look Ahead Research Group (2007) Reduction in weight and cardiovascular disease risk factors in individuals with type 2 diabetes: one-year results of the Look AHEAD trial. *Diabetes Care* 30(6), 1374–1383. https://doi.org/10.2337/dc07-0048

Martenstyn, J., King, M. and Rutherford, C. (2020) Impact of weight loss interventions on patient-reported outcomes in overweight and obese adults with type 2 diabetes: a systematic review. *Journal of Behavioral Medicine* 43(6), 873–891. https://doi.org/10.1007/s10865-020-00140-7

McInnes, N., Smith, A., Otto, R., Vandermey, J., Punthakee, Z., *et al.* (2017) Piloting a remission strategy in type 2 diabetes: results of a randomized controlled trial. *Journal of Clinical Endocrinology and Metabolism* 102, 1595–1605.

Mielke, G.I., Bailey, T.G., Burton, N.W. and Brown, W.J. (2020) Participation in sports/recreational activities and incidence of hypertension, diabetes, and obesity in adults. *Scandinavian Journal of Medicine and Science in Sports* 30(12), 2390–2398. https://doi.org/10.1111/sms.13795

Mutie, P.M., Drake, I., Ericson, U., Teleka, S., Schulz, C.-A., *et al.* (2020) Different domains of self-reported physical activity and risk of type 2 diabetes in a population-based Swedish cohort: the Malmö Diet and Cancer Study. *BMC Public Health* 20, 261. https://doi.org/10.1186/s12889-020-8344-2

Naci, H., Salcher-Konrad, M., Dias, S., Blum, M.R., Sahoo, S.A., *et al.* (2019) How does exercise treatment compare with antihypertensive medications? A network meta-analysis of 391 randomised controlled trials assessing exercise and medication effects on systolic blood pressure. *British Journal of Sports Medicine* 53, 859–869. https://doi.org/10.1136/bjsports-2018-099921

Orozco, L.J., Buchleitner, A.M., Gimenez-Perez, G., Figuls, M.R.I., Richter, B. and Mauricio, D. (2008) Exercise or exercise and diet for preventing type 2 diabetes mellitus. *Cochrane Database of Systematic Reviews* (3), CD003054. https://doi.org/10.1002/14651858.CD003054.pub3

Pi-Sunyer, X. (2014) The Look AHEAD Trial: a review and discussion of its outcomes. *Current Nutrition Reports* 3(4), 387–391.

Redberg, R.F., Vittinghoff, E. and Katz, M.H. (2021) Cycling for health. *JAMA Internal Medicine* 181(9), 1206. https://doi.org/10.1001/jamainternmed.2021.3830

Saeedi, P., Salpea, P., Karuranga, S., Petersohn, I., Malanda, B., *et al.* (2020) Mortality attributable to diabetes in 20–79 years old adults, 2019 estimates: results from the International Diabetes Federation Diabetes Atlas, 9th edition. *Diabetes Research and Clinical Practice* 162, 108086.

Sbraccia, P., D'Adamo, M. and Guglielmi, V. (2021) Is type 2 diabetes an adiposity-based metabolic disease? From the origin of insulin resistance to the concept of dysfunctional adipose tissue. *Eating and Weight Disorders – Studies on Anorexia, Bulimia and Obesity* 26, 2429–2441. https://doi.org/10.1007/s40519-021-01109-4

Sigal, R.J., Kenny, G.P., Boule, N.G., Wells, G.A., Prud'homme, D., *et al.* (2007) Effects of aerobic training, resistance training, or both on glycemic control in type 2 diabetes – a randomized trial. *Annals of Internal Medicine* 147(6), 357–369.

Tuomilehto, J., Lindström, J., Eriksson, J.G., Valle, T.T., Hämäläinen, H., *et al.* (2016) Prevention of type 2 diabetes mellitus by changes in lifestyle among subjects with impaired glucose tolerance. *New England Journal of Medicine* 344, 1343–1350. https://doi.org/10.1056/NEJM200105033441801

Yerramalla, M.S., Fayosse, A., Dugravot, A., Tabak, A.G., Kivimäki, M., *et al.* (2020) Association of moderate and vigorous physical activity with incidence of type 2 diabetes and subsequent mortality: 27 year follow-up of the Whitehall II study. *Diabetologia* 63(3), 537–548. https://doi.org/10.1007/s00125-019-05050-1

Zhao, F., Wu, W., Feng, X., Li, C., Han, D., *et al.* (2020) Physical activity levels and diabetes prevalence in US adults: findings from NHANES 2015–2016. *Diabetes Therapy* 11(6), 1303–1316. https://doi.org/10.1007/s13300-020-00817-x

14 The Metabolic Syndrome

The Nature of the Metabolic Syndrome

The metabolic syndrome, sometimes known as 'Syndrome X' or abbreviated to MetSyn, is an important cluster of some of the conditions that have been described in Chapters 10–13 (this volume) (NHS, 2019). Individually they can make a person particularly prone to arterial problems, especially coronary disease. There are five components of the metabolic syndrome: abdominal or central obesity, raised BP, insulin resistance (pre-diabetes), raised blood triglycerides and low HDL-C (see 'Dyslipidaemia', Chapter 12, this volume). Individuals with three or more of these are designated to be suffering from metabolic syndrome (Grundy *et al.*, 2004). Insulin resistance (see Chapter 13, this volume) appears to be its major component.

The metabolic syndrome has been recognized for the past 50 years or so. It is caused by a combination of unhealthy (over-)eating, lack of exercise, sedentary behaviour, increasing age and being under stress. It is common, affecting about one in four adults in the UK. Approximately 50% of heart attack patients have the syndrome and it increases the risk of dying from heart disease about threefold (Galassi *et al.*, 2006).

Exercise in the Prevention of the Metabolic Syndrome

Lack of exercise is an important risk factor for developing the metabolic syndrome. Conversely, exercise is an excellent way to prevent the condition, and this has been demonstrated experimentally.

In the Ely Study, 604 healthy, middle-aged men and women were followed up for 5.6 years and, during this time, their physical activity was measured objectively. The amount of physical activity predicted the development of the metabolic syndrome in a dose-dependent way. This means that the less exercise that was taken, the higher the risk of the syndrome (Ekelund *et al.*, 2005). The beneficial effect of exercise in reducing the risk of metabolic syndrome has been found at all levels of obesity (Berentzen *et al.*, 2007).

Similarly, the level of physical fitness, which itself is largely determined by levels of physical activity, is a strong predictor of the metabolic syndrome. In a study of fitness levels in 9666 men aged 20–69, the overall prevalence of the syndrome was 25%. The unfit men were twice as likely to have metabolic syndrome as the fit men (Ingle *et al.*, 2016). When the same association had been studied in older men and women aged 57 to 79, it was found to be even more dramatic. Metabolic syndrome is up to ten times more common in the unfit compared with a very fit group (Hassinen *et al.*, 2008).

Exercise in the Treatment of the Metabolic Syndrome

Exercise is effective in improving each one of the components of the metabolic syndrome, as shown in Chapters 10–13 (this volume). It is therefore not surprising that exercise has been shown to be effective in treating the whole syndrome.

One trial of exercise in 621 apparently healthy but sedentary individuals found that 105 had the metabolic syndrome at the start of the programme. At the end of the exercise programme, 32 of these were free of the syndrome, with significant improvements in all components (Katzmarzyk *et al.*, 2003). There is clear evidence of a relationship with exercise dose, with high-dose, vigorous-intensity exercise, such as hard running, cycling or swimming, being more effective than lower doses (Johnson *et al.*, 2007).

© H.J.N. Bethell and D. Brodie 2023. *Exercise: A Scientific and Clinical Overview*
(H.J.N. Bethell and D. Brodie)
DOI: 10.1079/9781800621855.0014

Summary

The metabolic syndrome is the combination of three or more of the following: abdominal or central obesity, raised BP, insulin resistance (pre-diabetes), raised blood triglycerides and low HDL-C. Insulin resistance is the most important component of the metabolic syndrome. It is caused by a combination of unhealthy (over-)eating, lack of exercise, sedentary behaviour, increasing age and being under stress. It is common, affecting about one in four adults in the UK. The main ill effect is a greatly increased risk of arterial disease, particularly heart attacks.

References

Berentzen, T., Petersen, L., Pedersen, O., Black, E., Astrup, A. and Sørensen, T.I.A. (2007) Long term effects of leisure time physical activity on risk of insulin resistance and impaired glucose tolerance, allowing for body weight history, in Danish men. *Diabetes Medicine* 24, 63–72.

Ekelund, U., Brage, S., Franks, P.W., Hennings, S., Emms, S. and Wareham, N.J. (2005) Physical activity energy expenditure predicts progression toward the metabolic syndrome independently of aerobic fitness in middle-aged healthy Caucasians: the Medical Research Council Ely Study. *Diabetes Care* 28, 1195–1200. https://doi.org/10.2337/diacare.28.5.1195

Galassi, A., Reynolds, K. and He, J. (2006) Metabolic syndrome and risk of cardiovascular disease: a meta-analysis. *American Journal of Medicine* 119(10), 812–819.

Grundy, S.M., Brewer, H.B. Jr, Cleeman, J.I., Smith, S.C. Jr and Lenfant, C. (2004) Definition of metabolic syndrome: report of the National Heart, Lung, and Blood Institute/American Heart Association conference on scientific issues related to definition. *Circulation* 109, 433–443.

Hassinen, M., Lakka, T.A., Savonen, K., Litmanen, H., Kiviaho, L., *et al.* (2008) Cardiorespiratory fitness as a feature of metabolic syndrome in older men and women. *Diabetes Care* 31, 1242–1247.

Ingle, L., Mellis, M., Brodie, D. and Sandercock, G.R. (2016) Associations between cardiorespiratory fitness and the metabolic syndrome in British men. *Heart* 103, 524–528. https://doi.org/10.1136/heartjnl-2016-310142

Johnson, J.L., Slentz, C.A., Houmard, J.A., Samsa, G.P., Duscha, B.D., *et al.* (2007) Exercise training amount and intensity effects on metabolic syndrome (from Studies of a Targeted Risk Reduction Intervention through Defined Exercise). *American Journal of Cardiology* 100, 1759–1766.

Katzmarzyk, P.T., Leon, A.S., Wilmore, J.H., Skinner, J.S., Rao, D.C., *et al.* (2003) Targeting the metabolic syndrome with exercise: evidence from the HERITAGE family study. *Medicine and Science in Sports and Exercise* 35, 1703–1709.

NHS (2019) Metabolic syndrome. Available at: https://www.nhs.uk/conditions/metabolic-syndrome/ (accessed 18 January 2023).

15 Coronary Heart Disease (CHD)

The coronary arteries are the vessels that take blood to the heart muscle. They arise from the root of the aorta, the body's main artery, and wind round the surface of the heart in the shape of an upside-down crown or corona (Fig. 15.1) – hence their name. Their function is to supply the heart muscle with oxygen and nutrition.

Coronary artery disease is the narrowing of one or more of the coronary arteries, thus reducing the rate at which blood can flow through the artery. Coronary artery disease, more usually referred to as coronary heart disease or CHD, was until very recently the commonest cause of death in most developed societies. For women, but not for men, death from CHD has recently been narrowly overtaken in the UK by dementia (see Chapter 20, this volume). In the UK approximately 2.3 million people are currently diagnosed with CHD, with around 300,000 new cases every year.

About 200 people in the UK die of CHD every day, mainly from heart attacks (Townsend *et al.*, 2015). It is also a major cause of extensive morbidity – the symptoms and limitations resulting from the disease.

Causes of Coronary Artery Disease

CHD is the result of atheroma of the coronary arteries (see also 'Dyslipidaemia', Chapter 12, this volume). As people age, they develop patchy narrowing of the arteries due to fatty plaques composed of cholesterol being laid down in the arterial wall. The narrowing is compounded by overlying thin layers of blood clots. This gradually restricts the flow of blood to the heart muscle (Fig. 15.2).

There is no single cause of coronary atheroma, but a number of risk factors contribute to its development. Some are irreversible. These include age, gender and family history.

Susceptibility to CHD is directly related to age, with older people having a higher incidence. Gender also impacts on the disease, with men developing CHD on average 10 years younger than women. There is some evidence to suggest that this gender difference is narrowing as more women work for a greater proportion of their life. Family history also impacts on the susceptibility to CHD, with individuals being at greater risk if they have a close relative with the disease – the younger the relative presents with the disease, the greater the risk.

These risk factors are uncontrollable, but it is possible to influence dramatically the reversible risk factors. These include cigarette smoking, high BP, diabetes, high blood cholesterol and obesity. The combination of these, particularly the metabolic syndrome, as discussed in Chapter 14 (this volume), is especially capable of control.

Overshadowing all of these, because it contributes to most of them, is *lack of exercise*. It is a critical risk factor and will be discussed more fully later in this chapter.

Measuring Risk

There are several tools for predicting the risk of developing CHD in any individual. The best validated is the Q-Risk 3 (further details can be obtained at https://qrisk.org/three/ (accessed 18 January 2023)). The Q-Risk 3 algorithm requires details of age, sex, height, weight, total cholesterol/HDL-C ratio, BP, presence or absence of diabetes, ethnicity, smoking status, family history, deprivation, BMI, presence of rheumatoid arthritis or kidney disease, and postcode. If any of this information is not available, the risk-scoring system will use average values for missing data. From this information, the tool will calculate the risk of developing both CHD and CVD over the next 10 years. CVD (cardiovascular disease) is a more general term for conditions affecting the heart or blood vessels. CVD includes all heart and circulatory diseases, including CHD, angina, heart attack, congenital heart disease, hypertension, stroke and vascular

© H.J.N. Bethell and D. Brodie 2023. *Exercise: A Scientific and Clinical Overview* (H.J.N. Bethell and D. Brodie)
DOI: 10.1079/9781800621855.0015

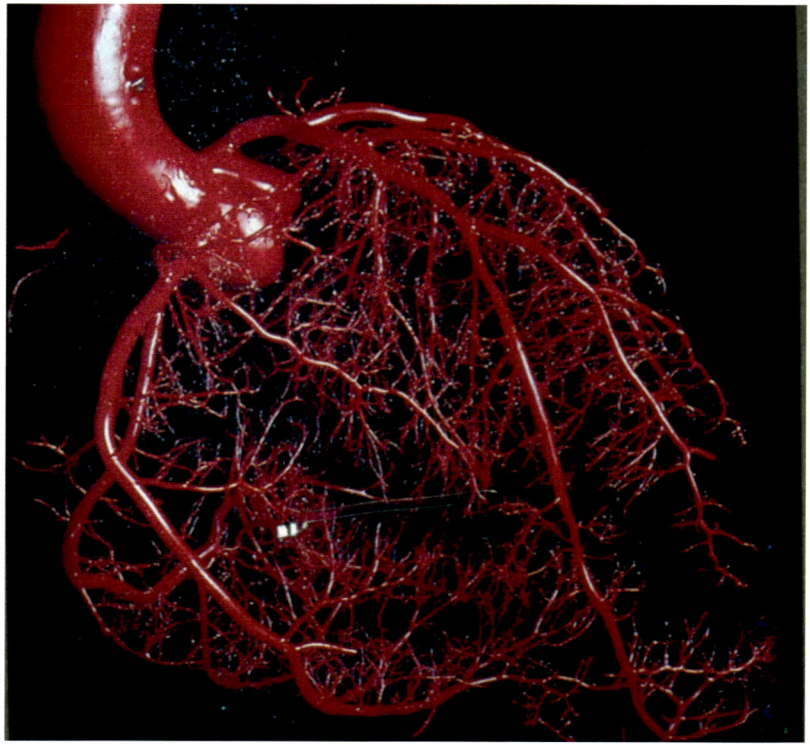

Fig. 15.1. Wax cast of the coronary arteries.

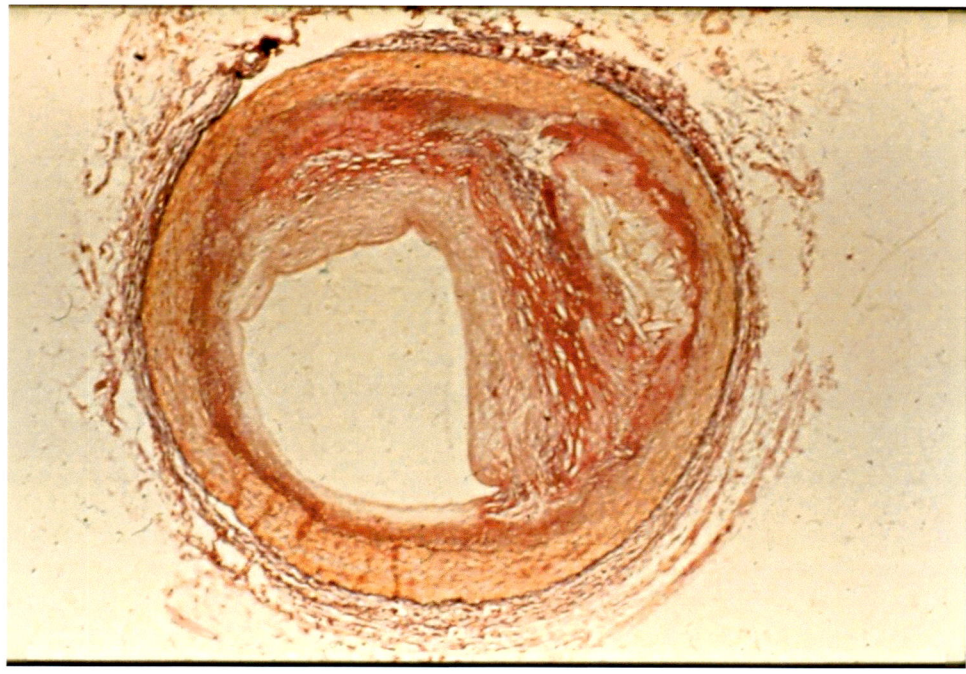

Fig. 15.2. Histology of severe coronary atheroma.

dementia. These will all be discussed in this and the following chapters of this book.

Angina

With progressive arterial narrowing a point may be reached when the artery is unable to supply the needs of the heart muscle during exercise. Consequently the muscle lacks a sufficient supply of oxygen to be able to continue to contract effectively. This produces pain during exertion, known as angina pectoris. It is felt as a tight, strangling pain across the centre of the chest, often radiating into the throat, jaws or left arm. It forces the sufferer to stop exercising but will usually settle over the next few minutes.

Heart Attack

The atheroma plaques are delicate creatures and may break, crack or burst. If this happens, the body's repair mechanisms are initiated, and a clot forms. This is a *coronary thrombosis* and may be large enough to block the artery. The result is death of the area of heart muscle supplied by that artery, called a *myocardial infarction*. This is what most people usually call a heart attack.

The immediate danger is sudden death due to abnormal cardiac rhythm and not related to the size of the infarct. For those who survive to reach hospital, the outlook is the same as for those who do not suffer this complication.

Heart Failure

The modern treatment of heart attacks is extremely effective in limiting the damage. Even so, if there is enough loss of myocardium (heart muscle), particularly after more than one attack, the ability of the heart to perform its full function is damaged. This can lead to heart failure. The term 'heart failure' sounds dire, but it does not mean the end of life. It simply means that the heart is too weak to deliver all its potential output during daily activities. This causes fatigue, poor circulation with cold hands and feet, breathlessness on exertion and inability to carry out the tasks of daily living. If inadequately treated, it may cause ankle-swelling and breathlessness while at rest or when lying down at night.

Exercise in the Prevention of CHD

In the 1950s and 1960s, studies of bus drivers (Morris *et al.*, 1953) and Whitehall civil servants (Morris

et al., 1990) were led by Professor Jerry Morris. Morris was a Scottish doctor working at University College, London, and these studies became epidemiological classics. In the former study, he and his colleagues compared the rates of heart disease in London bus drivers with those of bus conductors. While the drivers sat all day long, fuming at annoying taxi drivers and other road-users, the conductors scurried up and down stairs getting plenty of exercise. They found that the drivers had more than a 40% higher rate of CHD than the conductors.

The Whitehall civil servant study looked at leisure-time physical activity. It again found that the rate of fatal heart attacks in those who took vigorous exercise as recreation was about 40% that of the inactive. The rate of non-fatal heart attacks was reduced by an even greater proportion – 50%.

Morris made several discoveries: (i) that intermittent heavy exercise is more effective than lower-level activity, even with equivalent totals of exercise; (ii) that there is a threshold for the protective effect; and (iii) there is dose-response relationship above this level, i.e. the more exercise you take, the better will be the effect. The application of these trial data to mortality will be considered again in Chapter 27 (this volume).

In the USA, similar studies were carried out on the San Francisco longshore men (stevedores) and on university graduates (Paffenbarger and Hale, 1975; Paffenbarger *et al.*, 1978). In a study of nearly 17,000 Harvard graduates aged 35–74, they found that taking exercise was inversely related to mortality – the more exercise taken, the greater reduction in mortality. A further study from the USA followed over 26,000 men and women who had performed an exercise test to determine their levels of physical fitness (Sui *et al.*, 2007). They divided the subjects by fitness level – high, moderate and low. Over an average follow-up of 10 years, the rate of coronary disease was 11% lower in the moderate-fitness group and 25% lower in the high-fitness group when compared to the low-fitness group.

Since then numerous studies have confirmed the association between regular exercise, physical fitness and protection from CHD (Eckel *et al.*, 2014). Tanasescu *et al.* (2002) have shown that the greater the total volume of physical activity, which included running, weight training and rowing, the greater the reduction in the risk of CHD. Improving fitness level from unfit to fit nearly halves the risk compared with remaining unfit (Blair *et al.*, 1995).

A meta-analysis of 33 trials included over 100,000 subjects who were followed up for an average of 11 years after an exercise test. They were divided into low-, intermediate- and high-fitness categories. The low-fitness group had a 56% higher chance of suffering a heart attack than the high-fitness group (Kodama *et al.*, 2009). Another meta-analysis of 18 prospective studies covered almost 460,000 people over a period of 11.3 years (Hamer and Chida, 2008). All of these people were free of CVD at the start of the study. The researchers, from University College London, calculated that walking reduced the risk of heart problems by almost one-third and the risk of death by any cause by a similar amount. They found that walking just 6 miles per week at only 2 mph offered some protection, but longer, faster walking was more effective.

In the section on the causes of coronary artery disease above, reference was made to one of the uncontrollable factors, i.e. family history or genetics. It is estimated that one person in five has a combination of genes that puts them at a higher risk of suffering a heart attack. A major study from Harvard University and Massachusetts General Hospital, involving 50,000 people, found that such people still have some control of their fate (Khera *et al.*, 2016). Not smoking, keeping slim and, most importantly, keeping fit, reduced the risk of suffering a major heart attack by nearly a half over the next decade. Dr Kathiresan, the lead author, states 'people may feel they cannot escape a genetically determined risk for a heart attack, but the findings indicate that following a healthy lifestyle can powerfully reduce genetic risk.'

Another uncontrollable risk is that of gender. A study at Loughborough University examined the blood vessels of middle-aged men and postmenopausal women, 1 hour after a brisk walk (Craig and O'Donnell, 2018). Both groups had an improved arterial stiffness and BP, but the stiffness was higher in the women. This was only a small study (see Chapter 9, this volume) but it might imply that postmenopausal women do not gain quite the same benefit as similar-aged men. The important element is that they gain some benefit and will still reduce their risk of developing heart disease.

The beneficial effects of exercise hold for all age groups that have been investigated (Franco *et al.*, 2005; Mozaffarian *et al.*, 2015; Barbiellini Amidei *et al.*, 2022). It has been estimated that if everyone were physically active, 6% of coronary disease worldwide would be eliminated and life expectancy of the world population would be increased by 0.68 years (Lee *et al.*, 2012). A study based at the University of Cambridge tracked nearly 15,000 British people aged from 40 to 79 over 8 years to gauge their changing exercise levels (Mok *et al.*, 2019). Their health was then monitored for another 13 years. Even the people who only started to exercise over the initial 8 years of the study saw their subsequent risk of dying fall by 24% and the risk of a cardiac death fell by 29%. Those who were already active lowered their risk by as much as 42%. This demonstrates the value of exercising in middle age, even if previous exercise experience is lacking.

Regular exercise also protects against the future risk of heart failure. A meta-analysis, which looked at the combined effects of 12 studies with 370,000 people, recorded their exercise habits over an average of 15 years (Berry *et al.*, 2013). Those who completed the 150 minutes per week as recommended in Chapter 6 (this volume) had a 10% lower incidence of heart failure. Those who undertook four times that amount had a 35% lower chance of heart failure. Clearly the risk is related to the quantity of exercise, but this has to be balanced with realism. An individual would need to be highly dedicated to exercise for 10 hours per week. The incidence of heart failure is undoubtedly worryingly high, but the most important message for most people is to exercise more. A similar study in Sweden looked at 33,000 men who did not start exercising until their sixties (Rahman *et al.*, 2015). Once again, the results pointed to the benefit of *current* exercise levels, compared with the *past*. The current exercisers reduced their risk of heart failure by 21%. The investigators concluded that 'recent activity may be more important for heart failure protection than past activity levels.'

Even the rather limited doses of exercise recommended by national bodies (see Chapter 6, this volume) are protective. In a study of nearly half a million adults in the USA, compliance with exercise guidelines was compared with mortality over 9 years. For those following the recommendations for strength building, the death rate was 82% of that expected. For those following the aerobic exercise recommendations it was 65% of that expected. Most impressively, for those following both aerobic and strength building, the reduction in mortality was 50% of the expected level (Zhao *et al.*, 2020).

Some of the ways in which exercise prevents CHD are obvious. Most of the reversible risk factors are reduced. Regular exercisers are thinner than non-exercisers. They have lower BP, lower blood cholesterol and are less likely to develop diabetes. It is incontrovertible that, apart from stopping smoking, there is no more effective way of avoiding a heart attack than regular vigorous exercise.

Exercise in the Treatment of CHD

The use of exercise for treating CHD preceded its use for treating any other non-communicable disease (often abbreviated to NCD). Back in the 18th century, Dr William Heberden recognized angina and in 1768 he described one of his patients who had been cured by sawing wood for half an hour a day (Heberden, 1772).

CHD, however, was infrequently diagnosed over the next 150 years and by the time it became accepted as a serious health problem, early in the 20th century, this lesson had been forgotten. When a heart attack was diagnosed, prolonged bed rest was thought to be essential if the patient's life was to be saved. At the time, it was believed that exertion too soon after the attack risked rupturing the damaged heart. Doctors and nurses went to absurd lengths to keep the patient at complete 'rest' for several weeks, spoon-feeding them and insisting on the use of that most exercise-intensive utensil, the bedpan! When the patient was eventually released from hospital, the advice was for exercise to be restricted in favour of a peaceful, sedentary life.

In the 1940s and 1950s some of the undesirable consequences of bed rest were being appreciated. These included deconditioning, boredom, depression, venous thrombosis and chest infections. The notion of early mobilization was slowly gaining credibility. In Cleveland, Ohio, a far-seeing cardiologist called Herman Hellerstein and his colleagues developed a comprehensive rehabilitation programme with graduated exercise training as its centrepiece. The idea was to 'add life to years and perhaps years to life'. It was designed for 'habitually sedentary, lazy, hypokinetic, sloppy, endo-mesomorphic overweight males' through a programme of enhanced physical activity (Hellerstein and Goldston, 1954). Dr Hellerstein seems to have had little respect for the lifestyles of his patients! They showed that patients who had recovered from a heart attack could improve their physical fitness by a course of exercise. They also showed that electrocardiogram (ECG) changes recorded during and after exertion were reduced and psychological status was raised. In addition, they noted an improvement in nutrition, giving up smoking, the continuation of gainful employment and maintenance of a normal social life (Hellerstein, 1968).

Over the past 50 years there have been numerous controlled trials of cardiac rehabilitation in patients recovering from such events as heart attacks or heart surgery. Meta-analyses of the results have indicated a fall in the region of 25% in the mortality rate in treated groups over the subsequent 3 years. Interestingly, when exercise-only programmes have been compared with more comprehensive programmes, the exercise-only treatments fare as well as those also offering counselling, education and risk-factor advice (Taylor *et al.*, 2004; Clark *et al.*, 2005). This does not suggest that the more comprehensive programme has limited value but does suggest that exercise is easily the most effective element of cardiac rehabilitation for improving survival. It is extremely difficult to change the behaviour of middle-aged people.

These studies reinforce that the best advice which is likely to make a significant impact is that concerning exercise. This is particularly so when it is incorporated into patient management. Retrospective observations confirm the importance of all forms of physical activity in long-term prognosis of coronary patients. Compared with non-exercisers, those who take up exercise after an event have a mortality reduction of between 27 and 45%. Those who were active before the event have a mortality reduction of between 50 and 53% (Gonzalez-Jaramillo *et al.*, 2022; Kang *et al.*, 2022).

In patients with established CHD, exercise capacity remains a powerful predictor of prognosis. For every 1 MET reduction in fitness there is an increased risk of death of 13% (Hung *et al.*, 2014). One study of more than 12,000 CHD patients for an average of 8 years found that those with a VO_{2max} of less than 15 ml/min/kg had more than double the risk of death than those with a VO_{2max} of more than 22 ml/min/kg (Kavanagh *et al.*, 2002). Indeed, physical fitness in CHD patients is a better predictor of future mortality than any other measure. This effect is partly because low fitness reflects greater heart damage. None the less, increasing fitness by exercise training will reduce the mortality risk to the same level as that of untrained subjects with an equivalent fitness level.

Unfortunately, the application of this knowledge is not at the level that should be expected. The intensity of exercise and the length of the exercise component of cardiac rehabilitation in the UK are well below the levels that research has used to demonstrate their benefits. A recent study examined a sample of 70 coronary patients receiving the usual twice-weekly exercise course for 8 weeks. There was no increase in fitness level and no reduction in 5-year mortality (Nichols *et al.*, 2020). A further failure of the care of heart patients was shown by a study of 4000 people recovering from a coronary event from the previous 2 years. Forty-five per cent were still smoking, 36% were obese, 53% had central obesity and 52% were still classified as inactive (Jennings *et al.*, 2020).

Exercise in the Treatment of Heart Failure

As discussed above, one important consequence of cardiac damage from coronary disease is heart failure. In this condition the ability of the heart to pump out sufficient blood for daily living is impaired, with the resulting tiredness, breathlessness and restriction of activities. Currently, there are about 900,000 people living with heart failure in the UK.

The more the heart is damaged, the less effect any physical training has on its function. With heart failure, it is still possible to increase physical fitness, but this is mediated by peripheral training effects rather than improved cardiac performance. This is largely through improved muscular efficiency and blood-flow distribution. The effect of exercise training of patients with heart failure is further restricted by the limited exercise intensity and dose that can be sustained. Exercise training of heart-failure patients can be helpful but must be increased slowly and carefully. The resulting benefits are modest.

A meta-analysis of RCTs of exercise training for 4400 heart-failure patients found an increase in timed walking distance of about 6%. This was considered enough to be beneficial (Cook *et al.*, 2019). Quality-of-life scores increased slightly and there was no increase in either hospital admission or mortality.

Summary

Coronary artery disease is a narrowing of the coronary arteries, reducing the rate at which blood flows through the artery. It can result in angina, a heart attack or heart failure. Exercise has been shown conclusively to reduce heart disease, with fitness being an excellent indicator of future incidence. Exercise is also a valuable method of treating heart disease and is a central component of clinical cardiac rehabilitation programmes.

References

Barbiellini Amidei, C., Trevisan, C., Dotto, M., Ferroni, E., Noale, M., *et al.* (2022) Association of physical activity trajectories with major cardiovascular diseases in elderly people. *Heart* 108(5), 360–366. https://doi.org/10.1136/heartjnl-2021-320013

Berry, J.D., Pandey, A., Gao, A., Leonard, D., Farzaneh-Far, R., *et al.* (2013) Physical fitness and risk for heart failure and coronary artery disease. *Circulation: Heart Failure* 6(4), 627–634. https://doi.org/10.1161/CIRCHEARTFAILURE.112.000054

Blair, S.N., Kohl, H.W. 3rd, Barlow, C.E., Paffenbarger, R.S. Jr, Gibbons, L.W. and Macera, C.A. (1995) Changes in physical fitness and all-cause mortality. A prospective study of healthy and unhealthy men. *JAMA* 273, 1093–1098.

Clark, A.M., Hartling, L., Vandermeer, B. and McAlister, F.A. (2005) Meta-analysis: secondary prevention programs for patients with coronary disease. *Annals of Internal Medicine* 143, 659–672.

Cook, R., Davidson, P. and Martin, R. (2019) Cardiac rehabilitation for heart failure can improve quality of life and fitness. *BMJ* 367, l5456. https://doi.org/10.1136/bmj.l5456

Craig, J. and O'Donnell, E. (2018) Regular exercise may be more beneficial for men than post-menopausal women. Available at: https://www.lboro.ac.uk/internal/news/2018/june/regular-exercise-may-be-more-beneficial-for-men-than-post-menopausal-women.html (accessed 18 January 2023).

Eckel, R.H., Jakicic, J.M., Ard, J.D., de Jesus, J.M., Houston Miller, N., *et al.* (2014) 2013 AHA/ACC guideline on lifestyle management to reduce cardiovascular risk: a report of the American College of Cardiology/American Heart Association Task Force on Practice Guidelines. *Circulation* 129, S76–S99. https://doi.org/10.1161/01.cir.0000437740.48606.d1

Franco, O.H., de Laet, C., Peeters, A., Jonker, J., Mackenbach, J. and Nusselder, W. (2005) Effects of physical activity on life expectancy with cardiovascular disease. *Archives of Internal Medicine* 165, 2355–2360.

Gonzalez-Jaramillo, N., Wilhelm, M., Arango-Rivas, A.M., Gonzalez-Jaramillo, V., Mesa-Vieira, C., *et al.* (2022) Systematic review of physical activity trajectories and mortality in patients with coronary artery disease. *Journal of the American College of Cardiology* 79(17), 1690–1700. https://doi.org/10.1016/j.jacc.2022.02.036

Hamer, M. and Chida, Y. (2008) Walking and primary prevention: a meta-analysis of prospective cohort studies. *British Journal of Sports Medicine* 42(4), 238–243. https://doi.org/10.1136/bjsm.2007.039974

Heberden, W. (1772) Some account of a disorder of the breast. *Medical Transactions, The Royal College of Physicians of London* 2, 59–67.

Hellerstein, H.K. (1968) Exercise therapy in coronary disease. *Bulletin of the New York Academy of Medicine* 44, 1028–1047.

Hellerstein, H.K. and Goldston, E. (1954) Rehabilitation of patients with heart disease. *Postgraduate Medicine* 15, 265–278.

Hung, R.K., Al-Mulla, M.H., McEvoy, J.W., Whelton, S.P., Blumenthal, R.S., *et al.* (2014) Prognostic value of exercise capacity in patients with coronary artery disease: the FIT (Henry Ford Exercise Testing) project. *Mayo Clinic Proceedings* 89(12), 1644–1654.

Jennings, C.S., Kotseva, K., Bassett, P., Adamska, A. and Wood, D. (2020) A SPIRE-3-PREVENT: a cross-sectional survey of preventive care after a coronary event across the UK. *Open Heart* 7(1), e001196. https://doi.org/10.1136/openhrt-2019-001196

Kang, D.-S., Sung, J.-H., Kim, D., Jin, M.-N., Jang, E., *et al.* (2022) Association between exercise habit changes and mortality following a cardiovascular event. *Heart* 108, 1945–1951. https://doi.org/10.1136/heartjnl-2022-320882

Kavanagh, T., Mertens, T.J., Hamm, L.F., Beyene, J., Kennedy, J., *et al.* (2002) Prediction of long-term prognosis in 12,169 men referred for cardiac rehabilitation. *Circulation* 106, 666–671.

Khera, A.V., Emdin, C.A., Drake, I., Natarajan, P., Bick, A.G., *et al.* (2016) Genetic risk, adherence to a healthy lifestyle, and coronary disease. *New England Journal of Medicine* 375(24), 2349–2358. https://doi.org/10.1056/NEJMoa1605086

Kodama, S., Saito, K., Tanaka, S., Maki, M., Yachi, Y., *et al.* (2009) Cardiorespiratory fitness as a quantitative predictor of all-cause mortality and cardiovascular events in healthy men and women: a meta-analysis. *JAMA* 301(19), 2024–2035. https://doi.org/10.1001/jama.2009.681

Lee, I.-M., Shiroma, E.J., Lobelo, F., Puska, P., Blair, S.N., *et al.* (2012) Effect of physical inactivity on major non-communicable diseases worldwide: an analysis of burden of disease and life expectancy. *Lancet* 380, 219–229. https://doi.org/10.1016/S0140-6736(12)61031-9

Mok, A., Khaw, K.T., Luben, R., Wareham, N. and Brage, S. (2019) Physical activity trajectories and mortality: population based cohort study. *BMJ* 365, l2323. https://doi.org/10.1136/bmj.l2323

Morris, J.N., Heady, J.A., Raffle, P.A., Roberts, C.G. and Parks, J.W. (1953) Coronary heart-disease and physical activity of work. *Lancet* 262, 1053–1057.

Morris, J.N., Clayton, D.G., Everitt, M.G., Semmence, A.M. and Burgess, E.H. (1990) Exercise in leisure time: coronary attack and death rates. *British Heart Journal* 63, 325–334.

Mozaffarian, D., Benjamin, E.J., Go, A.S., Arnett, D.K., Blaha, M.J., *et al.* (2015) Heart disease and stroke statistics – 2015 update: a report from the American Heart Association. *Circulation* 131, e29–e322.

Nichols, S., Taylor, C., Goodman, T., Page, R., Kallvikbacka-Bennett, A., *et al.* (2020) Routine exercise-based cardiac rehabilitation does not increase aerobic fitness: a CARE CR study. *International Journal of Cardiology* 305, 25–34. https://doi.org/10.1016/j.ijcard.2020.01.044

Paffenbarger, R.S. and Hale, W.E. (1975) Work activity and coronary heart mortality. *New England Journal of Medicine* 292, 545–550.

Paffenbarger, R.S. Jr, Wing, A.L. and Hyde, R.T. (1978) Physical activity as an index of heart attack risk in college alumni. *American Journal of Epidemiology* 108, 161–175.

Rahman, I., Bellavia, A., Wolk, A. and Orsini, N. (2015) Physical activity and heart failure risk in a prospective study of men. *JACC: Heart Failure* 3(9), 681–687. https://doi.org/10.1016/j.jchf.2015.05.006

Sui, X., LaMonte, M.J. and Blair, S.N. (2007) Cardiorespiratory fitness as a predictor of nonfatal cardiovascular events in asymptomatic women and men. *American Journal of Epidemiology* 165, 1413–1423.

Tanasescu, M., Leitzmann, M.F., Rimm, E.B., Willett, W.C., Stampfer, M.J. and Hu, F.B. (2002) Exercise type and intensity in relation to coronary heart disease in men. *JAMA* 288, 1994–2000. https://doi.org/10.1001/jama.288.16.1994

Taylor, R.S., Brown, A., Ebrahim, S., Jolliffe, J., Noorani, H., *et al.* (2004) Exercise-based rehabilitation for patients with coronary heart disease: systematic review and meta-analysis of randomized controlled trials. *American Journal of Medicine* 116, 682–692. https://doi.org/10.1016/j.amjmed.2004.01.009

Townsend, N., Bhatnagar, P., Wilkins, E., Wickramasinghe, K. and Rayner, M. (2015) *Cardiovascular Disease Statistics 2015*. British Heart Foundation, London. Available at: https://www.bhf.org.uk/informationsupport/publications/statistics/cvd-stats-2015 (accessed 30 January 2023).

Zhao, M., Veeranki, S.P., Magnussen, C.G. and Xi, B. (2020) Recommended physical activity and all cause and cause specific mortality in US adults: prospective cohort study. *BMJ* 370, m2031. https://doi.org/10.1136/bmj.m2031

16 Peripheral Vascular Disease (PVD)

Atheroma can cause narrowing of any part of the vascular tree. When it involves any arteries apart from those to the heart or brain it is called peripheral vascular disease or PVD. Disease of the arteries supplying the legs is easily the commonest manifestation of PVD. The main risk factors are diabetes (see Chapter 13, this volume), cigarette smoking, high BP (see Chapter 11, this volume) and dyslipidaemia (see Chapter 12, this volume). In a minority there is a strong inherited predisposition.

PVD affects about 10% of diabetics at 10 years after diagnosis, rising to 45% at 20 years. The incidence in non-diabetics is between 5 and 10% for over 65-year-olds. Rather like coronary disease, PVD initially causes muscle pain on exertion. This is usually felt as pain in the calf when walking, resolving rapidly on stopping. This is similar to angina, but in the leg muscles instead of the heart muscle. This is called intermittent claudication (IC), or intermittent limping, named after the emperor Claudius, a famous limper.

Progression of the arterial narrowing may lead to blockage and severe lack of blood to the feet. The lower parts of the legs may develop ulcers, which may never heal. Toes become painful, then white and ultimately black and gangrenous, requiring amputation. For people who suffer from diabetes, it is essential not to be a smoker.

Penile blood supply may also be affected by PVD, causing erectile dysfunction (see Chapter 24, this volume). Erections are absent, weak or cannot be sustained. This is likely to cause much distress and frustration to those so afflicted.

Exercise in the Prevention of PVD

Regular exercise improves arterial elasticity and lessens arterial stiffness. This was shown in a study of middle-aged first-time marathon runners. By the end of their training the improvement in the state of their arteries was enough to make them appear, at least in cardiovascular terms, 4 years younger (Bhuva et al., 2020).

PVD is closely linked to other forms of arterial disease. About 60% of PVD sufferers have concurrent coronary artery disease (see Chapter 15, this volume) and 30% have cerebrovascular disease (see Chapter 17, this volume) (Morley et al., 2018). Preventive measures for all these diseases are very similar. Regular exercise and high levels of physical fitness reduce three out of the four most important risk factors for PVD. These are diabetes, high BP and abnormal blood lipids. Regular exercisers rarely suffer from PVD.

A study of Japanese men has shown that both low fitness and muscular weakness predict an increased likelihood of erectile dysfunction (Kumagai et al., 2019).

Exercise in the Treatment of PVD

There are operations to restore blood supply – either bypass grafting or angioplasty. This is a similar process to that required for coronary artery disease but easier because the heart is not stopped. Such surgery is only normally required when symptoms are severe or when the limb is threatened.

The only other effective treatment is exercise, particularly walking. The best results are obtained when the sufferer walks to the greatest degree of calf pain tolerable for more than 30 minutes on three or more days per week for at least 6 months (Gardner and Poehlman, 1995). A more recent study by Hodges et al. (2008) showed that a 12-week supervised exercise programme resulted in a significant increase in walking time for people with PVD and also increased all of the measured cardiovascular variables. Supervised walking is more effective than unsupervised (Frazzitta et al., 2015) and usually consists of walking on a treadmill under the guidance of a physiotherapist. The Cochrane Review of this treatment covered 1837 adults in 32 trials

DOI: 10.1079/9781800621855.0016

(Lane *et al.*, 2017). The treated groups showed significant increases in both pain-free walking distance and maximum walking distance.

Unfortunately this treatment is made available to very few PVD patients, and even among those enrolled only a minority complete the programme (McDermott, 2022). Advice to increase walking distance without supervision is relatively ineffective in increasing exercise tolerance but when reinforced by a motivational approach can produce significant improvement (Bearne *et al.*, 2022).

The way in which walking improves IC is probably by provoking muscle ischaemia (inadequate blood supply). This encourages the growth of new, small blood vessels (collaterals) to bypass the narrowed or occluded arteries. Structural changes in the walking muscles also contribute to the improvement (Lane *et al.*, 2017).

Certain medication, such as naftidrofuryl oxalate, can assist in increasing the range of pain-free walking. A small study by Mary McDermott and co-workers at Northwestern University in Chicago suggested that drinking flavanol-rich cocoa can also improve walking distance, but this should not be seen as a replacement for exercise therapy (McDermott *et al.*, 2020).

In summary, a supervised exercise programme for at least 3 months should be the first line of treatment for people with PVD. This should be undertaken in conjunction with an examination of other CVD prevention strategies.

Summary

Peripheral vascular disease (PVD) is disease of any of the peripheral arteries except those supplying the heart or brain. The ones most usually affected are those supplying the legs – resulting in pain, mainly in the calves, on walking, and known as intermittent claudication (IC). Gangrene leading to amputation is a risk from severe PVD. Other effects include erectile dysfunction and abdominal 'angina'. An effective treatment for IC is walking, preferably to the point of pain. This encourages the growth of collateral vessels and increases walking distance.

References

Bearne, L.M., Volkmer, B., Peacock, J., Sekhon, M., Fisher, G., *et al.* (2022) Effect of a home-based, walking exercise behavior change intervention vs usual care on walking in adults with peripheral artery disease: the MOSAIC randomized clinical trial. *JAMA* 327(14), 1344–1355. https://doi.org/10.1001/jama.2022.3391

Bhuva, A.N., D'Silva, A., Torlasco, C., Jones, S., Nadarajan, N., *et al.* (2020) Training for a first-time marathon reverses age-related aortic stiffening. *Journal of the American College of Cardiology* 75(1), 60–71. https://doi.org/10.1016/j.jacc.2019.10.045

Frazzitta, G., Maestri, R., Bertotti, G., Riboldazzi, G., Boveri, N., *et al.* (2015) Intensive rehabilitation treatment in early Parkinson's disease: a randomised pilot study with a 2-year follow up. *Neurorehabilation and Neural Repair* 29, 123–131.

Gardner, A.W. and Poehlman, E.T. (1995) Exercise rehabilitation programmes for the treatment of claudication pain. A meta-analysis. *JAMA* 274, 975–980.

Hodges, L.D., Sandercock, G.R.H., Das, S.K. and Brodie, D.A. (2008) Randomized controlled trial of supervised exercise to evaluate changes in cardiac function in patients with peripheral atherosclerotic disease. *Clinical Physiology and Functional Imaging* 28(1), 32–37. https://doi.org/10.1111/j.1475-097X.2007.00770.x

Kumagai, H., Yoshikawa, T., Myoenzono, K., Kosaki, K., Akazawa, N., *et al.* (2019) Role of high physical fitness in deterioration of male sexual function in Japanese adult men. *American Journal of Men's Health* 13(3), 1557988319849171. https://doi.org/10.1177/1557988319849171

Lane, R., Harwood, A., Watson, L. and Leng, G.C. (2017) Exercise for intermittent claudication. *Cochrane Database of Systematic Reviews* 12(12), CD000990. https://doi.org/10.1002/14651858.CD000990.pub4

McDermott, M.M. (2022) Home-based walking exercise for peripheral artery disease. *JAMA* 327(14), 1339–1340. https://doi.org/10.1001/jama.2022.2457

McDermott, M.M., Criqui, M.H., Domanchuk, K., Ferrucci, L., Gurainik, J.M., *et al.* (2020) Cocoa to improve walking performance in older people with peripheral artery disease. *Circulation Research* 125, 589–599.

Morley, R.L., Sharma, A., Horsch, A.D. and Hinchliffe, R.J. (2018) Peripheral artery disease. *BMJ* 360, j5842.

17 Stroke

There are three main causes of strokes – cerebral thrombosis (*c.*70%), cerebral embolus (*c.*17%) and cerebral haemorrhage (*c.*13%). Exercise has a large role in prevention of cerebral thrombosis and is vital in the management of all forms of stroke.

The cause of cerebral thrombosis is nearly always atheroma of the cerebral arteries. Sudden blocking of one of the arteries to the brain deprives the area supplied of blood, oxygen and nutrition. Rapid death of the brain tissue results, the most recognizable result being hemiplegia which is a one-sided paralysis or weakness. However, any region of the brain can be involved and result in such disparate damage as loss of speech, severe giddiness, changed behaviour, numbness, loss of sight and loss of cognition.

Stroke survivors often report long-term problems. The most common include poor mobility (58%), fatigue (52%), loss of concentration (45%) and falls (44%). Damage to the brain can be limited by rapid introduction of a stent into the damaged artery or by giving blood-clot-dissolving drugs – hence the public health campaign 'FAST' designed to promote rapid diagnosis and transfer to hospital. FAST stands for Face, Arms, Speech (all unusual symptoms) and Time.

According to the Stroke Association, there are more than 100,000 strokes in the UK each year and more than 1.2 million stroke survivors, many with severe ongoing disabilities. Stroke is the fourth biggest killer in the UK and costs the country about £26 billion annually.

Damage to the brain can be minor and repeated and can result in 'vascular' dementia (see Chapter 20, this volume).

Exercise in the Prevention of Stroke

As discussed in earlier chapters, regular exercise reduces several of the factors that are known to be the most important risk factors associated with strokes. These include obesity, high BP, dyslipidaemia and type 2 diabetes (see Chapters 10–13, this volume). It would be impossible to carry out a long-term, large-scale RCT of exercise for stroke prevention. However, observational studies confirm that the incidence of stroke is between 20 and 70% lower in those who are physically active compared with those who are not (Sacco *et al.*, 1998; Lee *et al.*, 1999). Moreover, these studies have shown that there is a dose-response relationship between the amount of exercise taken and the reduction in risk. Both duration and frequency of exercise are related to the reduction in risk. The longer and more often a person exercises, the greater the reduction in stroke risk.

Too much sedentary behaviour is also a risk. A study of more than 7000 US adults, mean age 63, used accelerometers to measure both physical activity and sedentary time with a mean follow-up time of 7.4 years (Hooker *et al.*, 2022). One-third of the participants who performed at least 14 minutes of moderate or vigorous exercise daily had a 43% lower risk of stroke compared with the third of participants who managed less than 2.7 minutes. Greater time spent being sedentary and longer bouts of sedentary time were associated with a higher risk of stroke.

As might be expected, therefore, physical fitness is also closely related to stroke risk. One study of over 16,000 healthy men showed a striking relationship between greater CRF and lower stroke mortality. Those in the high-fitness group had less than one-third the risk of dying from stroke compared with those in the low-fitness group (Lee and Blair, 2002). A study from the Cooper Institute in Dallas, Texas, followed 20,000 adults who had been fitness-tested and found a similar dose-response relationship between physical fitness and stroke risk – the fitter the subject, the lower the risk (Pandey *et al.*, 2016).

An indication of physical fitness is walking pace. A slow walking pace in the over-65s is associated with an increased risk of stroke (Hayes *et al.*,

DOI: 10.1079/9781800621855.0017

2020). The study used the UK Biobank and concluded that self-reported walking pace could be a useful additional screening tool for stroke risk in primary care.

Increasing age is usually associated with decreasing physical activity and this may play some part in increasing stroke risk. However, older people who do increase their activity levels decrease this risk. An Oslo study of more than 2000 middle-aged men followed for 35 years confirmed the tendency to take less exercise at this age but found 35% who increased their activity (Prestgaard *et al.*, 2018). This group had a 56% reduction of stroke risk.

Exercise in the Treatment of Stroke

Restoration of function

Exercise is vital to the restoration of muscle function. Rehabilitation after a stroke should start as soon as the blood supply to the brain has been re-established to the best possible level. It is usually provided by inpatient physiotherapy, which often takes place in a specialist stroke rehabilitation ward. Treatment is focused on strengthening the weakened muscles to improve arm and leg function and restore mobility (Harris and Eng, 2010). Balance exercises are an important part of this treatment.

There has been little research into the optimal frequency and duration of physiotherapy for post-stroke rehabilitation. What evidence there is, indicates that more is better. Unfortunately, stroke rehabilitation is usually under-resourced, with patients seldom receiving adequate physiotherapy. A period of time in a hospital bed is almost designed to reduce strength and mobility. Ten days in hospital is said to be equivalent to 10 years of ageing.

Hospital culture encourages lying and sitting rather than being active. This is in part driven by the desire to prevent falls in often under-staffed wards. The sitting patient is in less personal danger than the mobile patient. Rehabilitation therefore has to be intense to overcome the deconditioning effects of being in hospital. Probably most of the gains are from the spontaneous recovery that is characteristic of strokes. The sooner the patient can go home and return to normal daily activities, the better.

A model of stroke rehabilitation was provided by Roald Dahl. In 1965 his wife, actress Patricia Neal, had a disabling stroke caused by a brain haemorrhage. She was left with a severe speech impediment and one-sided weakness. Dahl feared she would become an 'enormous pink cabbage', so with his friends and neighbours he set up an intensive 6-hours-a-day regimen of physical activity and speech retraining. Some professionals warned this was too much, but he ignored them. Pat was coached back to normality, 'slowly, insidiously and quite relentlessly'. She eventually resumed her acting career, even getting another Oscar nomination.

Secondary prevention

This hugely important part of the long-term care of the stroke patient is seldom applied. A low level of physical fitness is one of the risk factors for stroke. Regular exercise reduces BP, improves blood lipids, gives better diabetic control and helps with weight loss. A suitable regimen has been suggested as 50 minutes or so of moderate-intensity exercise three or four times per week. A meta-analysis on combined forms of training after stroke concludes that a training programme of moderate intensity, three days per week, for at least 20 weeks had the greatest effect on CRF, muscle strength and walking capacity in stroke patients (Lee and Stone, 2020).

A study of physical activity in first-ever ischaemic stroke survivors looked at type, frequency, intensity and duration of exercise in this group (Hou *et al.*, 2021). Those who engaged in long-term, regular, mild exercises had a lower recurrence rate. A salutary warning from this study was that if irregular exercise was taken, it increased the risk of stroke recurrence.

There is also evidence that exercise is as effective as medication in delaying mortality from strokes and may be more effective. A study explored the effects of exercise on 14,716 people who were part of 57 different trials. Physical activity interventions were found to be about 10% more effective than drug treatments such as anticoagulation or antiplatelet agents in reducing long-term stroke mortality (Naci and Ioannidis, 2013).

Although there are very few long-term rehabilitation programmes for stroke patients, modified cardiac rehabilitation could fill this void. More than 1600 stroke patients have been treated in this way in the USA (Cuccurullo *et al.*, 2022). In a subgroup of 449 closely matched patients, 246 completed the programme. Of these completers four died within a year of the stroke compared with 14 in the non-participants. The participants' fitness level improved as did mobility, self-care and communication skills.

Other benefits of physical training

Post-stroke physical training has also been shown to reinforce the gains of early rehabilitation. It further increases CRF and muscle strength, with improved walking capacity. Immobility, unilateral limb weakness, poor balance, cognitive impairment, reduced ADL and quality of life, plus the risk of stroke recurrence, all benefit.

Greater self-confidence and independence are additional rewards, as are the amelioration of boredom and frustration (Luker *et al.*, 2015). A systematic study of 30 RCTs of exercise for stroke patients showed that exercise can lead to a moderately beneficial effect on health-related quality of life and concluded that exercise should become an integral part of stroke rehabilitation (Ali *et al.*, 2021).

It is difficult to overstate the multiple benefits of fitness training for stroke patients. It is just as effective as standard drug treatments, and maybe more effective in reducing the risk of recurrence and subsequent stroke-related death. The rationale for this is that decreased fitness is one of the risk factors for stroke. Like other consequences of arterial disease, the prospect of further episodes must be increased by failing to try to remedy this lack of fitness (Saunders *et al.*, 2014).

A Cochrane Review examined many of the problems faced by recovering stroke patients in a meta-analysis of 45 trials involving 2188 subjects. The report concluded that cardiorespiratory training reduces disability after a stroke, improves the speed and tolerance of walking, and probably improves balance (Saunders *et al.*, 2013). A recent study (Greb, 2021) has implied that walking speed after a stroke may help predict which patients will show greater post-rehabilitation improvement in performing a secondary task while walking. The study had a number of limitations, but additionally showed the benefits to overall walking distance following exercise intervention. Other benefits of exercise training for stroke victims include improved cognitive function, self-confidence and independence (Reed *et al.*, 2010; Cumming *et al.*, 2012).

Summary

Stroke is caused by a cerebral thrombosis, a cerebral embolus or a cerebral haemorrhage. It can result in a variety of outcomes, but most commonly hemiplegia. Observational studies show the incidence of stroke to be between 20 and 70% lower in those who are physically active. By the same token, physical fitness is closely related to stroke risk. Exercise is used in the treatment of stroke by restoring function and for secondary prevention.

References

Ali, A., Tabassum, D., Baig, S.S., Moyle, B., Redgrave, J., et al. (2021) Effect of exercise interventions and health-related quality of life after stroke and transient ischemic attack: a systematic review and meta-analysis. *Stroke* 52(7), 2445–2455.

Cuccurullo, S.J., Fleming, T.K., Zinonos, S., Park, M.O., Gizzi, M., et al. (2022) Stroke recovery program with modified cardiac rehabilitation improves mortality, functional & cardiovascular performance. *Journal of Stroke & Cerebrovascular Diseases* 31(5), 106322. https://doi.org/10.1016/j.jstrokecerebrovasdis.2022.106322

Cumming, T.B., Tyedin, K., Churilov, L., Morris, M.E. and Bernhardt, J. (2012) The effect of physical activity on cognitive function after stroke: a systematic review. *International Journal of Psychogeriatrics* 24, 557–567.

Greb, E. (2021) Walking speed following stroke a good predictor of recovery? *Medscape*, 2 July 2021. Available at: https://www.medscape.com/viewarticle/954181 (accessed 18 January 2023).

Harris, J.E. and Eng, J.J. (2010) Strength training improves upper-limb function in individuals with stroke: a meta-analysis. *Stroke* 41, 136–140.

Hayes, S., Forbes, J.F., Celis-Morales, C., Anderson, J., Ferguson, L., et al. (2020) Association between walking pace and stroke incidence: findings from the UK Biobank prospective cohort study. *Stroke* 51(5), 1388–1395. https://doi.org/10.1161/STROKEAHA.119.028064

Hooker, S.P., Diaz, K.M., Blair, S.N., Colabianchi, N., Hutto, B., et al. (2022) Association of accelerometer-measured sedentary time and physical activity with risk of stroke among US adults. *JAMA Network Open* 5(6), e2215385. https://doi.org/10.1001/jamanetworkopen.2022.15385

Hou, L., Mi, M., Wand, J., Li, Y., Zheng, Q., et al. (2021) Association between physical exercise and stroke recurrence among first-ever ischemic stroke survivors. *Scientific Reports* 11, 13372.

Lee, C.D. and Blair, S.N. (2002) Cardiorespiratory fitness and stroke mortality in men. *Medicine and Science in Sports and Exercise* 34, 592–595.

Lee, I.-M., Hennekens, C.H., Berger, K., Buring, J.E. and Manson, J.E. (1999) Exercise and risk of stroke in male physicians. *Stroke* 30, 1–6.

Lee, J. and Stone, A.J. (2020) Combined aerobic and resistance training for cardiorespiratory fitness, muscle strength and walking capacity after stroke: a systematic review and meta-analysis. *Journal of Stroke & Cerebrovascular Diseases* 29(1), 104498. https://doi.org/10.1016/j.jstrokecerebrovasdis.2019.104498

Luker, J., Lynch, E., Bernhardsson, S., Bennett, L. and Bernhardt, J. (2015) Stroke survivors' experiences of physical rehabilitation: a systematic review of qualitative studies. *Archives of Physical Medicine and Rehabilitation* 96(9), 1698–1708.e10. https://doi.org/10.1016/j.apmr.2015.03.017

Naci, H. and Ioannidis, J.P.A. (2013) Comparative effectiveness of exercise and drug interventions on mortality outcomes: metaepidemiological study. *BMJ* 347, f5577. https://doi.org/10.1136/bmj.f5577

Pandey, A., Patel, M.R., Willis, B., Gao, A., Leonard, D., *et al.* (2016) Association between midlife cardiorespiratory fitness and risk of stroke. The Cooper Center Longitudinal Study. *Stroke* 47, 1720–1726. https://doi.org/10.1161/STROKEAHA.115.011532

Prestgaard, E., Hodnesdal, C., Engeseth, K., Erikssen, J., Bodegård, J., *et al.* (2018) Long-term predictors of stroke in healthy middle-aged men. *International Journal of Stroke* 13(3), 292–300. https://doi.org/10.1177/1747493017730760

Reed, M., Harrington, R., Duggan, A. and Wood, V.A. (2010) Meeting stroke survivors' perceived needs: a qualitative study of a community-based exercise and education scheme. *Clinical Rehabilitation* 24, 16–25.

Sacco, R.L., Gan, R., Boden-Albala, B., Lin, I.F., Kargman, D.E., *et al.* (1998) Leisure-time physical activity and ischemic stroke risk: the Northern Manhattan Stroke Study. *Stroke* 29, 380–387.

Saunders, D.H., Sanderson, M., Brazzelli, M., Greig, C.A. and Mead, G.E. (2013) Physical fitness training for stroke patients. *Cochrane Database of Systematic Reviews* (10), CD003316. https://doi.org/10.1002/14651858.CD003316.pub5

Saunders, D.H., Greig, C.A. and Mead, G.E. (2014) Physical activity and exercise after stroke. *Stroke* 45, 3742–3747.

18 Parkinson's Disease (PD)

Parkinson's disease (PD) was originally described as 'the shaking palsy' by James Parkinson in 1817. The main features of PD are stiffness, difficulty with movements and a characteristic so-called pill-rolling tremor. Affected individuals have increasing problems with physical activities such as walking, writing and some social functions, like holding a teacup.

The prevalence of the condition is about one in 600 in the over-65s, so with an increasing population of older people it will undoubtedly become more common. PD progresses with age and may in time completely incapacitate the sufferer. Thought disorder and behavioural problems may occur, and dementia is common later in the disease. More than one-third of sufferers become depressed.

Exercise in the Prevention of PD

Only recently has evidence emerged that regular physical exercise can reduce the risk of PD. A number of smaller studies had failed to prove the link, but a meta-analysis of eight of these studies, involving over half a million subjects, did confirm the relationship. The review compared habitual exercise level with the risk of developing PD and found that those in the highest exercise category had 80% the risk of PD compared with those in the lowest category (Fang et al., 2018).

A Korean study of almost 11,000 people with PD showed that there was a dose-response relationship between self-reported physical activity and all-cause mortality (Yoon et al., 2021). This clearly supports the benefit of maintaining physical activity throughout life. A major review by Crotty and Schwarzschild (2020) has shown that people who engage in moderate to high levels of physical activity show a lower risk for developing PD later in life. They do accept that 'many outstanding questions remain, including whether exercise is truly neuroprotective and disease-modifying versus symptomatically but reversibly beneficial.' The benefit of a more active lifestyle was supported in older adults participating in the Rush Memory and Aging Project (Oveisgharan et al., 2020). The physically active participants were found to have a reduced risk for PD and a slower rate of its progression by as much as 20%.

Furthermore, levels of physical fitness also predict the risk of PD and considerably strengthen the evidence for inactivity as a risk factor for the disease. A cohort of 7347 US veterans were exercise-tested and followed up for up to 18 years. Men with high levels of physical fitness (VO_{2max} > 42 ml/min/kg) had only 25% the risk for developing PD compared to those in the lowest fitness group (VO_{2max} < 28 ml/min/kg) (Müller and Myers, 2018).

Exercise in the Treatment of PD

Intensive exercise programmes have been shown to improve mobility and reduce disability in PD patients. A 2010 meta-analysis found that exercise, mainly physiotherapy, improves physical functioning and quality of life, leg strength, balance and walking in PD patients (Goodwin et al., 2008). A more recent Cochrane Review of treadmill training in patients with PD found that this intervention does improve stride length and gait speed, although curiously does not improve walking distance (Mehrholz et al., 2015). Other benefits from exercise training have included improvements in various scales that measure severity of PD symptoms, and also improved balance, increased preferred walking speed and faster timed get-up-and-go tests (Choi et al., 2020). Depression may be improved, along with cognitive function and health-related quality of life (Schootemeijer et al., 2020). Schootemeijer et al.'s extensive review of 17 RCTs concluded that aerobic exercise has generic health benefits for people with PD, including a reduced incidence of CVD, lower mortality and improved bone health. A study in the USA (Schenkman et al.,

2018) involved 128 people, aged 40 to 80, who were all in the early stages of the disease, but not taking medication for it. They compared the participants who did high-intensity cardio exercise with those who took no exercise. Using a symptom scale, they found there was no change in the exercise group after 6 months, whereas the non-exercise group showed a worsening of their symptoms. One finding of the study was that people with early-stage PD could tolerate a high-intensity level of exercise. A rather unusual form of exercise, namely singing, was used in a small study on PD (Shirtcliff and Zaman, 2018). Heart rate, BP and cortisol levels were shown to be reduced following an hour of group singing. Participants also reported feeling less sad and anxious. That small study additionally noticed an improvement in symptoms such as finger-tapping and the manner of walking. A recent study (Tsukita *et al.*, 2022) suggests that people with early-stage PD who regularly undertake 2 hours of moderate exercise twice weekly, like walking or gardening, may have less trouble balancing, walking and engaging in daily activities.

Although it is now some 10 years old, the position paper presented by the Michigan Parkinson Foundation (2013) summarizes the situation well. It states:

> studies indicate that exercise benefits physical and mental function, health-related quality of life, strength, balance and gait speed. The choice of any particular exercise regimen is not generally as important as the time devoted to exercise and the regularity of the exercise sessions.

An important finding of all these studies is the wide variability in response. Exercise can be very helpful to some, but by no means to all sufferers of PD. An example of this is given in an 8-year follow-up study of fitness levels (Cancela-Carral *et al.*, 2021). Men showed a trend towards deterioration in fitness over the 8 years, whereas the women showed a trend towards improvement.

Several trials have tested different forms of exercise, including gait and balance training, progressive resistance training, treadmill exercise, strength training, aerobic exercise, and music and dancing (Armstrong and Okun, 2020). Non-contact boxing is used in 871 sites across the world with some 43,500 participants (Anderson, 2020). Table tennis also has its advocates (Sasser, 2020).

Finally, a word of caution. Parkinson's patients, with inherent balance problems, are vulnerable to falls sustained during exercise programmes. So far, however, this risk has not been shown to outweigh the benefits of regular exercise. This concern can be mitigated by using the numerous types of exercise equipment currently available which avoid a reliance on balance. An example of this would be an exercise cycle. Scientists at the University of Pennsylvania asked patients with PD to pedal on an exercise cycle every day for 8 weeks. The results showed that brain activity associated with movement increased. This was particularly so with those who cycled the fastest (Shah *et al.*, 2016). The reason for this is uncertain, but one theory is that exercise has an effect on dopamine, a brain chemical that helps control movement.

Summary

Parkinson's disease (PD) is a moderately common affliction of later life, characterized by stiffness, reduced body movements and a characteristic tremor. There is good evidence that regular exercise slows the onset and reduces the severity of PD. Once PD has developed, exercise can slow progression and has a modest effect on reducing some of the symptoms.

References

Anderson, P. (2020) Boxing helps knock out nonmotor Parkinson's symptoms. *Medscape*, 4 March 2020. Available at: https://www.medscape.com/viewarticle/926229 (accessed 19 January 2023).

Armstrong, M.J. and Okun, M. (2020) Diagnosis and treatment of Parkinson disease: a review. *JAMA* 323(6), 548–560. https://doi.org/10.1001/jama.2019.22360

Cancela-Carral, J.M., Mollinedo-Cardalda, I., López-Rodríguez, A. and Vila-Suárez, H. (2021) Exercise, physical fitness, and Parkinson's disease: an 8-year follow-up study. *Journal of Sports Medicine and Physical Fitness* 62(9), 1228–1236. https://doi.org/10.23736/S0022-4707.21.12483-1

Choi, H.-Y., Cho, K.-H., Jin, C., Lee, J., Kim, T.-H., *et al.* (2020) Exercise therapies for Parkinson's disease: a systematic review and meta-analysis. *Parkinson's Disease* 2020, 2565320. https://doi.org/10.1155/2020/2565320

Crotty, G.F. and Schwarzschild, M.A. (2020) Chasing protection in Parkinson's disease: does exercise reduce risk and progression? *Frontiers in Aging Neuroscience* 12, 186. https://doi.org/10.3389/fnagi.2020.00186

Fang, X., Han, D., Cheng, Q., Zhang, P., Zhao, C., *et al.* (2018) Association of levels of physical activity with risk of Parkinson's disease. A systematic review and meta-analysis. *JAMA Network Open* 1(5), e182421.

Goodwin, V.A., Richards, S.H., Taylor, R.S., Taylor, A.H. and Campbell, J.L. (2008) The effectiveness of exercise interventions for people with Parkinson's disease: a systematic review and meta-analysis. *Movement Disorders* 23(5), 631–640. https://doi.org/10.1002/mds.21922

Mehrholz, J., Kugler, J., Storch, A., Pohl, M., Elsner, B. and Hirsch, K. (2015) Treadmill training for patients with Parkinson's disease. *Cochrane Database of Systematic Reviews* (8), CD007830. https://doi.org/10.1002/14651858.CD007830.pub3

Michigan Parkinson Foundation (2013) Exercise as a component in the management of Parkinson's disease: a position paper. Presented by the Professional Advisory Board, May 2013. Available at: https://parkinsonsmi.org/treatment/entry/exercise-as-a-component-in-the-management-of-parkinson-s-disease-a-position-paper (accessed 19 January 2023).

Müller, J. and Myers, J. (2018) Association between physical fitness, cardiovascular risk factors, and Parkinson's disease. *European Journal of Preventive Cardiology* 25(13), 1409–1415. https://doi.org/10.1177/2047487318771168

Oveisgharan, S., Yu, L., Dawe, R.J., Bennett, D.A. and Buchman, A.S. (2020) Total daily physical activity and the risk of Parkinsonism in community-dwelling older adults. *The Journals of Gerontology: Series A* 75(4), 704–711. https://doi.org/10.1093/gerona/glz111

Sasser, L. (2020) Picking up a pingpong paddle may benefit people with Parkinson's. *Science Daily*, 25 February 2020. Available at: https://www.sciencedaily.com/releases/2020/02/200225171757.htm (accessed 19 January 2023).

Schenkman, M., Moore, C.G., Kohrt, W.M., Hall, D.A., Delitto, A., *et al.* (2018) Effect of high-intensity treadmill exercise on motor symptoms in patients with de novo Parkinson disease. *JAMA Neurology* 75(2), 219–226. https://doi.org/10.1001/jamaneurol.2017.3517

Schootemeijer, S., van der Kolk, N.M., Bloem, B.R. and de Vries, N.M. (2020) Current perspectives on aerobic exercise in people with Parkinson's disease. *Neurotherapeutics* 17(4), 1418–1433. https://doi.org/10.1007/s13311-020-00904-8

Shah, C., Beall, E.B., Frankemolle, A.M., Penko, A., Phillips, M.D., *et al.* (2016) Exercise therapy for Parkinson's disease: pedaling rate is related to changes in motor connectivity. *Brain Connectivity* 6(1), 25–36. https://doi.org/10.1089/brain.2014.0328

Shirtcliff, E.B. and Zaman, A. (2018) Singing for Parkinson's? Improvement in gait and finger tapping reported. *Rehab Management*, 13 November 2018. Available at: https://rehabpub.com/conditions/neurological/parkinsons-disease/singing-touted-rehab-aid-parkinsons-patients/ (accessed 30 January 2023).

Tsukita, K., Sakamaki-Tsukita, H. and Takahashi, R. (2022) Long-term effect of regular physical activity and exercise habits in patients with early Parkinson's disease. *Neurology* 98(8), e859–e871. https://doi.org/10.1212/WNL.0000000000013218

Yoon, S.Y., Suh, J.H., Yang, S.N., Han, K. and Kim, Y.W. (2021) Association of physical activity, including amount and maintenance, with all-cause mortality in Parkinson's disease. *JAMA Neurology* 78(12), 1446–1453. https://doi.org/10.1001/jamaneurol.2021.3926

19 Psychological Ill Health

Psychological illnesses are extremely common. The most frequent examples are depression and anxiety. A European study of depression found prevalence rates varying from 2.5% in Santander, Spain, to 17% in Liverpool, UK (Ayuso-Mateos *et al.*, 2001), while a worldwide study found rates of up to 29.5% (Goldberg and Lecrubier, 1995). Anxiety is almost as common, affecting as many as 16% of the population over a lifetime. There is a plethora of other mental illnesses, but only the major ones will be considered in this chapter.

The Impact of Psychological Illness

The severity of anxiety varies from low-level disquiet to a state of panic or permanent terror. Depression can progress from mild unhappiness to profound despair. In their worst forms these illnesses can be totally incapacitating and sometimes fatal. Depression is the main cause of suicide, which is commonest among men aged 40 to 50. There are about 6500 deaths by suicide annually in the UK and the rate is rising.

Mental health problems are associated with enormous direct costs for individuals and society, including the provision of health and social care, and indirect costs such as lost employment. They are the third most important cause of sick leave. They account for about 18 million days' sick leave, or 12.7% of the total sick days taken each year in the UK. The UK's gross domestic product (GDP) could be over £25 billion higher if it were not for the economic consequences of mental health problems both to individuals and to businesses.

Exercise and Stress

One of the most effective and satisfying ways of combating stress is 'letting off steam', a process which usually involves exertion in one form or another. The release of endorphins mediates this, the

so-called, 'feel-good' experience. Indeed, the state of anxiety or emotional arousal prepares us for effort. The heart rate, BP and blood sugar all increase. This was the natural response for our wild ancestors fighting for survival. Nowadays we seldom have the option of exerting ourselves when placed under stress. There is no opportunity to dissipate the metabolic consequences of the 'fight or flight' response. We tend to do little more than sit and worry.

The relationship between a healthy body and a healthy mind has been known for centuries, often illustrated by the quote: *Mens sana in corpore sano* (Juvenal, *c*.AD 100) (see also Chapter 1, this volume). Bodily movements affect the mind positively in a number of ways, which are well presented in a *New Scientist* feature article (Williams, 2021).

Exercise in the Prevention of Psychological Ill Health

The preventive effects of exercise are more apparent for depression than for anxiety. A number of well-conducted studies have confirmed the definite, if modest, reduction in risk of depression in regular exercisers (Hassmén *et al.*, 2000; De Moor *et al.*, 2006; Snehal *et al.*, 2014). A 2012 meta-analysis of the association between regular exercise and subsequent depression included some 30 studies, 25 of which confirmed the association with a reduction in depression of between 8 and 67% in those doing less than 150 minutes of exercise per week and 19–27% in those doing more than 150 minutes (Mammen and Faulkner, 2013). A more recent study from Norway (Harvey *et al.*, 2018) included 34,000 people without either mental or physical illness who were followed up for 11 years. Their exercise habits were compared with the risk of developing psychological symptoms. Undertaking regular leisure-time exercise was associated with reduced incidence of future depression but not anxiety. The majority of this protective effect occurred at low levels of exercise and was observed regardless of intensity. The findings suggested that about 12% of future cases of depression could have been prevented if all participants had engaged in at least 1 hour of physical activity each week, an estimate very closely supported by Pearce *et al.* (2022). They analysed 15 studies comprising 191,130 participants and 2,110,588 person-years and found 'an inverse curvilinear dose-response association between physical activity and depression'. That meant that the association of incident depression was steeper at lower activity volumes. Relative to adults not reporting any activity, those accumulating half the recommended volume of physical activity had 18% lower risk of depression. Adults accumulating the fully recommended volume of physical activity had 25% lower risk, with diminishing potential benefits and higher uncertainty observed beyond that exposure level. Their estimate concluded that if underactive adults had achieved the current physical activity recommendations, 11.5% of depression cases could have been prevented.

A survey of more than a million adults in the USA found that people who said they took exercise experienced more than 50% fewer days of poor mental health (Chekroud *et al.*, 2018). The effect was greatest in those with diagnosed depression and the optimal exercise dose was 45 minutes, three to five times per week. Exercising for more than 3 hours daily produced no further benefit.

The most effective type of exercise for reducing risk of depression was explored in a combined analysis of 1.5 million people from four US health surveillance surveys (2011–2017). Of the participants, 286,325 had depression and their exercise patterns were compared with the non-depressed group (Bennie *et al.*, 2020). Almost all physical activity combinations were associated with lower depression prevalence. The lowest prevalence of depression was shown for those combining moderate or vigorous physical activity with muscle-strengthening exercise. At the higher levels (up to 300 minutes of moderate or vigorous physical activity + 2 hours of muscle-strengthening exercise per week), the reduction of risk of depression was about 40%.

An Australian study of 14,000 men confirmed that just meeting the minimal recommendation for exercise decreased the risk of future depression. Higher levels were even more effective, but the study did not include extremely high levels (Pirkis *et al.*, 2017).

As might be expected, too much sedentary behaviour increases the chance of becoming depressed, particularly in young people (Kandola *et al.*, 2020). Hemmeter *et al.* (2021) also considered depression and cognitive decline. They argued that the assessment of exercise habits with individual recommendations for physical activity should be standard procedure in the therapy of affective disorders. They suggest that this should begin as early as possible, irrespective of age.

Regular exercise has also been found to reduce the risk of developing anxiety by about 25%, agoraphobia by 58% and post-traumatic stress disorder by 43% (Schuch *et al.*, 2019).

Finally, the effectiveness of physical activity is confirmed by the dose-response relationship between the level of CRF and the risk of becoming mentally unwell (Kandola *et al.*, 2019). The fitter a person, the lower the risk. The Maastricht Study, which tracked 1730 people for 5 years, also found an association between higher CRF and depression. This relationship was maintained, independent of the level of MVPA at baseline (Gianfredi *et al.*, 2021).

Exercise in the Treatment of Psychological Ill Health

There is a general belief that physical activity and exercise have positive effects on mood and anxiety. A large number of publications describe an association between physical activity and general wellbeing, improved mood and lessened anxiety. Some intervention studies describe exercise as lessening anxiety and depression in healthy subjects and patients. Recent well-controlled studies suggest that exercise training may be clinically effective. This certainly applies in major depression and panic disorder. There is also an acute effect of exercise. Research by the University of Missouri (Marshall, 1983) found that anxious women who exercised at a high intensity for 30 minutes on an exercise cycle felt considerably better after their workout. The benefits lasted for up to 90 minutes afterwards, compared with just 30 minutes after a moderate workload.

The Cochrane Review of the effect of exercise in the treatment of depression, involving some 1356 participants, showed exercise to have a moderate clinical effect. The same report found that exercise also appeared to be as effective as either psychological therapies or antidepressant drug treatment (Cooney *et al.*, 2013). When targeted specifically at depressed adolescents, exercise also has a moderate effect (Carter *et al.*, 2016). Even light levels of exercise are beneficial (Helgadóttir *et al.*, 2017), but the response to exercise is related to the degree of increase in CRF achieved (Perez-Sousa *et al.*, 2020). Exercise may also work for resistant depression that has failed to respond to other treatments (Mota-Pereira *et al.*, 2011).

The evidence for the positive effects of exercise and exercise training on depression and anxiety is growing. Yet its clinical use, at least as an adjunct to established treatments like psychotherapy or medication, is still at a very early stage (Ströhle, 2009). Exercise on its own, though clearly useful as an antidepressant, may not work so well as cognitive behavioural therapy (CBT) (Hallgren *et al.*, 2016). The ideal approach would be to combine both methods. There was concern that publication bias may influence meta-analyses on exercise as a treatment for depression. This was considered by Schuch *et al.* (2016). Their data strongly supported the claim that exercise is a beneficial treatment for depression.

The Faculty of Sport and Exercise Medicine recommends regular exercise as part of the treatment of anxiety and depression and explains some possible reasons why it is beneficial. The Faculty has produced a guide on the role that physical activity has in treating mental illness for health professionals, sports participants, schools, parents and carers (Faculty of Sport and Exercise Medicine, 2018).

The possible mechanism for the effect of physical activity is summarized by Meeusen and De Meirleir. In their abstract they state:

> Physical exercise influences the central dopaminergic, noradrenergic and serotonergic systems. A number of studies have examined brain noradrenaline (norepinephrine), serotonin (5-hydroxytryptamine; 5-HT) and dopamine with exercise. Although there are great discrepancies in experimental protocols, the results indicate that there is evidence in favour of changes in synthesis and metabolism of monoamines during exercise. There is a possibility that the interactions between brain neurotransmitters and their specific receptors could play a role in the onset of fatigue during prolonged exercise.
> (Meeusen and De Meirleir, 1995)

The complete mechanism for the reduction of stress through exercise is unclear. In part it may be because during exercise negative thoughts are diverted to focus on the exercise. A high level of physical fitness also has the benefit of raising self-esteem, often lacking in those with depression. One unusual application has been the inclusion of parkruns into prison regimes in the UK and Australia, which has resulted in a great improvement in the morale of inmates (parkrun.com, 2023).

Children with attention deficit hyperactivity disorder (ADHD) can benefit from physical activity. A systematic review (Villa-González *et al.*, 2020) concluded that physical activity may become an alternative, or at least complementary, to medicine in children with ADHD.

The physiological effect of exercise, as shown above, is to increase levels of neurotrophic factors in the brain. This, in turn, encourages the growth of new cells in the hippocampus, the area that controls mood. It is also known that exercise lowers the level of inflammation in body tissues, and this probably has an impact on depressive symptoms.

Mental Health

Just as physical health is much more than the absence of physical illness, so it is for mental health. There are a large number of instruments for assessing mental well-being from a variety of different perspectives (Parkinson, 2008). These include emotional well-being, life satisfaction, optimism and hope, self-esteem, resilience and coping, spirituality, social functioning and emotional intelligence.

The Covid-19 pandemic has highlighted the importance of mental health to the well-being of the population, with an emphasis on young people. The prevalence of poor mental health is higher in girls than boys and the level of physical activity seems to be the deciding factor (Halliday *et al.*, 2019). Exercising for between 2.5 and 7.5 hours per week has been shown to be protective (Kim *et al.*, 2012; Qu, 2020). Even in healthy college students, it was found that reasonable physical exercise (as little as 1 hour, twice weekly) had a positive impact on maintaining or promoting good mental health (Qu, 2020). The same outcome applied to the overall mental state of inpatients, although it took at least 3 months for the effect to become noticeable (Mazyarkin *et al.*, 2019). In adults, there is also a relationship between physical activity and self-reported days of poor mental health – the more exercise taken, the less the problem of psychological ill health (Fluetsch *et al.*, 2019).

Active commuting, such as walking or cycling to work, also helps, while sedentary time makes things worse (Tamminena *et al.*, 2020). A small study of 123 Canadian commuters compared the association between transport type and stress and mood at work (Brutus *et al.*, 2017). Those who cycled to work had stress levels 14% lower than those who drove and 11% lower than people who used public transport. Others have confirmed the beneficial effects of active transport (Teychenne *et al.*, 2021) and also the greater effect of leisure-time exercise rather than work-related activity.

When it comes to exercise mode, team sports seem to be most beneficial, reducing the time spent in poor mental health by 22% (Chekroud *et al.*, 2018). Next best modes are cycling, giving a reduction of 21%, attending the gym at 20%, jogging at 19% and walking by 18%. It is thought that the socialization associated with team sports promotes resilience and subsequently reduces depression. There is fresh evidence (de Lange, 2022) showing that time spent near water can provide a powerful boost to mental health. This may explain why many people choose to exercise near water.

The combination of being outdoors and engaging in physical activity has been shown to promote positive mental health in young people (Bélanger *et al.*, 2019). It is believed that it is the physical activity that mediates the relationship between outdoor time and mental health. All age groups can be beneficiaries, including the young, whose mental health is improved largely through the reduction in symptoms of anxiety and depression (Pascoe *et al.*, 2020).

A further often-neglected group is those people who provide care for persons living with chronic illnesses. A systematic review by researchers from Atlanta, Georgia, showed that exercise training improved the mental and physical health of this group (Epps *et al.*, 2019).

Summary

Psychological illness is extremely common, causing almost 13% of total sick days taken each year. Exercise can reduce stress and contribute considerably to the prevention of psychological ill health. Various studies have shown the preventive benefits of exercise, including the impact on depression and anxiety. Exercise can also be used to treat psychological ill health, with the mechanism likely to be via certain chemicals in the brain. The issue of mental health is being discussed more and the role of exercise should be part of this debate.

References

Ayuso-Mateos, J.L., Vázquez-Barquero, J.L., Dowrick, C., Lehtinen, V., Dalgard, O.S., *et al.* (2001) Depressive disorders in Europe: prevalence figures from the ODIN study. *British Journal of Psychiatry* 179, 308–316. https://doi.org/10.1192/bjp.179.4.308

Bélanger, M., Gallant, F., Doré, I., O'Loughlin, J.L., Sylvestre, M.-P., *et al.* (2019) Physical activity mediates the relationship between outdoor time and mental health. *Preventive Medicine Reports* 16, 101006. https://doi.org/10.1016/j.pmedr.2019.101006

Bennie, J.A., De Cocker, K., Biddle, S.J.H. and Teychenne, M.J. (2020) Joint and dose-dependent associations between aerobic and muscle-strengthening activity with depression: a cross-sectional study of 1.48 million adults between 2011 and 2017. *Depression and Anxiety* 37(2), 166–178. https://doi.org/10.1002/da.22986

Brutus, S., Javadian, R. and Panaccio, A.J. (2017) Cycling, car, or public transit: a study of stress and mood upon arrival at work. *International Journal of Workplace Health Management* 10, 13–24. https://doi.org/10.1108/IJWHM-10-2015-0059

Carter, T., Morres, I.D., Meade, O. and Callaghan, P. (2016) The effect of exercise on depressive symptoms in adolescents: a systematic review and meta-analysis. *Journal of the American Academy of Child & Adolescent Psychiatry* 55(7), 580–590. https://doi.org/10.1016/j.jaac.2016.04.016

Chekroud, S.R., Gueorguiva, R., Zheutlin, A.B., Paulus, M., Krumholz, H.M., *et al.* (2018) Association between physical exercise and mental health in 1.2 million individuals in the USA between 2011 and 2015: a cross-sectional study. *Lancet Psychiatry* 9, 739–746.

Cooney, G.M., Dwan, K., Greig, C.A., Lawlor, D.A., Rimer, J., *et al.* (2013) Exercise for depression. *Cochrane Database of Systematic Reviews* (9), CD004366. https://doi.org/10.1002/14651858.CD004366.pub6

de Lange, C. (2022) Why spending time near water gives us a powerful mental health boost. *New Scientist* issue 3395(16 July).

De Moor, M.H.M., Beem, A.L., Stubbe, J.H., Boomsma, D.I. and De Geus, E.J.C. (2006) Regular exercise, anxiety, depression and personality: a population-based study. *Preventive Medicine* 42, 273–279.

Epps, F., To, H., Liu, T.T., Karanjit, A. and Warren, G. (2019) Effect of exercise training on the mental and physical well-being of caregivers for persons living with chronic illnesses: a systematic review and meta-analysis. *Journal of Applied Gerontology* 40(1), 18–27. https://doi.org/10.1177/0733464819890753

Faculty of Sport and Exercise Medicine (2018) The role of physical activity and sport in metal health. Available at: https://www.fsem.ac.uk/position_statement/the-role-of-physical-activity-and-sport-in-mental-health/ (accessed 30 January 2023).

Fluetsch, N., Levy, C. and Tallon, L. (2019) The relationship of physical activity to mental health: a 2015 behavioral risk factor surveillance system data analysis. *Journal of Affective Disorders* 253, 96–101. https://doi.org/10.1016/j.jad.2019.04.086

Gianfredi, V., Koster, A., Eussen, S.J.M.P., Odone, A., Amerio, A., *et al.* (2021) The association between cardio-respiratory fitness and incident depression: The Maastricht Study. *Journal of Affective Disorders* 279, 484–490.

Goldberg, D. and Lecrubier, Y. (1995) Form and frequency of mental disorders across centres. In: Sartorius, N. and Ustun, T.B. (eds) *Mental Illness in General Health Care: An International Study*. Wiley (on behalf of WHO), Chichester, UK, pp. 323–334.

Hallgren, M., Helgadóttir, B., Herring, M.P., Zeebari, Z., Lindefors, N., *et al.* (2016) Exercise and internet-based cognitive-behavioural therapy for depression: multicentre randomised controlled trial with 12-month follow-up. *British Journal of Psychiatry* 209(5), 414–420. https://doi.org/10.1192/bjp.bp.115.177576

Halliday, A.J., Kern, M.L. and Turnbull, D.A. (2019) Can physical activity help explain the gender gap in adolescent mental health? A cross-sectional exploration. *Mental Health and Physical Activity* 16, 8–18. https://doi.org/10.1016/j.mhpa.2019.02.003

Harvey, S.B., Overland, S., Hatch, S.L., Wessely, S., Mykletun, A. and Hotopf, M. (2018) Exercise and the prevention of depression: results of the HUNT Cohort Study. *American Journal of Psychiatry* 175, 28–36. https://doi.org/10.1176/appi.ajp.2017.16111223

Hassmén, P., Koivula, N. and Uutela, A. (2000) Physical exercise and psychological well-being: a population study in Finland. *Preventive Medicine* 30, 17–25.

Helgadóttir, B., Forsell, Y., Hallgren, M., Möller, J. and Ekblom, Ö. (2017) Long-term effects of exercise at different intensity levels on depression: a randomized controlled trial. *Preventive Medicine* 105, 37–46. https://doi.org/10.1016/j.ypmed.2017.08.008

Hemmeter, U., Ngamsri, T. and Henkel, K. (2021) The role of exercise for prevention and treatment of depression and cognitive decline in the elderly. *Deutsche Zeitschrift für Sportmedizin* 72, 300–306.

Juvenal (*c*.AD 100) *Satires, Book IV, Satire X: Wrong Desire is the Source of Suffering*, tr. G.G. Ramsay (Heinemann, 1928).

Kandola, A., Ashdown-Franks, G., Stubbs, B., Osborn, D.P.J. and Hayes, J.F. (2019) The association between cardiorespiratory fitness and the incidence of common mental health disorders: a systematic review and meta-analysis. *Journal of Affective Disorders* 257, 748–757. https://doi.org/10.1016/j.jad.2019.07.088

Kandola, A., Lewis, G., Osborn, D.P.J., Stubbs, B. and Hayes, J.F. (2020) Depressive symptoms and objectively measured physical activity and sedentary behaviour throughout adolescence: a prospective cohort study. *Lancet Psychiatry* 7(3), 262–271. https://doi.org/10.1016/S2215-0366(20)30034-1

Kim, Y.S., Park, Y.S., Allegrante, J.P., Marks, R., Ok, H., *et al.* (2012) Relationship between physical activity and general mental health. *Preventive Medicine* 55(5), 458–463. https://doi.org/10.1016/j.ypmed.2012.08.021

Mammen, G. and Faulkner, G. (2013) Physical activity and the prevention of depression: a systematic review of prospective studies. *American Journal of Preventive Medicine* 45, 649–657.

Marshall, M.P. (1983) The relationship of aerobic exercise training and workouts to lower levels of anxiety and depression. PhD thesis, University of Missouri, Kansas City, Missouri.

Mazyarkin, Z., Pelegi, T., Golani, I., Sharony, L., Kremer, I. and Shamir, A. (2019) Health benefits of a physical exercise program for inpatients with mental health; a pilot study. *Journal of Psychiatric Research* 113(1), 10–16. https://doi.org/10.1016/j.jpsychires.2019.03.002

Meeusen, R. and De Meirleir, K. (1995) Exercise and brain neurotransmission. *Sports Medicine* 20(3), 160–188.

Mota-Pereira, J., Silverio, J., Carvalho, S., Ribeiro, J.C., Fonte, D. and Ramos, J. (2011) Moderate exercise improves depression parameters in treatment-resistant patients with major depressive disorder. *Journal of Psychiatric Research* 45(8), 1005–1111. https://doi.org/10.1016/j.jpsychires.2011.02.005

Parkinson, J. (2008) *Review of Scales of Positive Mental Health Validated for Use with Adults in the UK: Technical Report*. Health Scotland, Edinburgh.

parkrun.com (2023) Blog. Available at: https://blog.parkrun.com/uk/tag/prison-parkruns/ (accessed 19 January 2023).

Pascoe, M., Bailey, A.P., Craike, M., Carter, T., Patten, R., *et al.* (2020) Physical activity and exercise in youth mental health promotion: a scoping review. *BMJ Open Sport & Exercise Medicine* 6(1), e000677. https://doi.org/10.1136/bmjsem-2019-000677

Pearce, M., Garcia, L., Abbas, A., Strain, T., Schuch, F.B., *et al.* (2022) Association between physical activity and risk of depression: a systematic review and meta-analysis. *JAMA Psychiatry* 79(6), 550–559. https://doi.org/10.1001/jamapsychiatry.2022.0609

Perez-Sousa, M.A., Olivares, P.R., Gonzalez-Guerrero, J.L. and Gusi, N. (2020) Effects of an exercise program linked to primary care on depression in elderly: fitness as mediator of the improvement. *Quality of Life Research* 29, 1239–1246. https://doi.org/10.1007/s11136-019-02406-3

Pirkis, J., Currier, D., Carlin, J., Degenhardt, L., Dharmage, S.C., *et al.* (2017) Cohort profile: Ten to Men (the Australian Longitudinal Study on Male Health). *International Journal of Epidemiology* 46(3), 793–794i. https://doi.org/10.1093/ije/dyw055

Qu, X. (2020) Empirical analysis of the influence of physical exercise on psychological stress of college students. *Revista Argentina de Clínica Psicológica* XXIX(2), 1443–1451.

Schuch, F.B., Vancampfort, D., Richards, J., Rosenbaum, S., Ward, P.B. and Stubbs, B. (2016) Exercise as a treatment for depression: a meta-analysis adjusting for publication bias. *Journal of Psychiatric Research* 77, 42–51.

Schuch, F.B., Stubbs, B., Meyer, J., Heissel, A., Zech, P., *et al.* (2019) Physical activity protects from incident anxiety: a meta-analysis of prospective cohort studies. *Depression and Anxiety* 36(9), 846–858. https://doi.org/10.1002/da.22915

Snehal, M., Pereira, P., Geoffroy, M.-C. and Power, C. (2014) Depressive symptoms and physical activity during 3 decades in adult life. *JAMA Psychiatry* 71, 1373–1380.

Ströhle, A. (2009) Physical activity, exercise, depression and anxiety disorders. *Journal of Neural Transmission (Vienna)* 116(6), 777–784. https://doi.org/10.1007/s00702-008-0092-x

Tamminena, N., Reinikainen, J., Appelqvist-Schmidlechner, K., Borodulin, K., Mäki-Opas, T. and Solin, P. (2020) Associations of physical activity with positive mental health: a population-based study. *Mental Health and Physical Activity* 18, 100319.

Teychenne, M., White, R.L., Richards, J., Schuch, F.B., Rosenbaum, S. and Bennie, J.A. (2021) Do we need physical activity guidelines for mental health: what does the evidence tell us? *Mental Health and Physical Activity* 20, 10037.

Villa-González, R., Villalba-Heredia, L., Crespo, I., Del Valle, M. and Olmedillas, H. (2020) A systematic review of acute exercise as a coadjuvant treatment of ADHD in young people. *Psicothema* 32(1), 67–74.

Williams, C. (2021) Mind-altering moves. *New Scientist*, 20 May, 34–38.

20 Dementia and Cognition

Dementia is an advancing modern scourge and has recently been reported to have overtaken CHD as the most frequent cause of death for women in the UK. There are a number of different types of dementia. The two most common are Alzheimer's disease and vascular dementia, which between them make up 80% of cases. About 47 million people in the world live with dementia and this number is projected to rise to about 130 million by 2050. The current figures for the UK are 850,000, rising to 2 million over that same period (Alty *et al.*, 2019). About 10% of over-65s have dementia and a further 20% suffer mild cognitive impairment. Recently there has been a large rise in the number of people with dementia admitted to hospital as emergencies. Many of them remain as inpatients for much longer than necessary because of a lack of social-care support in the community. In 2017/18 there were 379,000 such admissions, up 35% over 5 years, and 40,000 of these remained in hospital for between 1 and 12 months.

The devastation caused by this epidemic is hard to overstate, as the ill effects are seen in every aspect of our lives. Most families will sooner or later have to face the emotional, financial and social problems brought by a relative with dementia. The cost to the health service and to social services of this rising tide of dependence is astronomical. The London School of Economics estimated in 2019 that the cost to the UK is £34.74 billion annually. Health care accounts for 14% (£4.9 billion) of the total costs in the UK, whereas social care (publicly and privately funded) and unpaid care account for 45% (£15.7 billion) and 40% (£13.9 billion), respectively, of the total costs (Wittenberg *et al.*, 2019). The economic impact of caring for each sufferer is currently some £28,500 per annum.

Curiously, for any particular age group dementia is getting less common. This is perhaps the result of a steady decline of vascular disease, with less smoking and better treatment of raised BP and lipid levels. However, this effect is overwhelmed by the steady increase in the age of the population. Thus demented people are becoming more numerous, although not as numerous as might be expected.

There are several known contributors to the development of dementia. These include smoking, hypertension, obesity and that cause of so many problems – lack of exercise. About one-third of dementia cases are attributable to these modifiable risk factors. A rather worrying study in midlife subjects (Greb, 2020) shows that the relationship between cardiovascular risk factors and cognition becomes evident much earlier than previously realized. Individuals in their fifties who smoked were 65% more likely to have accelerated cognitive decline. Those with hypertension were 87% more likely to show such decline, and individuals with diabetes had a nearly threefold increased risk.

Beta-amyloid plaques have been implicated in the disease for a long time and most drug treatments have been aimed at reducing these. However, a recent feature article in *New Scientist* (Thomasy, 2021) has questioned whether the focus should be elsewhere. Another correlate of dementia severity is the build-up of a protein called tau. This, along with genetic analysis, infections, sleep issues and insulin resistance are all promising lines of research into what now appears to be a disease with multiple contributing factors. This chapter will concentrate on exercise as one of the modifiable risk factors.

Exercise in the Prevention of Dementia

The evidence that dementia is delayed and reduced in severity by regular exercise is growing. Meta-analyses of all the prospective studies of the effects of midlife exercise have confirmed a significantly reduced risk of dementia and of milder forms of cognitive impairment in later life (Ahlskog *et al.*, 2011).

As an example, a Scandinavian study used the Swedish Twin Registry to identify 264 individuals with dementia. They were compared with 2870 unimpaired controls, matched for age, sex and a number of other features. All were normal at baseline, with a mean age of 49, and were followed up for an average of 30 years. Compared with those who did virtually no exercise, those who performed light exercise had less than half the risk of developing dementia, while those who performed moderate exercise had one-third the risk (Andel *et al.*, 2008). A meta-analysis involving 164,000 subjects found a risk reduction of 28% for dementia – and 55% for Alzheimer's – for those who were physically active (Hamer and Chida, 2009). Higher levels of exercise are more protective and there is more evidence for the effectiveness of aerobic exercise than resistance training.

A major study in Korea, which included 62,286 participants, demonstrated that an increased physical activity level, including a low amount of light-intensity activity, was associated with a reduced risk of dementia in older adults (Yoon *et al.*, 2021).

Higher levels of physical fitness in midlife are also associated with a lower risk of dementia in later life. Those in the upper 20% for fitness had two-thirds the risk of dementia compared with those in the lowest 20%. This was based on a long-term study of nearly 20,000 middle-aged Americans (Defina *et al.*, 2013). A number of studies have confirmed that having a high level of physical fitness delays the onset of dementia by around a decade. The Gothenburg Study of fitness and dementia included cycle-exercise testing of 200 women aged 38–60 and followed them for 44 years. By this time only 5% of the fittest group had developed dementia compared with 32% in the least-fit group (Hörder *et al.*, 2018).

The importance of CRF rather than self-reported physical activity level was emphasized by a study of nearly 7000 subjects. It found that both CRF and physical activity are associated with quality of life over time, but only CRF was associated with preservation of cognitive function. This particularly applied to language ability, attention and processing speed (Damiel *et al.*, 2020).

An overall healthy lifestyle seems to be the best option for reducing the risk of developing dementia in old age. The more aspects of healthy behaviour that are adopted, the better will be the outcome. The Caerphilly Cohort Study looked at five different behaviours: exercise, maintaining normal weight, eating a healthy diet, not smoking and avoiding excess alcohol. It examined the rate of dementia over the following decades. Adhering to all five of these behaviours was associated with just one-third the risk of dementia. Unfortunately, less than 1% of subjects followed all five behaviours and only 5% followed four out of the five behaviours. The biggest contributor to lowering the risk of dementia was regular exercise. This, on its own, reduced the risk by about 60% (Elwood *et al.*, 2013).

Both aerobic exercise and resistance training play a part in the prevention of dementia. A meta-analysis of 39 trials involving nearly 13,000 individuals aged 50 or more compared aerobic exercise, strength training and a mixture of the two. It found that there was a clear benefit to cognitive function from taking the usually recommended level of exercise needed for health gain. The conclusion was:

> The findings suggest that an exercise programme with components of both aerobic and resistance-type training, of at least moderate intensity and at least 45 min per session, on as many days of the week as possible, is beneficial to cognitive function in adults aged >50 years.
>
> (Northey *et al.*, 2018)

Almost any form of exercise of almost any intensity may contribute to dementia prevention. Dr Eric Larson, from the National Institute of Aging in Maryland, USA, notes that 'elderly people who only exercised gently for 15 minutes at a time, three times per week, were 32% less likely to get Alzheimer's' (Larson *et al.*, 2006). Gardening, according to the influential King's Fund thinktank, has been shown to reduce depression, loneliness, anxiety and stress. Trials have shown that 6 months of gardening resulted in a slowing down of cognitive decline over the next 18 months (Buck, 2016).

Not all studies support the idea that exercise prevents dementia. A meta-analysis of 19 studies involving more than 400,000 subjects followed up for an average of 15 years found no such protective effect (Kivimäki *et al.*, 2019). They did, however, find some protection for a subgroup suffering from dementia associated with conditions such as diabetes, hypertension and other causes of vascular dementia. It was suggested that the apparent protection by exercise from dementia may be due to 'reverse causality'. This means that the diminished physical activity observed before the onset of dementia might be due to a preclinical reduction in brain efficiency reducing the urge to exercise. This possibility was allowed for in a systematic review and meta-analysis of midlife physical activity and the risk of subsequently developing dementia (Iso-Markku et al., 2022). After allowing for possible reverse causation, midlife physical activity was associated with a decreased risk of 20% for all-cause dementia, 14% for Alzheimer's disease and 21% for vascular dementia.

Early intervention may be important. Researchers from Boston University tracked nearly 1000 people for 20 years. Poor fitness at an early age was correlated with brain volume decades later. Another study, London based, of 9000 people, showed that those who exercised regularly performed better in tests of memory, attention, reasoning and learning, even at the age of 50 (Dregan and Gulliford, 2013). This gives further support for the benefit of high levels of cardiovascular health throughout life.

Mechanisms

The understanding of brain function is developing rapidly but is still at a very early stage. Clinicians and medical scientists are beginning to explore the possible mechanisms by which exercise mediates preservation of normal cognitive function. The region of the brain responsible for memory and spatial awareness is the hippocampus, which sits at the base of the brain. This area is one of the first to show loss of tissue in Alzheimer's disease. Regular exercise in older subjects is associated with a slowing of the rate of loss of substance within the hippocampus (Erickson et al., 2012). One year of aerobic exercise in a large RCT of seniors was associated with significantly larger hippocampal volumes and better spatial memory. Other RCTs in seniors have documented a reduction of age-related loss of grey-matter volume with aerobic exercise (Thomas et al., 2012). Cross-sectional studies similarly reported significantly larger hippocampal or grey-matter volumes among physically fit seniors compared with unfit people of the same age (Ahlskog et al., 2011). The relationship of hippocampal volume with peak oxygen consumption (see Chapter 3, this volume) supports the notion of the benefits of fitness in old age (Petersen et al., 2019).

An interesting observation from the Rush Memory and Aging Project is that physical exercise appears to be associated with a reduced activation of microglia, the primary immune cells of the brain. These immune cells, which make up 15% of all brain cells, could well be a fruitful area of future research into the aetiology of dementia (Bennett et al., 2012). A most detailed review of the pathophysiological molecular pathways of the disease and its association with physical exercise is by Susana López-Ortiz et al. (2021). The detail is well outside the scope of this book, but it is recommended for anyone interested in the detailed molecular pathways.

Brain cognitive networks, studied with functional magnetic-resonance imaging (MRI), display improved connectivity after 6–12 months of exercise. The ability of the brain to increase activity and functional nerve connections is known as neuroplasticity and this can be increased by bouts of exercise. The harder the exercise, the greater the effect (Andrews et al., 2020). These studies support the belief that regular exercise can prevent dementia. Importantly, they also suggest that physical activity could be effective for treating this otherwise fairly untreatable condition. Both diabetes and obesity, conditions which are prevented by regular exercise, are associated with increased risk of dementia. This effect must play a part in reducing dementia in the physically active. The epidemiological relationship between obesity and dementia has been observed more recently in 6582 participants. They concluded that having an increased body weight or abdominal obesity was associated with an increased incidence of dementia (Ma et al., 2020). A study of 518 participants over a 30-year period showed that lifestyle habits formed as young as 20 years will impact on brain function in early life and onwards to middle age. Even young children can improve their ability to learn by being physically active. Studies in Japan at both Kobe University and Tsukuba University have demonstrated superior cognitive abilities in young people who are regular exercisers (Ishihara et al., 2021).

Exercise in the Treatment of Dementia

The 2015 Cochrane Review of trials of exercise as an intervention for dementia examined 17 trials involving more than 1000 patients. The main positive finding was that those treated with exercise were more capable of performing ADL, but there was no evidence of improved cognitive function. The results, however, were very variable and the authors found the quality of the trials to be very low (Forbes et al., 2015). A 2018 review of the findings in 1100 adults, average age 73, who had taken part in RCTs of exercise found that long-term exercise (at least 52 hours over 6 months) improved the brain's processing speeds in both healthy individuals and those with cognitive impairment (Gomes-Osman *et al.*, 2018). Memory was not improved. A recent study on cognition over a period of 5 years showed that those who achieved a good level of CRF over the age of 70 were able to maintain cognition. It appeared that the mode of exercise was less important (Sokolowski *et al.*, 2021). These findings were confirmed by a cross-sectional study whose authors state:

> better physical fitness is important for cognition and autonomous functional capacity and that it has positive repercussions on the QoL [quality of life] in institutionalized older adults with dementia. Consequently, exercise-based therapeutic strategies aiming to improve physical fitness should be implemented.
>
> (Sampaio *et al.*, 2020)

The age at which exercise is beneficial was explored at University College London (Hollamby *et al.*, 2017). The study suggests that it is never too late to benefit from exercise, with the more active showing fewer signs of memory loss. Researchers led by Columbia University in the USA showed that just 6 months of regular exercise helped 40-year-olds achieve the thinking skills of a 30-year-old. The study, published in the journal *Neurology*, even showed an improvement in those in their twenties (Stern *et al.*, 2019).

Subjects with mild cognitive impairment have been shown to respond to aerobic exercise with an improvement in cognitive ability and a small improvement in memory (Zheng *et al.*, 2016; Biazus-Sehn *et al.*, 2020). The severity of the disease is probably relevant, and those with mild cognitive impairment seem to be more treatable than those with well-established dementia. Multicomponent training, which combines aerobic exercise, strength training, postural and balance exercises, has been used to treat the symptoms of dementia and to delay the progression of the disease. A systematic review by Ribeiro *et al.* (2019) found the results were unclear for the effects of multicomponent training on cognition and ADL, although the control group showed a decline. One of the reasons for this uncertainty is that inter-individual differences occur. These differences in cognitive responses to aerobic exercise in older people will be the basis for inconsistent cognitive benefits (Yu *et al.*, 2021). Mental decline was reported in an interesting study that compared 150 pairs of female twins.

The researchers, at King's College London, found that the sibling with the strongest legs at the start of the study tended to have fewer age-related brain changes at the end (Steves *et al.*, 2016).

A major review from Germany and Switzerland concludes that 'individual recommendations for physical activity should be implemented as a standard procedure in the therapy of affective disorders and dementia. It should begin as early as possible but also at older ages' (Hemmeter *et al.*, 2021). As shown in Chapter 9 (this volume), systematic reviews and meta-analyses are very powerful ways to consider a topic. In one of the most complete undertaken, the conclusions were:

> Collectively, the evidence indicated that exercise can improve cerebrovascular function, cognition and neuroplasticity through areas of the brain associated with executive function and memory in adults 50 years or older, irrespective of their health status. However, more research is required to ascertain the mechanisms of action.
>
> (Bliss *et al.*, 2021)

No lesser an authority than the World Health Organization considers that increasing physical activity reduces cognitive decline, which in itself could improve mobility, reduce the risk of falls and help people with dementia to live independently for longer (World Health Organization, 2019).

As in the prevention of dementia, the effect of exercise in its treatment may be partly mediated by hippocampal function. The hippocampus shrinks in late adulthood, leading to impaired memory and an increased risk for dementia. Hippocampal volumes are larger in higher-fitness adults. An RCT with 120 older adults found that aerobic exercise training increased the size of the anterior hippocampus, leading to improvements in spatial memory. Exercise training increased hippocampal volume by 2%, effectively reversing age-related loss in volume by 1 to 2 years. This leads to the possibility that exercise might reverse some of the effects of dementia (Erickson *et al.*, 2011).

The management of dementia is a bleak and unrewarding field and individuals must do everything in their power to prevent this disease. The most promising approach is regular exercise. Once dementia has become established, it seems that it may be too late for exercise to have too much effect on cognitive ability. However, there are still important quality-of-life attributes to be gained for affected individuals. Symptoms like depression, an extremely common complaint in demented people, can respond well to increased physical activity. A systematic review showed that 'non-drug approaches were associated with a meaningful reduction in symptoms of depression in people with dementia and without a diagnosis of a major depressive disorder' (Watt et al., 2021).

Other important effects include improvements in strength, balance, mobility, endurance and quality of life (Lam et al., 2018; Sampaio et al., 2020). A particularly valuable advantage is improvement in ADL, which helps individuals to maintain their independence (Borges-Machado et al., 2021).

Cognition and Exercise

Cognition is defined as 'the mental action or process of acquiring knowledge and understanding through thought, experience and the senses'. People who suffer from dementia are most likely to have the symptoms associated with poor cognition and the two are closely related. There will be examples of cognitive impairment prior to a diagnosis of dementia and there are also studies which examine cognition as a separate entity. Both these will be explored below.

As people age, it is not uncommon to show signs of mild cognitive impairment unrelated to dementia. There is evidence that weekly physical activity can help prevent this mild cognitive impairment progressing to dementia (Kim et al., 2020). The authors suggest that regular exercise may increase the production of molecules that support the growth and survival of neurons or increase blood flow to the brain. This, in turn, could prevent a reduction in brain volume often associated with dementia. Exercise also has an acute effect. A Dutch study divided 72 students into three groups (van Dongen et al., 2016). All three groups were shown images and were asked to study and recall them. The first group exercised after 4 hours, the second exercised immediately after the lesson, and the third group did not exercise. MRI scans of the first group scored an average of 87% compared to the other two groups, which scored 80% on average. The researchers concluded that appropriately timed exercise could improve long-term memory and highlight the potential of exercise as an intervention in education and clinical settings.

Exercise will improve physical fitness (see Chapter 5, this volume) and a study at the University of Birmingham's School of Psychology showed how fitness is related to mental health. They used a name-recall test to compare aerobic fitness with ability to find words and concluded that 'the higher the older adults' aerobic fitness level, the lower the probability of experiencing a tip-of-the-tongue state' (Segaert et al., 2018). A systematic review and meta-analysis has shown that aerobic exercise improves episodic memory in late adulthood (Aghjayan et al., 2022). These results demonstrate the clinical and public health importance of exercise as an accessible intervention to improve memory in late adulthood.

The type and dose of exercise have been analysed in another large meta-analysis, which found a non-linear dose-response association between overall exercise and cognition (Gallardo-Gómez et al., 2022). The estimated minimal exercise dose to give clinically relevant changes in cognition was 724 MET minutes per week and doses beyond 1200 MET minutes per week provided less clear benefit. The findings also highlighted the greater impact of resistance exercise over other modalities.

Exercise appears to increase blood flow into two key regions of the brain associated with memory, including the anterior cingulate cortex and the hippocampus (Thomas et al., 2020). A recent study shows that low and high exercise intensities influence brain function differently. Resting-state functional MRI was used to study brain connectivity. Low-intensity exercise activates brain networks involved in cognition control and attention processing, while high-intensity exercise primarily activates networks involved in affective/emotion processing (Schmitt et al., 2019). A further clue to the mechanism comes from a study by Gaitán et al. (2021), which examined the role of specific biomarkers during exercise. They found plasma myokine cathepsin B (CTSB) levels were increased following this 26-week structured aerobic exercise training in older adults. Verbal learning and memory correlated positively with change in CTSB. The present correlation between CTSB and verbal learning and memory suggests that CTSB may be useful as a marker for cognitive changes relevant to hippocampal function after exercise in a population at risk for dementia.

Recent research published in Nature (Islam et al., 2021) suggests that irisin, a chemical secreted during exercise, can protect the brain by reducing inflammation. A group of men with cognitive impairment were given exercise sessions and chemical changes in the brain suggested that exercise can 'kick-start' beneficial chemical changes.

Summary

Dementia is an increasingly prevalent condition that is the commonest cause of death in women and second commonest in men. It is also a huge social and financial cost to both individuals and society as a whole. Regular exercise delays the onset of dementia by several years. Once dementia has developed, regular exercise can slow the progression of mild dementia and improve ability to perform activities of daily living. Physical activity does not improve cognition in advanced dementia but does provide social benefits.

References

Aghjayan, S.L., Bournias, T., Kang, C., Zhou, X., Stillman, C.M., *et al*. (2022) Aerobic exercise improves episodic memory in late adulthood: a systematic review and meta-analysis. *Communications Medicine* 2, 15.

Ahlskog, J.E., Geda, Y.E., Graff-Radford, N.R. and Petersen, R.C. (2011) Physical exercise as a preventive or disease-modifying treatment of dementia and brain aging. *Mayo Clinical Proceedings* 86(9), 876–884. https://doi.org/10.4065/mcp.2011.0252

Alty, J., Farrow, M. and Lawler, K. (2019) Exercise and dementia prevention. *Practical Neurology* 20(3), 234–240. https://doi.org.10.1136/practneurol-2019-002335

Andel, R., Crowe, M., Pedersen, N.L., Fratiglioni, L., Johansson, B. and Gatz, M. (2008) Physical exercise at midlife and risk of dementia three decades later: a population-based study of Swedish twins. *The Journals of Gerontology: Series A* 63(1), 62–66.

Andrews, S.C., Curtin, D., Hawi, Z., Wongtrakun, J., Stout, J.C. and Coxon, J.P. (2020) Intensity matters: high-intensity interval exercise enhances motor cortex plasticity more than moderate exercise. *Cerebral Cortex* 30(1), 101–112. https://doi.org/10.1093/cercor/bhz075

Bennett, D.A., Schneider, J.A., Buchman, A.S., Barnes, L.L., Boyle, P.A. and Wilson, R.S. (2012) Overview and findings from the Rush Memory and Aging Project. *Current Alzheimer Research* 9(6), 646–663.

Biazus-Sehn, L.F., Schuch, F.B., Firth, J. and Stigger, F.S. (2020) Effects of physical exercise on cognitive function of older adults with mild cognitive impairment: a systematic review and meta-analysis. *Archives of Gerontology and Geriatrics* 89; 104048. https://doi.org/10.1016/j.archger.2020.104048

Bliss, E.S., Wong, R.H.X., Howe, P.R.C. and Mills, D.E. (2021) Benefits of exercise training on cerebrovascular and cognitive function in ageing. *Journal of Cerebral Blood Flow & Metabolism* 41(3), 447–470. https://doi.org/10.1177/0271678X20957807

Borges-Machado, F.B., Silva, N., Farinatti, P., Poton, R., Ribeiro, Ó. and Carvalho, J. (2021) Effectiveness of multi-component exercise interventions in older adults with dementia: a meta-analysis. *The Gerontologist* 61(8), e449–e462. https://doi.org/10.1093/geront/gnaa091

Buck, D. (2016) *Gardening and Health. Implications for Policy and Practice.* The Kings Fund, London.

Damiel, L., Martínez-González, M.A., Corella, D., Salas-Salvadó, J., Schröder, H., *et al*. (2020) Physical fitness and physical activity association with cognitive function and quality of life: baseline cross-sectional analysis of the PREDIMED-Plus trial. *Scientific Reports* 10(1), 3472. https://doi.org/10.1038/s41598-020-59458-6

Defina, L.F., Willis, B.L., Radford, N.B., Gao, A., Leonard, D., *et al*. (2013) The association between midlife cardio-respiratory fitness levels and later-life dementia: a cohort study. *Annals of Internal Medicine* 158, 162–168.

Dregan, A. and Gulliford, M.C. (2013) Leisure-time physical activity over the life course and cognitive functioning in late mid-adult years: a cohort-based investigation. *Psychological Medicine* 43(11), 2447–2458. https://doi.org/10.1017/S0033291713000305

Elwood, P., Galante, J., Pickering, J., Palmer, S., Bayer, A., *et al*. (2013) Healthy lifestyles reduce the incidence of chronic diseases and dementia: evidence from the Caerphilly Cohort Study. *PLoS One* 8(12), e81877. https://doi.org/10.1371/journal.pone.0081877

Erickson, K.I., Voss, M.W., Prakash, R.S., Basak, C., Szabo, A., *et al*. (2011) Exercise training increases size of hippocampus and improves memory. *Proceedings of the National Academy of Sciences USA* 108, 3017–3022.

Erickson, K.I., Weinstein, A.M. and Lopez, O.L. (2012) Physical activity, brain plasticity, and Alzheimer's disease. *Archives of Medical Research* 43(8), 615–621.

Forbes, D., Forbes, S.C., Blake, C.M., Thiessen, E.J. and Forbes, S. (2015) Exercise programs for people with dementia. *Cochrane Database of Systematic Reviews* (4), CD006489.

Gaitán, J.M., Moon, H.Y., Stremlau, M., Dubal, D.B., Cook, D.B., *et al*. (2021) Effects of aerobic exercise training on systemic biomarkers and cognition in late middle-aged adults at risk for Alzheimer's disease. *Frontiers in Endocrinology* 12, 660181. https://doi.org/10.3389/fendo.2021.660181

Gallardo-Gómez, D., Del Pozo-Cruz, J., Noetel, M., Álvarez-Barbosa, F., Alfonso-Rosa, R.M. and Del Pozo Cruz, B. (2022) Optimal dose and type of exercise to improve cognitive function in older adults: a systematic review and Bayesian model-based network meta-analysis of RCTs. *Ageing Research Reviews* 76, 101591. https://doi.org/10.1016/j.arr.2022.101591

Gomes-Osman, J., Cabral, D.F., Morris, T., McInerney, K., Cahalin, L.P., *et al.* (2018) Exercise for cognitive brain health in aging. A systematic review for an evaluation of dose. *Neurology: Clinical Practice* 8(3), 257–265.

Greb, E. (2020) Cardiovascular risk factors tied to midlife cognitive decline. *Medscape*, 15 July 2020. Available at: https://www.medscape.com/viewarticle/933988 (accessed 20 January 2023).

Hamer, M. and Chida, Y. (2009) Physical activity and risk of cognitive decline. *Psychological Medicine* 39, 3–11.

Hemmeter, U., Ngamsri, T. and Henkel, K. (2021) The role of exercise for prevention and treatment of depression and cognitive decline in the elderly. *Deutsch Zeitschrift für Sportsmedizin* 72, 300–306.

Hollamby, A., Davelaar, E.J. and Cadar, D. (2017) Increased physical fitness is associated with higher executive functioning in people with dementia. *Frontiers in Public Health* 5, 346. https://doi.org/10.3389/fpubh.2017.00346

Hörder, H., Johansson, L., Guo, X., Grimby, G., Kern, S., *et al.* (2018) Midlife cardiovascular fitness and dementia: a 44-year longitudinal population study in women. *Neurology* 90(15), e1298–e1305. https://doi.org/10.1212/WNL.0000000000005290

Ishihara, T., Miyazaki, A., Tanaka, H., Fujii, T., Takahashi, M., *et al.* (2021) Childhood exercise predicts response inhibition in later life via changes in brain connectivity and structure. *NeuroImage* 237, 118196. https://doi.org/10.1016/j.neuroimage.2021.118196

Islam, M.R., Valaris, S., Young, M.F., Haley, E.B., Luo, R., *et al.* (2021) Exercise hormone irisin is a critical regulator of cognitive function. *Nature Metabolism* 3, 1058–1070.

Iso-Markku, P., Kujala, U.M., Knittle, K., Polet, J., Vuoksimaa, E. and Waller, K. (2022) Physical activity as a protective factor for dementia and Alzheimer's disease: systematic review, meta-analysis and quality assessment of cohort and case–control studies. *British Journal of Sports Medicine* 56, 701–709.

Kim, Y.J., Han, K.-D., Baek, M.S., Cho, H., Lee, E.J. and Lyou, C.H. (2020) Association between physical activity and conversion from mild cognitive impairment to dementia. *Alzheimer's Research & Therapy* 12(1), 136. https://doi/.org/10.1186/s13195-020-00707-1

Kivimäki, M., Singh-Menoux, A., Pentti, J., Sabia, S., Nyberg, S.T., *et al.* (2019) Physical inactivity, cardio-metabolic disease, and risk of dementia: an individual-participant meta-analysis. *BMJ*, 365, l1495.

Lam, F.M., Huang, M.Z., Liao, L.-R., Chung, R.C., Kwok, T.C. and Pang, M.Y. (2018) Physical exercise improves strength, balance, mobility, and endurance in people with cognitive impairment and dementia: a systematic review. *Journal of Physiotherapy* 64(1), 4–15. https://doi.org/10.1016/j.jphys.2017.12.001

Larson, E.B., Wang, L., Bowen, J.D. McCormick, W.C., Teri, L., *et al.* (2006) Exercise is associated with reduced risk for incident dementia among persons 65 years of age and older. *Annals of Internal Medicine* 144(2), 73–81.

López-Ortiz, S., Pinto-Fraga, J., Valenzuela, P.L., Martín-Hernández, J., Seisdedos, M.M., *et al.* (2021) Physical exercise and Alzheimer's disease: effects on pathophysiological molecular pathways of the disease. *International Journal of Molecular Sciences* 22, 2897. https://doi.org/10.3390/ijms22062897

Ma, Y., Ajnakina, O., Steptoe, A. and Cadar, D. (2020) Higher risk of dementia in English older individuals who are overweight or obese. *International Journal of Epidemiology* 49(4), 1353–1365. https://doi.org/10.1093/ije/dyaa099

Northey, J.M., Cherbuin, N., Pumpa, K., Smee, D.J. and Rattray, B. (2018) Exercise interventions for cognitive function in adults older than 50: a systematic review with meta-analysis. *British Journal of Sports Medicine* 52(3), 154–160. https://doi.org/10.1136/bjsports-2016-096587

Petersen, R.C., Joyner, M.J. and Jack, C.R. (2019) Cardiorespiratory fitness and brain volumes. *Mayo Clinic Proceedings* 95(1), 6–8. https://doi.org/10.1016/j.mayocp.2019.11.011

Ribeiro, O., Borges-Machado, F., Lima, N., Farinatti, P. and Carvalho, J. (2019) Effectiveness of multicomponent exercise interventions in dementia patients: a systematic review. *Innovations in Aging* 3(Suppl. 1), S909.

Sampaio, A., Marques-Aleixo, I., Seabra, A., Mota, J., Marques, E. and Carvalho, J. (2020) Physical fitness in institutionalized older adults with dementia: association with cognition, functional capacity and quality of life. *Aging Clinical and Experimental Research* 32, 2329–2338. https://doi.org/10.1007/s40520-019-01445-7

Schmitt, A., Upadhyay, N., Martin, J.A., Rojas, S., Strüder, H.K. and Boecker, H. (2019) Modulation of distinct intrinsic resting state brain networks by acute exercise bouts of differing intensity. *Brain Plasticity* 5(1), 39–55. https://doi.org/10.3233/BPL-190081

Segaert, K., Lucas, S.J.E., Burley, C.V., Segaert, P., Milner, A.E., *et al.* (2018) Higher physical fitness levels are associated with less language decline in healthy ageing. *Science Reports* 8, 6715. https://doi.org/10.1038/s41598-018-24972-1

Sokolowski, D.R., Hansen, T.I., Rise, H.H., Reitlo, L.S., Wisløff, U., *et al.* (2021) 5 years of exercise intervention did not benefit cognition compared to the physical activity guidelines in older adults, but higher cardiorespiratory fitness did. A Generation 100 substudy. *Frontiers in Aging Neuroscience* 13, 742587. https://doi.org/10.3389/fnagi.2021.742587

Stern, Y., MacKay-Brandt, A., Lee, S., McKinley, P., McIntyre, K., *et al.* (2019) Effect of aerobic exercise on cognition in younger adults: a randomized clinical trial. *Neurology* 92(9), e905–e916. https://doi.org/10.1212/WNL.0000000000007003

Steves, C.J., Mehta, M.M., Jackson, S.H.D. and Spector, T.D. (2016) Kicking back cognitive ageing: leg power predicts ageing after ten years in older female twins. *Gerontology* 62(2), 138–149.

Thomas, A.G., Dennis, A., Bandettini, P.A. and Johansen-Berg, H. (2012) The effects of aerobic activity on brain structure. *Frontiers in Psychology* 3, 86.

Thomas, B.P., Tarumi, T., Sheng, M., Tseng, B., Womack, K.B., *et al.* (2020) Brain perfusion change in patients with mild cognitive impairment after 12 months of aerobic exercise training. *Journal of Alzheimer's Disease* 75(2), 617–631. https://doi.org/10.3233/JAD-190977

Thomasy, H. (2021) Piecing it together. *New Scientist* 6 November, 46–50.

van Dongen, E.V., Kersten, I.H.P., Wagner, I.C., Morris, R.G.M. and Fernández, G. (2016) Physical exercise performed four hours after learning improves memory retention and increases hippocampal pattern similarity during retrieval. *Current Biology* 26(13), 1722–1727. https://doi.org/10.1016/j.cub.2016.04.071

Watt, J.A., Goodarzi, Z., Veroniki, A.A., Nincic, V., Khan, P.A., *et al.* (2021) Comparative efficacy of interventions for reducing symptoms of depression in people with dementia: systematic review and network meta-analysis. *BMJ* 372, n532. https://doi.org/10.1136/bmj.n532

Wittenberg, R., Hu, B., Barraza-Araiza, L. and Rehill, A. (2019) *Projections of Older People with Dementia and Costs of Dementia Care in the United Kingdom, 2019–2040*. CPEC Working Paper No. 5. Care Policy and Evaluation Centre, London School of Economics and Political Science, London.

World Health Organization (2019) Motion for your mind: physical activity for mental health promotion, protection and care. Available at: https://apps.who.int/iris/handle/10665/346405#:~:text=World%20Health%20Organization.%20Regional%20Office%20for%20Europe.%20%28%E2%80%8E2019%29%E2%80%8E.,activity%20for%20mental%20health%20promotion%2C%20protection%20and%20care (accessed 30 January 2023).

Yoon, M., Yang, P.-S., Jin, M.-N., Yu, H.T., Kim, T.-H., *et al.* (2021) Association of physical activity level with risk of dementia in a nationwide cohort in Korea. *JAMA Network Open* 4(12), e2138526. https://doi.org/10.1001/jamanetworkopen.2021.38526

Yu, F., Salisbury, D. and Mathiason, M.A. (2021) Inter-individual differences in responses to aerobic exercise in Alzheimer's disease: findings from the FIT-AD trial. *Journal of Sport and Health Science* 10, 65–72.

Zheng, G., Xia, R., Zhou, W., Tao, J. and Chen, L. (2016) Aerobic exercise ameliorates cognitive function in older adults with mild cognitive impairment: a systematic review and meta-analysis of randomised controlled trials. *British Journal of Sports Medicine* 50, 1443–1450.

21 Lung Disease

Lung disease encompasses a large collection of widely varying chest conditions. The commonest include chronic obstructive pulmonary disease (COPD – previously referred to as chronic bronchitis and/or emphysema), asthma and pulmonary fibrosis. They share the feature of causing more than usual breathlessness at levels of exertion that would normally be tolerated well.

COPD is caused by a combination of progressive narrowing of the airways and loss of a proportion of the air sacs that make up the bulk of lung tissue. The main causes are cigarette smoking, asthma over many years and exposure to air pollution. There are more than a million people with COPD in the UK and each year there are about 30,000 deaths.

About 12% of the population has been diagnosed with asthma. It is more common in children and young adults, but it may continue into old age by when it has often morphed into COPD. There are about 1200 deaths from asthma annually in the UK.

Pulmonary fibrosis is caused by progressive increases in fibrous (scarring) tissue in the lungs, interfering with the ability of the lungs to absorb the oxygen upon which life depends. It is a condition of later life; there are several different forms, and the cause is often unknown. There are about 35,000 sufferers in the UK with an annual death toll of about 5000.

Exercise and Lung Disease

There is no lung disease that is caused by or aggravated by lack of exercise (except when this has resulted in obesity). However, any loss of lung function has effects which can be improved by being active and physically fit. When lung function is impaired, the supply of oxygen from the lungs to the blood is compromised. As explained in Chapter 4 (this volume), lung function is not normally a limiting factor in exercise tolerance. The oxygen saturation of arterial blood is still high at maximal exercise. This is not true of exercise for patients with lung disease. As they increase the intensity or duration of exercise, the oxygen saturation of their blood falls progressively until breathlessness prevents further effort.

Exercise in the Management of Lung Disease

Patients with chronic lung disease inevitably have low levels of physical fitness. This is a consequence of their limited exercise tolerance and their inability over a long period of time to take sufficient exercise. Pulmonary rehabilitation (PR) has developed over the past 20 years or so. It aims to reverse this loss of fitness by providing a programme of graduated exercise within the limits of the patient's breathlessness. It works by increasing 'peripheral' fitness – more efficient blood flow to the working muscles and more efficient muscular performance. These changes allow better physical functioning despite the limited rate of oxygen provision.

PR has been shown to improve symptoms, provide greater exercise tolerance and lengthen life for COPD patients (Rochester and Holland, 2020). A Cochrane systematic review of PR included 64 RCTs with 3822 participants. The conclusions were that:

> pulmonary rehabilitation relieves dyspnoea [breathlessness] and fatigue, improves emotional function and enhances the sense of control that individuals have over their condition. These improvements are moderately large and clinically significant. Rehabilitation serves as an important component of the management of COPD and is beneficial in improving health related quality of life and exercise capacity.
>
> (McCarthy *et al.*, 2015)

The report found that hospital-based programmes were more effective than community programmes, but that the complexity of the intervention made no difference – it was just the exercise that resulted

© H.J.N. Bethell and D. Brodie 2023. *Exercise: A Scientific and Clinical Overview* (H.J.N. Bethell and D. Brodie)
DOI: 10.1079/9781800621855.0021

in the successful outcome. PR works better if it is started as soon as possible after the episode of the lung problem that initiated it. Among 2700 COPD patients who started their PR programme within 30 days of an episode, the mortality at 1 year was 7.3% compared with 19.6% who started later or not at all (Rochester and Holland, 2020). One study with stable COPD patients found that different training programmes could bring benefits to such patients in both exercise endurance and quality of life. Interestingly, strength training brought about more lasting improvements in symptoms (Cui et al., 2020). Another systematic analysis found that exercise training in adults with asthma reduced the risk of CVD mortality by 9% (Valkenborghs et al., 2021). A comprehensive study was undertaken to compare the mortality of US adults who undertook the recommended amount of physical activity with those who were insufficiently active. Those with chronic lower respiratory tract disease had a hazard ratio (HR) of only 0.3 when both aerobic exercise and muscle strengthening were involved (Zhao et al., 2020), indicating superior survival benefits. For patients who were hospitalized for COPD and started a PR programme, a significantly lower risk of mortality was observed after 1 year (Lindenauer et al., 2020).

A worrying respiratory condition for many is obstructive sleep apnoea. Promoting physical activity can prevent this condition (Liu et al., 2021), especially if it is combined with reducing the number of sedentary hours.

Patients with lung disease benefit from exercise but PR programmes are underfunded, under-resourced and under-provided both in the UK and the USA. Also, NICE recommends PR for patients with COPD but not routinely for asthma or other lung diseases (Bolton et al., 2013). Fortunately, pulmonary patients can gain the considerable benefits of exercise from any source.

This appears to apply equally to children, although most studies have been small in the number of participants. Lu and Forno (2020) report that 'assessing physical activity, fitness levels, sedentary time, and nutritional status is important in the management of children with asthma as they are all modifiable factors.'

A questionnaire study of asthmatic patients found a correlation between control of symptoms and exercise frequency and intensity. It showed an improvement from low-to-medium to high exercise loads but decreasing slightly for very-high exercise loads (Jaakkola et al., 2020). Both aerobic and muscle-strengthening exercises are effective (Nici et al., 2005).

Regular exercise does not reduce the risk of catching respiratory infections, but it does reduce the severity and duration of the resulting symptoms. Finally, regular exercise does protect against premature death from these conditions (Geidl et al., 2020).

An excellent source of information on activity, exercise and pulmonary rehabilitation can be found in the British Lung Foundation (2022) publication.

Summary

Lung disease includes chronic obstructive pulmonary disease, asthma and pulmonary fibrosis. Lack of exercise does not cause these conditions, but the effects of any loss of lung function can be improved by being active and physically fit.

Pulmonary rehabilitation can provide graduated exercise within the limits of a person's breathlessness. Exercise-based pulmonary rehabilitation will improve symptoms, resulting in better survival and a lower mortality.

References

Bolton, C.E., Bevan-Smith, E.F., Blakey, J.D., Crowe, P., Elkin, S.L., et al.; British Thoracic Society Pulmonary Rehabilitation Guideline Development Group; British Thoracic Society Standards of Care Committee (2013) British Thoracic Society guideline on pulmonary rehabilitation in adults: accredited by NICE. Thorax 68(Suppl. 2), ii1–ii30. https://doi.org/10.1136/thoraxjnl-2013-203808

British Lung Foundation (2022) Your exercise handbook: For people living with a lung condition. Available at: https://www.blf.org.uk/sites/default/files/EH1_Exercise%20Handbook_v5_onlinePDF.pdf (accessed 30 January 2023).

Cui, S., Zhu, H., Li, X., Zhou, Y., Jiang, W., et al. (2020) Study of different physical training programs for stable COPD patients. *American Journal for Respiratory and Critical Care Medicine* 201, A2209.

Geidl, W., Schlesinger, S., Mino, E., Miranda, L. and Pfeifer, K. (2020) Dose–response relationship between physical activity and mortality in adults with noncommunicable diseases: a systematic review and meta-analysis of prospective observational studies. *International Journal of Behavioral Nutrition and Physical Activity* 17, 109. https://doi.org/10.1186/s12966-020-01007-5

Jaakkola, M.S., Aalto, S.A.M., Hyrkäs-Palmu, H. and Jaakkola, J.J.K. (2020) Association between regular exercise and asthma control among adults: the population-based Northern Finnish Asthma Study. *PLoS One* 15(1), e0227983.

Lindenauer, P.K., Stefan, M.S., Pekow, P.S., Mazor, K.M., Priya, A., et al. (2020) Association between initiation of pulmonary rehabilitation after hospitalization for COPD and 1-year survival among Medicare beneficiaries. *JAMA* 323(18), 1813–1823. https://doi.org/10.1001/jama.2020.4437

Liu, Y., Yang, L., Stampfer, M.J., Redline, S., Tworoger, S.S. and Huang, T. (2021) Physical activity, sedentary behaviour, and incidence of obstructive sleep apnoea in three prospective US cohorts. *European Respiratory Journal* 59(2), 2100606. https://doi.org/10.1183/13993003.00606-2021

Lu, K.D. and Forno, E. (2020), Exercise and lifestyle changes in pediatric asthma. *Current Opinion in Pulmonary Medicine* 26(1), 103–111.

McCarthy, B., Casey, D., Devane, D., Murphy, K., Murphy, E. and Lacasse, Y. (2015) Pulmonary rehabilitation for chronic obstructive pulmonary disease. *Cochrane Database of Systematic Reviews* (2), CD003793. https://doi.org/10.1002/14651858.CD003793.pub3

Nici, L., Donner, C., Wouters, E., Zuwallack, R., Ambrosino, N., et al. (2005) American Thoracic Society/European Respiratory Society statement on pulmonary rehabilitation. *American Journal of Respiratory and Critical Care Medicine* 173(12), 1393–1413. https://doi.org/10.1164/rccm.200508-1211ST

Rochester, C.L. and Holland, A.E. (2020) Pulmonary rehabilitation and improved survival for patients with COPD. *JAMA* 323(18), 1783–1785. https://doi.org/10.1001/jama.2020.4436

Valkenborghs, S., Anderson, S., Scott, H. and Callister, R. (2021) The characteristics and effects of exercise interventions on improving physical fitness in adults with asthma: a systematic review and meta-analysis. *Journal of Science and Medicine in Sport* 24(Suppl. 1), S71. https://doi.org/10.1016/j.jsams.2021.09.175

Zhao, M., Veeranki, S.P., Magnussen, C.G. and Xi, B. (2020) Recommended physical activity and all cause and cause specific mortality in US adults: prospective cohort study. *BMJ* 370, m2031.

22 Cancer

Cancers form a very large group of conditions that are extremely common causes of disease, disability, suffering and death. Nearly 40% of people will be diagnosed with one or another type of cancer in their lifetime and cancer causes nearly 30% of all deaths in the UK. Cancers are also very disparate, varying from minor skin excrescences to devastatingly fast-spreading and fatal malignancies. The place of exercise in the prevention and management of such a wide spread of conditions is likewise very variable.

Exercise in the Prevention of Cancer

It has been known for many years that some cancers are more common in physically inactive people (World Cancer Research Fund/American Institute for Cancer Research, 2007) and that the risk can be reduced by following the standard recommendation of about 30–60 minutes of MVPA per day. Cancers involved include colon, breast, uterus, gullet, gall bladder, pancreas and kidney. Physically active men and women have about a 30–40% reduction in the risk of developing colon cancer compared with inactive persons and there is a dose-response relationship, with the risk declining further at higher levels of physical activity. With breast cancer, physically active women have about a 20–30% reduction in risk compared with inactive women (Lee, 2003). A more recent study (Lee, 2020) reviewed 30 previous studies. The author concludes that the benefits of exercise to physical functioning and quality of life are well established for cancer patients and survivors. The often recommended 30–60 minutes of MVPA daily is also the exercise dose needed to decrease the risk of breast cancer. It is likely that there is a dose-response relationship.

Scientists at Harvard Medical School looked at 136,000 health records and concluded that all cases of cancer would fall by 20–40% and deaths would drop by a half if everyone adopted a healthy lifestyle (Song and Giovannucci, 2016). This goes beyond just exercise and includes giving up smoking, losing weight and consuming low levels of alcohol. Unfortunately few people follow all the lifestyle advice, but if they did, deaths from lung cancer would drop by 80%, bowel cancer by up to 30%, prostate cancer by 21% and breast cancer by 12%. The American Cancer Society engaged in a study that looked at the benefits of moderate exercise for 2½ hours per week (Matthews et al., 2020). The risk of liver cancer dropped by 18% and breast cancer by 6%. If the amount of exercise per week is doubled, then the benefits are even greater. These benefits are also seen in cancer cases later in life, when the subjects exercised as teenagers. Researchers from Vanderbilt University in the USA showed that regular exercise in the teens can result in a 16% reduction in cancer cases when aged 40–70 (Nechuta et al., 2015).

Endometrial (the lining of the womb) cancer is also less common in physically active women by a factor of about 20% (Voskuil et al., 2007; Parkin, 2011). A large meta-analysis of 1.44 million individuals found that regular physical activity reduced the risk of 13 different cancers – by 10% for breast cancer and up to 42% for the cancer of the gullet (Moore et al., 2016). Other cancers that were reduced by physical activity included liver, lung, kidney, stomach, womb, bone marrow (i.e. leukaemia), colon, rectum and bladder. The World Cancer Research Fund in 2009 estimated that 12% of colon cancers, 12% of breast cancers and 30% of endometrial cancers in the UK are related to inadequate physical activity (World Cancer Research Fund, 2010). Physical activity was the subject of a review by the Spanish Society of Medical Oncology (Pollán et al., 2020). It was concluded that regular physical activity is associated with major benefits to human health, including a reduced risk of some cancers.

© H.J.N. Bethell and D. Brodie 2023. *Exercise: A Scientific and Clinical Overview*
(H.J.N. Bethell and D. Brodie)
DOI: 10.1079/9781800621855.0022

A team from the University of Manchester in the UK reviewed 91,217 white postmenopausal women in the UK Biobank, an ongoing longitudinal study of the contribution of genetic, environmental and lifestyle risk factors in disease. There were 2728 women who developed breast cancer at a median follow-up of 10 years. The data showed an association between breast cancer and a BMI of 25 kg/m² or higher, *no regular physical activity*, alcohol intake at least three times per week and use of hormone replacement therapy for 5 years or more. The researchers conclude 'a healthier lifestyle ... appeared to be associated with a reduced level of risk for breast cancer, even if the women were at higher genetic risk' (Al Ajmi *et al.*, 2020). The combination of exercise and a healthy weight certainly seems to be highly desirable in women to avoid breast cancer. Dr La Vecchia of the International Agency for Research in Cancer claims that 25–30% of breast cancer cases could be avoided if women were thinner and exercised more (OregonLive, 2010). Exactly the same conclusions applied to Iranian women. Low levels of physical activity and being overweight or obese are major risk factors for breast cancer (Maleki *et al.*, 2020). Higher levels of physical activity in 65,000 premenopausal women in the USA were shown to reduce the prospect of developing breast cancer before the age of 50 (Maruit *et al.*, 2008). It is thought that the exercise lowers the levels of oestrogen, a hormone known to increase cancer risk.

As might be expected, there is also a relationship between CRF and cancer risk. A low level of CRF has been found to increase cancer risk by up to 50%. It has an even greater effect on cancer mortality (Vainshelboim *et al.*, 2019), reducing survival time free from cancer by as much as 7 years (Sui *et al.*, 2010). A smaller study of just 565 men showed that CRF was independently associated with lower risk of cancer mortality, although it was not associated with cancer incidence. Improving CRF through supervised exercise rehabilitation programmes could potentially serve as a cost-effective public-health strategy for secondary prevention and survivorship in men (Vainshelboim *et al.*, 2020).

Regular walking seems to lower the risk of prostate cancer. Men who walked for around 3 to 6 hours per week were two-thirds less likely to be diagnosed with prostate cancer compared with those who did nothing. The aggressive form of fast-growing cancer seems to be particularly affected, with an 86% less likely incidence. The reason for this is uncertain, but exercise may lower the blood levels of testosterone and other hormones linked to the growth of prostate tumours (Worthington, 2020).

Too much sedentary behaviour also plays a part in increasing cancer risk. A report in the *International Journal of Clinical Practice* claims that men who are more active at work, instead of just sitting at a desk, have lower rates of prostate cancer (Alford, 2010).

Mortality from cancer has also been linked to physical activity. A 17-year follow-up study of 480,000 adults related exercise with the risk of dying from cancer. It found the risk to be reduced by 30% for aerobic exercise, 22% for muscle strengthening and an amazing 50% for the two combined (Zhao *et al.*, 2020). A prospective cohort study by Li *et al.* (2020) observed that a healthier lifestyle was associated with a lower risk of cancer, CVD and diabetes as well as mortality. The study found an increased total life expectancy and number of years lived free of these diseases. A healthy lifestyle will therefore reduce the healthcare burdens through lowering the risk of developing multiple chronic diseases.

It is not exactly clear why exercise prevents some cancers, but there are several possibilities. These include reduction of inflammation, a potent cause of a number of conditions, and improved immune function with higher levels of natural antioxidants.

Closely related to lack of exercise, excess weight and obesity are among the commonest contributory causes of cancer. These include gullet, multiple myeloma, stomach, colon, rectum, biliary system, pancreas, breast, uterus, ovary and kidney (Kyrgiou *et al.*, 2017). Exercise clearly has a preventive role in this regard. In 2013, an estimated 4.5 million deaths worldwide were caused by overweight and obesity. On the basis of recent estimates, the obesity-related contribution to cancer represents up to 9% of the cancer burden among women in North America, Europe and the Middle East (Lauby-Secretan *et al.*, 2016). Body fatness and weight gain throughout the life course are largely determined by behaviour, including physical inactivity. Avoidance of weight gain has been shown to reduce the risk of cancers of the colon, gullet, kidney, breast and womb.

Weight loss is even more effective. An analysis of 180,000 women followed up for 10 years found that those who lost between 2 and 4.5 kg lowered their risk of developing breast cancer by 13%, while those who lost more than 9 kg lowered the risk by 26% (Teras *et al.*, 2020).

The best current estimate is that around 1% of all cancers in the UK may be related to physical inactivity. Physical inactivity is defined in this case as below a modest aspiration of 30 minutes, five times per week, meaning that around 3400 cases of cancer every year are linked to people doing less physical activity than outlined in government guidelines.

Exercise in the Treatment of Cancer

Prehabilitation

Prehabilitation is the use of healthy lifestyle changes before embarking on treatment – in this case before surgery, chemotherapy, radiotherapy or all three. An exercise programme can improve the patient's general health, physical fitness and ability to withstand the rigours of the treatment regime. In the case of surgery for lung cancer, for instance, physical and pulmonary function can be substantially improved with a pre-surgery exercise programme, reducing the complications of the operation and the recovery period (Himbert et al., 2020). Recovery is faster and more complete.

One study examined the impact of a home-based exercise prehabilitation programme. The outcome was a 40% increase in physical activity and significant reductions in self-reported measures of distress, anxiety, depression and anger. Health outcomes overall were equivalent to a clinic-based prehabilitation programme (Zaninotto et al., 2021). An Australian review (Edbrooke et al., 2020) found that increasing evidence supports the use of exercise prior to treatment to improve outcomes following surgery. This was supported by a paper in Exercise Oncology (Stout et al., 2020). They suggest that prehabilitation positively impacts on important disease-specific end points, such as adherence to cancer therapeutic modalities, and positively influences surgical and functional outcomes. A further systematic review by Ligibel et al. (2022) has recommended that oncology providers should recommend aerobic and resistance exercises during active treatment and also recommend pre-operative exercise for patients undergoing lung cancer surgery.

A major systematic review and meta-analysis demonstrated a significant association between superior pre-operative cardiorespiratory exercise test values, especially a high peak VO_2, and better post-operative outcomes. The assessment of pre-operative functional capacity in patients undergoing cancer surgery has the potential to facilitate improved treatment decision making (Steffens et al., 2021).

Such is the strong evidence for the benefits of prehabilitation exercise that the NHS in the UK is offering so-called 'bootcamps' to prepare patients physically and mentally for treatment. Simon Stevens, the former NHS chief executive, states 'it's really worth trying to get match fit ahead of chemo or major surgery. In effect you are "priming" your own recovery before your treatment even begins.'

Rehabilitation

When it comes to the treatment of cancers, exercise is attracting increasing attention. Evidence is emerging to show that regular exercise can reduce recurrence of treated cancers after medical and surgical treatment. It has also been shown to prolong life. In one study of breast cancer, exercise treatment was associated with double the rate of survival over 8 years and two-thirds the chance of recurrence (Hayes et al., 2017), and this was confirmed by Geidl et al. (2020). They found that higher levels of post-diagnosis physical activity are associated with lower mortality rates in breast cancer, with an indication of a no-threshold and non-linear dose-response pattern.

Patients recovering from cancer and its management have to deal not only with the effects of the disease itself but also with the toxic effects of treatment, which can include pain, nausea, vomiting, fatigue, anorexia, anxiety and depression. Reduction in physical capacity, muscle strength and quality of life are very common aftermaths. Chemotherapy and its side effects may affect the physical and functional capacity of patients negatively. The decrease in aerobic capacity affects muscle strength, endurance, body awareness and the quality of life. The practice of aerobic exercise programmes during the treatment of breast cancer is important for reducing the side effects, for physiological health and for physical functions. It should also prevent weight gain, and maintain muscle strength (Kocamaz and Düger, 2019). Cancer-related fatigue is a common symptom and a review by Olimat et al. (2021) indicated that exercise such as aerobic exercises, tai chi exercises and yoga can play an important role in decreasing this symptom and enhancing physical fitness.

A systematic review of the effects of exercise in breast-cancer patients found significant improvements in quality of life, CRF, physical functioning and fatigue (McNeely *et al.*, 2006). A meta-analysis of trials of exercise treatment in a wide variety of cancer types concluded that such treatment led to improvements in quality of life and fitness both during and after treatment. The main benefit found in the case of the active treatment was from moderate-intensity exercise. After treatment, benefits had been derived from all forms of exercise. These include running, brisk walking, cycling, weightlifting, and bodyweight or elastic-band exercises, all of which can produce similar benefits. So far, studies have not been designed to determine more exact exercise programmes for specific cancer types, nor the long-term effects of exercise. Segal *et al.* (2017) state that 'sufficient evidence is available to promote exercise for adults with cancer, and some evidence is available to promote exercise in a group or supervised setting and for a long period of time to improve QoL (quality of life) and muscular and aerobic fitness.'

A meta-analysis of patients with prostate cancer concluded that exercise was effective in improving metabolic health, with aerobic exercise as the superior modality. The effect of exercise on quality of life was small and was not affected by any particular exercise strategy (Andersen *et al.*, 2022). A study on men who were under surveillance with localized prostate cancer showed that high-intensity exercise resulted in increased CRF and a decrease in prostate-specific antigen (PSA) levels and prostate cancer cell growth (Kang *et al.*, 2021).

An examination of oesophageal cancer (May *et al.*, 2020) showed that patients were quite able to complete an intensive supervised exercise programme after treatment. This resulted in a small but significant improvement in several aspects of quality of life and CRF. Supervised exercise is a beneficial addition to routine care of patients with oesophageal cancer.

In the case of people with lung cancer, the previously mentioned Australian review (Edbrooke *et al.*, 2020), showed that exercise interventions are safe and effective. They improve physical fitness, muscle strength and patient-reported outcomes including cancer-related fatigue, dyspnoea and health-related quality of life.

A Cochrane Review reliably sums up the benefits of exercise programmes for patients with cancer. It concludes that exercise has beneficial effects at varying follow-up periods on health-related quality of life. There are improvements in physical functioning, role function, social functioning and fatigue. Positive effects of exercise interventions are more pronounced with moderate- or vigorous-intensity than with mild-intensity exercise programmes (Mishra, *et al.*, 2012). The mechanism by which exercise may benefit those with exercise is unclear but researchers have found a likely explanation of why exercise helps slow down cancer growth in mice (Rundqvist *et al.*, 2020). Physical activity changes the metabolism of the immune system's cytotoxic T cells and thereby improves their ability to attack cancer cells. It has yet to be shown if this mechanism applies to humans.

The benefits of exercise to support cancer patients are clear, and a structured rehabilitation programme has been designed under the heading 'Cancer Rehabilitation to Recreation' (Dennett *et al.*, 2020). This framework uses a tailored stepped approach to guide health services and clinicians on the design and implementation of interventions to promote physical activity among cancer survivors. A similar model has been proposed by Suderman *et al.* (2019).

Summary

Cancers comprise a very diverse range of different malignancies with an equally diverse range of fatality rates. Regular exercise reduces the risk of cancers of the colon, breast, uterus, gullet, gall bladder, pancreas and kidney by between 10 and 40%.

Exercise also improves the prognosis of extant cancers. Regular exercise has been found to reduce cancer mortality by 30% for aerobic exercise, by 22% for muscle strengthening and by 50% for the two combined.

References

Al Ajmi, K., Lophatanon, A., Mekli, K., Ollier, W. and Muir, K.R. (2020) Association of nongenetic factors with breast cancer risk in genetically predisposed groups of women in the UK Biobank cohort. *JAMA Network Open* 3(4), e203760. https://doi.org/10.1001/jamanetworkopen.2020.3760

Alford, L. (2010) What men should know about the impact of physical activity on their health. *International Journal of Clinical Practice* 64, 1731–1734. https://doi.org/10.1111/j.1742-1241.2010.02478.x

Andersen, M.F., Midtgaard, J. and Bjerra, E.D. (2022) Do patients with prostate cancer benefit from exercise interventions? A systematic review and meta-analysis. *International Journal of Environmental Research and Public Health* 19(2), 972. https://doi.org/10.3390/ijerph19020972

Dennett, A.M., Peiris, C.L., Shields, N. and Taylor, N.F. (2020) From cancer rehabilitation to recreation: a coordinated approach to increasing physical activity. *Physical Therapy* 100(11), 2049–2059. https://doi.org/10.1093/ptj/pzaa135

Edbrooke, L., Granger, C.L. and Denehy, L. (2020) Physical activity for people with lung cancer. *Australian Journal of General Practitioners* 49(4), 175–181.

Geidl, W., Schlesinger, S., Mino, E., Miranda, L. and Pfeife, K. (2020) Dose–response relationship between physical activity and mortality in adults with non communicable diseases: a systematic review and meta-analysis of prospective observational studies. *International Journal of Behavioral Nutrition and Physical Activity* 17, 109. https://doi.org/10.1186/s12966-020-01007-5

Hayes, S.C., Steele, M., Spence, R., Pyke, C., Saunders, C., *et al.* (2017) Can exercise influence survival following breast cancer: results from a randomised, controlled trial. *Journal of Clinical Oncology* 35(15_suppl), 10067.

Himbert, C., Klossner, N., Coletta, A.M., Barnes, C.A., Wiskemann, J., *et al.* (2020) Exercise and lung cancer surgery: a systematic review of randomized-controlled trials. *Critical Reviews in Oncology/Hematology* 156, 103086. https://doi.org/10.1016/j.critrevonc.2020.103086

Kang, D.-W., Fairey, A.S., Boulé, N.G., Field, C.J., Wharton, S.A. and Courneya, K.S. (2021) Effects of exercise on cardiorespiratory fitness and biochemical progression in men with localized prostate cancer under active surveillance: the ERASE randomized clinical trial. *JAMA Oncology* 7(10), 1487–1495. https://doi.org/10.1001/jamaoncol.2021.3067

Kocamaz, D. and Düger, T. (2019) Breast cancer and exercise. In: Afroze, D., Rah, B., Ali, S., Shehjar, F., Dar, M.I., *et al.* (eds) *Breast Cancer Biology*. IntechOpen, London. https://doi.org/10.5772/intechopen.85077

Kyrgiou, M., Kalliala, I., Markozannes, G., Gunter, M.J., Paraskevaidis, E., *et al.* (2017) Adiposity and cancer at major anatomical sites: umbrella review of the literature. *BMJ* 356, j477.

Lauby-Secretan, B., Scoccianti, C., Loomis, D., Grosse, Y., Bianchini, F. and Straif, K. (2016) Body fatness and cancer – viewpoint of the IARC working group. *New England Journal of Medicine* 375, 794–798. https://doi.org/10.1056/NEJMsr1606602

Lee, I.-M. (2003) Physical activity and cancer prevention – data from epidemiologic studies. *Medicine and Science in Sports and Exercise* 35(11), 1823–1827. https://doi.org/10.1249/01.MSS.0000093620.27893.23

Lee, N. (2020) The benefits of exercise on cancer: a review. *Exercise Science* 29(1), 4–9. https://doi.org/10.15857/ksep.2020.29.1.4

Li, Y., Schoufour, J., Wang, D.D., Dhana, K., Pan, A., *et al.* (2020) Healthy lifestyle and life expectancy free of cancer, cardiovascular disease, and type 2 diabetes: prospective cohort study. *BMJ* 368, l6669. https://doi.org/10.1136/bmj.l6669

Ligibel, J.A., Bohike, K., May, A.M., Clinton, S.K., Demark-Wahnefried, W., *et al.* (2022) Exercise, diet, and weight management during cancer treatment: ASCO guideline. *Journal of Clinical Oncology* 40(22), 2491–2507. https://doi.org/10.1200/JCO.22.00687

Maleki, F., Fotouhi, A., Ghiasvand, R., Harirchi, I., Talebi, G., *et al.* (2020) Association of physical activity, body mass index and reproductive history with breast cancer by menopausal status in Iranian women. *Cancer Epidemiology* 67, 101738.

Maruit, S.S., Willett, W.C., Feskanich, D., Rosner, B. and Colditz, G.A. (2008) A prospective study of age-specific physical activity and premenopausal breast cancer. *Journal of the National Cancer Institute* 100, 728–737.

Matthews, C.E., Moore, S.C., Arem, H., Cook, M.B., Trabert, B., *et al.* (2020) Amount and intensity of leisure-time physical activity and lower cancer risk. *Journal of Clinical Oncology* 38(7), 686–697. https://doi.org/10.1200/JCO.19.02407

May, A.M., van Vulpen, J., Heinsh, A.E., Ruurda, J.P., Nieuwenhuijzen, G., *et al.* (2020) Randomized clinical trial on the effect of a supervised exercise program on quality of life, fatigue, and fitness following esophageal cancer treatment (PERFECT study). *Journal of Clinical Oncology* 8(15_suppl), 12055. https://doi.org/10.1200/JCO.2020.38.15_suppl.12055

McNeely, M.L., Campbell, K.L., Rowe, B.H., Klassen, T.P., Mackey, J.R. and Courneya, K.S. (2006) Effects of exercise on breast cancer patients and survivors: a systematic review and meta-analysis. *Canadian Medical Association Journal* 175, 34–41.

Mishra, S.I., Scherer, R.W., Snyder, C., Geigle, P.M., Berlanstein, D.R. and Topaloglu, O. (2012) Exercise interventions on health-related quality of life for people with cancer during active treatment. *Cochrane Database of Systematic Reviews* 2012(8), CD008465.

Moore, S.C., Lee, I.-M., Weiderpass, E., Campbell, P.T., Sampson, J.N., *et al.* (2016) Association of leisure-time physical activity with risk of 26 types of cancer in 1.44 million adults. *JAMA Internal Medicine* 176, 816–825.

Nechuta, S.J., Shu, X.O., Yang, G., Cai, H., Gao, Y.T., *et al.* (2015) Adolescent exercise in association with mortality from all causes, cardiovascular disease, and cancer among middle-aged and older Chinese women. *Cancer Epidemiology, Biomarkers & Prevention* 24(8), 1270–1276. https://doi.org/10.1158/1055-9965.EPI-15-0253

Olimat, F., Bashtawy, M.A., Alkhawaldeh, A., Al Omari, O., ALBashtawy, B., *et al.* (2021) Effectiveness of exercise to reduce cancer-related fatigue: a literature review. *EC Emergency Medicine and Critical Care* 5.5. Available at: https://www.researchgate.net/publication/351523685_Effectiveness_of_Exercise_to_Reduce_Cancer_Related_Fatigue_A_Literature_Review (accessed 21 January 2023).

OregonLive (2010) Exercising more, eating less would cut breast cancer cases by up to a third. Available at: https://www.oregonlive.com/health/2010/03/exercising_more_eating_less_wo.html (accessed 31 January 2023).

Parkin, D.M. (2011) Cancers attributable to inadequate physical exercise in the UK in 2010. *British Journal of Cancer* 105(Suppl. 2), S38–S41.

Pollán, M., Barrio-Casla, S., Alfaro, J., Esteban, C., Segui-Palmer, M.A., *et al.* (2020) Exercise and cancer: a position statement from the Spanish Society of Medical Oncology. *Clinical and Translational Oncology* 22, 1710–1729. https://doi.org/10.1007/s12094-020-02312-y

Rundqvist, H., Veliça, P., Barbieri, L., Gameiro, P.A., Bargiela, D., *et al.* (2020) Cytotoxic T-cells mediate exercise-induced reductions in tumor growth. *eLife* 9, e59996. https://doi.org/10.7554/eLife.59996

Segal, R., Zwaal, C., Green, E., Tomasone, J.R., Loblaw, A., *et al.* (2017) Exercise for people with cancer: a systematic review. *Current Oncology* 24, e290–315.

Song, M. and Giovannucci, E. (2016) Preventable incidence and mortality of carcinoma associated with lifestyle factors among white adults in the United States. *JAMA Oncology* 2(9), 1154–1161. https://doi.org/10.1001/jamaoncol.2016.0843

Steffens, D., Ismail, H., Denehy, L., Beckenkamp, P.R., Solomon, M., *et al.* (2021) Preoperative cardiopulmonary exercise test associated with postoperative outcomes in patients undergoing cancer surgery: a systematic review and meta-analyses. *Annals of Surgical Oncology* 28, 7120–7146. https://doi.org/10.1245/s10434-021-10251-3

Stout, N.L., Silver, J.K., Baima, J., Knowlton, S.E. and Hu, X. (2020) Prehabilitation: an emerging standard in exercise oncology. In: Schmitz, K. (ed.) *Exercise Oncology*. Springer, Cham, Switzerland, pp. 111–143.

Suderman, K., McIntyre, C., Sellar, C. and McNeely, M.L. (2019) Implementing cancer exercise rehabilitation:

an update on recommendations for clinical practice *Current Cancer Therapy Reviews* 15(2), 100–109.

Sui, X., Lee, D.C., Matthews, C.E., Adams, S.A., Hébert, J.R., *et al.* (2010) Influence of cardiorespiratory fitness on lung cancer mortality. *Medicine and Science in Sports and Exercise* 42(5), 872–878. https://doi.org/10.1249/MSS.0b013e3181c47b65

Teras, L.R., Patel, A.V., Wang, M., Yaun, S.-S., Anderson, K., *et al.* (2020) Sustained weight loss and risk of breast cancer in women 50 years and older: a pooled analysis of prospective data. *Journal of the National Cancer Institute* 112(9), 929–937. https://doi.org/10.1093/jnci/djz226

Vainshelboim, B., Lima, R.M. and Myers, J. (2019) Cardiorespiratory fitness and cancer in women: a prospective pilot study. *Journal of Sport and Health Science* 8(5), 457–462. https://doi.org/10.1016/j.jshs.2019.02.001

Vainshelboim, B., Chan, K., Chen, Z. and Myers, J. (2020) Cardiorespiratory fitness and cancer in men with cardiovascular disease: analysis from the Veterans Exercise Testing Study. *European Journal of Preventive Cardiology* 28(7), 715–721. https://doi.org/10.1177/2047487320916595

Voskuil, D.W., Monninkhof, E.M., Elias, S.G., Vlems, F.A. and van Leeuwen, F.E. (2007) Physical activity and endometrial cancer risk, a systematic review of current evidence. *Cancer Epidemiology, Biomarkers & Prevention* 16, 639–648.

World Cancer Research Fund/American Institute for Cancer Research (2007) *Food, Nutrition, Physical Activity, and the Prevention of Cancer: A Global Perspective*. AICR, Washington, DC.

World Cancer Research Fund (2010) *Annual Review, 2009–10*. World Cancer Research Fund, London.

Worthington, J.F. (2020) Exercise is the turbo boost to a healthy prostate. Available at: https://www.pcf.org/c/exercise-is-the-turbo-boost-to-a-healthy-prostate/#:~:text=The%20brisk%20pace%20is%20important,Walking%20is%20so%20common (accessed 21 January 2023).

Zaninotto, F., Wynter-Blyth, V., Hug, A., Halley, M., Long, L., *et al.* (2021) Feasibility of implementing a digital prehabilitation service for cancer patients in the NHS. *Annals of Oncology* 32(5), S1179. https://doi.org/10.1016/j.annonc.08.1655

Zhao, M., Veeranki, S.P., Magnussen, C.G. and Xi, B. (2020) Recommended physical activity and all cause and cause specific mortality in US adults: prospective cohort study. *BMJ* 370, m2031. https://doi.org/10.1136/bmj.m2031

23 Osteoporosis

Osteoporosis is the loss of calcium from bone with consequent fragility and increased risk of fracture. Bone strength starts to be lost from the age of about 35 and the loss continues throughout life. It becomes more rapid in women after the menopause. From middle age about 1% of bone mass is lost annually. Globally, 137 million women and 21 million men have osteoporosis, and this prevalence is expected to double over the next 40 years (Brooke-Wavell *et al.*, 2022). Some 3 million people in the UK have osteoporosis and they suffer more than 300,000 fragility fractures annually. These include such horrors as broken wrists and hips. This can lead to temporary or sometimes permanent dependency (see Chapter 25, this volume) and often to shortening of life. Ten per cent will die within a month and about 30% within a year. Hip fractures alone occupy 1.3 million hospital bed days and cost the English economy £1.7 billion annually (National Osteoporosis Guideline Group, 2021). Postmenopausal women are particularly susceptible, though men are not immune.

Bones are not inert struts to support the human carcass. They are living structures, which continually renew themselves to maintain their functional strength. Old bone is continuously being replaced by new. Weight bearing is needed to promote this process. Weightlessness, as in space flight, leads rapidly to loss of bone strength and to osteoporosis.

Exercise in the Prevention of Osteoporosis

There are a number of ways of measuring bone strength, the most frequently used being bone mineral density (BMD). Logic suggests that the best way to prevent osteoporosis is to use weight-bearing exercises, particularly 'impact' exercises like running or skipping. Population studies involving athletes confirm this and indicate that high-impact sports, such as running, squash and weightlifting, lead to an increase in BMD, whereas low-impact sports such as swimming do not (Warburton *et al.*, 2001).

It is important to start this process early in life. The more time spent on MVPA in adolescence, the greater is bone mass by the age of 25. This is the age at which bone mass peaks and a low BMD at this age is a marker of risk of osteoporosis later in life (Elhakeem *et al.*, 2020).

For the spine and lower limbs, weight-bearing exercise is ideal to prevent osteoporosis. However, the really important question is whether exercise reduces the risk of osteoporosis-related fractures. This particularly applies to the hip or vertebrae, fractures of which can be so devastating for the sufferer. No intervention study has assessed the effect of exercise on the rate of osteoporotic fracture. No one to date has carried out an RCT of exercise versus no exercise to show whether the exercised group has a lower long-term risk of fracture. Such a trial would be extremely difficult to perform. However, observational epidemiological studies have indicated a strong protective effect. A study of 3262 healthy men (mean age 44 years) followed for 21 years found that intense physical activity at the start of the study was associated with a reduced incidence of hip fracture. The risk was just 38% of the risk for the non-exercisers (Kujala *et al.*, 2000). Another study from the USA reported that women who had a high frequency of participation in outdoor sports had just 30% the chance of suffering a hip fracture compared with those with a low frequency of participation (Paganini-Hill *et al.*, 1991). As one reviewer wrote in studies from Britain and Hong Kong: 'physical inactivity is currently proffered as the most salient explanatory factor for the increasingly high hip fracture rates reported by developing countries, as well as many first-world countries' (Marks, 2010).

As has been seen elsewhere, physical fitness is the outcome of exercise training. A study by Moradell *et al.* (2020) showed that bone mass seems to be more influenced by physical fitness in elderly males than in females. The components of agility and walking speed were the variables showing greater associations.

A clever way of showing the effect of exercise on BMD is to examine the effects on different limbs. Squash players from Finland showed a 15.6% higher BMD at the proximal humerus (upper arm) of the racquet hand than in the inactive arm (Haapasalo *et al.*, 1994).

A Cochrane Review in 2011 presented evidence for the role of exercise in preventing osteoporosis and related fractures in postmenopausal women. They found a small but important reduction in osteoporosis from exercise programmes. The authors found that resistance strength training was most effective in protecting the hip and combination exercises were best for the spine. For the women studied, the overall fracture rate was 11 per 100 in those who did not exercise, compared to seven per 100 in those who did, a saving of four fractures for every 100 exercisers (Howe *et al.*, 2011).

Frailty (see Chapter 25, this volume) is one of the predictors examined in a further systematic review (Kojima, 2021). This showed evidence that frailty and prefrailty are significant predictors of fractures among community-dwelling older people. Treating frailty has the potential to lower the risk of a subsequent fracture.

One strategy to reduce the incidence of fractures has been to send additional exercise advice by mail (Lamb *et al.*, 2020). Disappointingly, those receiving the mail gained no benefit. The authors commented: 'researchers and clinicians subsequently need to rethink the cause of fractures in later life and find more effective treatments.' They emphasize that people should not stop exercising since there is much evidence that exercise reduces falls (see Chapter 25, this volume). Indeed, fewer fractures may be the result of falling less rather than having stronger bones. It is likely that both are true.

It is recognized that load-bearing activities are ideal to protect against osteoporosis, but which type and how much is uncertain. Just 5 minutes of hopping per day can protect middle-aged females from osteoporosis. Bone density was improved when a group of healthy women aged from 55 to 70 were asked to hop 50 times a day (Hartley *et al.*, 2020). Jumping has a similar effect. A group of early postmenopausal women jumped down from a 20 cm box as well as performing other 'jumping'

activities for 1 year (Montgomery *et al.*, 2020). The exercises produced a net gain of around 2% in BMD in a year. This was considered to be sufficient to reduce the incidence of osteoporosis. The mechanisms for such improvements are not fully understood, but an experiment in Italy provided some clues. Researchers, from the Istituto Ortopedico Galeazzi in Milan, examined the hormone levels of ultra-distance runners and observed that after a run they had higher levels of procollagen type I N-propeptide (PINP), which is a protein essential for bone formation (Sansoni *et al.*, 2017).

Exercise in the Treatment of Osteoporosis

A definitive assessment of the effectiveness of exercise in treating osteoporosis was published in 2012 (Gómez-Cabello *et al.*, 2012). After an analysis of 74 trials, the authors concluded that both aerobic exercise and weight training increase bone mass. At the very least exercise reduces the rate of bone loss in osteoporotic (mostly postmenopausal) women. They found that the lower the BMD, the more effective was the exercise as a form of treatment. They quote Zehnacker and Bemis-Dougherty (2007) by stating 'the best improvements seem to be achieved through strength training of high-loading intensities with three sessions per week and 2–3 sets per session' and go on to state that although significant effects can be observed after 4 or 6 months in some parts of the body, the efficacy of the training programme is greater when it extends for at least 1 year (Gómez-Cabello *et al.*, 2012).

Another meta-analysis has shown a small positive effect of exercise on BMD at the lumbar spine and femoral neck. Findings from subgroup analyses suggest larger benefits in multicomponent interventions that include weight-bearing and resistance-training exercises compared to using a single mode of exercise (Shojaa *et al.*, 2020).

In May 2022 the first UK consensus statement on exercise benefits in osteoporosis was published (Brooke-Wavell *et al.*, 2022). Key recommendations, endorsed by the Royal Osteoporosis Society, include progressive resistance training and impact exercise involving major muscle groups to maximize bone strength. Resistance training ideally uses resistance machines or weights but if this is unavailable then Pilates or yoga, stair climbing, sit-to-stands, heavy housework, gardening or DIY may be good muscle-strengthening alternatives.

Impact exercise may include running, jumping, aerobics, Zumba and many ball games. Strength and balance exercises to reduce fall risk include tai chi, Pilates and yoga. Spinal extension exercises can improve posture and potentially curb the risk of falls and vertebral fractures. Vertebral fracture symptoms may benefit from exercise to reduce pain as well as improve mobility and quality of life, ideally with specialist advice to encourage return to normal activities.

The statement also advises against postures involving a high degree of forward bending of the spine, such as toe touches or activities in daily life such as picking up heavy objects without bending at the knees and hips. It also advises exercises only up to an impact equivalent to brisk walking in people who have previous low-trauma fractures, vertebral fractures, or who are frail/elderly.

For people at risk of falls, it is recommended to start with targeted strength and balance training and breathing, and pelvic-floor exercises are advised to help ease symptoms that may be worsened by severe curvature of the spine (spinal kyphosis).

The National Osteoporosis Society has produced a 60-page booklet of exercise advice for osteoporosis prevention and treatment (National Osteoporosis Guideline Group, 2021).

Summary

Osteoporosis is the loss of calcium from bone and is often more rapid in postmenopausal women. Weight-bearing exercise such as running and skipping is valuable in preventing osteoporosis. To prevent the hip from fracture, resistance exercise was found to be most effective. Osteoporosis can also be treated with exercise, with weight-bearing and resistance exercises being the most effective.

References

Brooke-Wavell, K., Skelton, D.A., Barker, K.L., Clark, E.M., De Biase. S., *et al.* (2022) Strong, steady and straight: UK consensus statement on physical activity and exercise for osteoporosis. *British Journal of Sports Medicine* 56, 837–846. https://doi.org/10.1136/bjsports-2021-104634

Elhakeem, A., Heron, J., Tobias, J.H. and Lawlor, D.A. (2020) Physical activity throughout adolescence and peak hip strength in young adults. *JAMA Network Open* 3(8), e2013463. https://doi.org/10.1001/jamanetworkopen.2020.13463

Gómez-Cabello, A., Ara, I., González-Agüero, A., Casajús, J.A. and Vicente-Rodríguez, G. (2012) Effects of training on bone mass in older adults: a systematic review. *Sports Medicine* 42, 301–325.

Haapasalo, H., Kannus, P., Sievänen, H., Heinonen, A., Oja, P. and Vuori, I. (1994) Long-term unilateral loading and bone mineral density and content in female squash players. *Calcified Tissue International* 54, 249–255.

Hartley, C., Folland, J.P., Kerslake, R. and Brooke-Wavell, K. (2020) High-impact exercise increased femoral neck bone density with no adverse effects on imaging markers of knee osteoarthritis in postmenopausal women. *Journal of Bone Mineral Research* 35(1), 53–63. https://doi.org/10.1002/jbmr.3867

Howe, T.E., Shea, B., Dawson, L.J., Downie, F., Murray, A., *et al.* (2011) Exercise for preventing and treating osteoporosis in postmenopausal women. *Cochrane Database of Systematic Reviews* (7), CD000333.

Kojima, G. (2021) Frailty as a predictor of fractures among community-dwelling older people: a systematic review and meta-analysis. *Bone* 90, 116–122. https://doi.org/10.1016/j.bone.2016.06.009

Kujala, U.M., Kaprio, J., Kannus, P., Sarna, S. and Koskenvuo, M. (2000) Physical activity and osteoporotic hip fracture risk in men. *Archives of Internal Medicine* 160, 705–708.

Lamb, S.E., Bruce, J., Hossain, A., Ji, C., Longo, R., *et al.* (2020) Screening and intervention to prevent falls and fractures in older people. *New England Journal of Medicine* 383(19), 1848–1859. https://doi.org/10.1056/NEJMoa2001500

Marks, R. (2010) Hip fracture epidemiological trends, outcomes, and risk factors, 1970–2009. *International Journal of Medicine* 3, 1–17.

Montgomery, G.J., Abt, G., Dobson, C.A., Evans, W.J., Aye, M. and Ditroilo, M. (2020) A 12-month continuous and intermittent high-impact exercise intervention and its effects on bone mineral density in early postmenopausal women: a feasibility randomized controlled trial. *Journal of Sports Medicine and Physical Fitness* 60(5), 770–778. https://doi.org/10.23736/S0022-4707.20.10412-2

Moradell, A., Gómez-Cabello, A., Gómez-Bruton, A., Muniz-Pardos, B., Marín Puyalto, J., et al. (2020) Associations between physical fitness, bone mass, and structure in older people. *BioMed Research International* 2020, 6930682. https://doi.org/10.1155/2020/6930682

National Osteoporosis Guideline Group (2021) Clinical guideline for the prevention and treatment of osteoporosis. Available at: https://www.nogg.org.uk/sites/nogg/download/NOGG-Guideline-2021-g.pdf (accessed 30 January 2023).

Paganini-Hill, A., Chao, A., Ross, R.K. and Henderson, B.E. (1991) Exercise and other factors in the prevention of hip fracture: the Leisure World study. *Epidemiology* 2(1), 16–25.

Sansoni, V., Vernillo, G., Perego, S., Barbuti, A., Merati, G., et al. (2017) Bone turnover response is linked to both acute and established metabolic changes in ultra-marathon runners. *Endocrine* 56, 196–204. https://doi.org/10.1007/s12020-016-1012-8

Shojaa, M., Von Stengel, S., Schoene, D., Kohl, M., Barone, G., et al. (2020) Effect of different types of exercise on bone mineral density in post-menopausal women: a systematic review and meta-analysis. *Frontiers in Physiology* 11, 652. https://doi.org/10.3389/fphys.2020.00652

Warburton, D.E., Glendhill, N. and Quinney, A. (2001) The effects of changes in musculoskeletal fitness on health. *Canadian Journal of Applied Physiology* 26(2), 161–216. https://doi.org/10.1139/h01-012

Zehnacker, C.H. and Bemis-Dougherty, A. (2007) Effect of weighted exercises on bone mineral density in post menopausal women: a systematic review. *Journal of Geriatric Physical Therapy* 30(2), 79–88.

24 Other Conditions

Pregnancy

In Victorian times, riding a horse was considered a form of exercise to induce labour, but such drastic measures are no longer necessary. Exercise has, however, been shown to be beneficial during pregnancy for both the mother and the developing baby.

Research in the USA has suggested that older women who exercise while pregnant can halve the risk of their baby being born with congenital heart disease (Schulkey *et al.*, 2015). Exercising while pregnant also has an effect on time spent in labour. In an RCT that used 1-hour classes involving aerobic dance and pelvic-floor exercises, three times per week throughout pregnancy, Barakat *et al.* (2018) showed a decrease in the duration of the first phase of labour, the combined first and second stages, and of total labour time of as much as an hour.

A team from the Norwegian School of Sports Sciences concluded that regular light-to-moderate activity lowered the risk of needing a caesarean section. The Norwegian researchers also found that mothers-to-be who stayed active had a 31% lower risk of having an overweight baby than women who did no exercise (Sanda *et al.*, 2018). A major study led by Queen Mary University of London showed that babies are not adversely affected by physical activity or dieting (International Weight Management in Pregnancy (i-WIP) Collaborative Group, 2017). The study of 12,000 women showed that those who had a healthy diet and regular moderate exercise were less likely to have a caesarean section. The Royal College of Obstetricians and Gynaecologists advises that pregnant women undertake up to 30 minutes of aerobic exercise per day (RCOG, 2022). A more recent study (Baena-García *et al.*, 2020) has examined how physical fitness during pregnancy impacts on maternal and neonatal outcomes. The results confirmed earlier studies that increased physical fitness is associated with a decreased risk of a caesarean section.

A study at the University of Oslo found that children of women who did little exercise were twice as likely to have poor lung function (Gudmundsdóttir *et al.*, 2021). They tested the lung function of 3-month-old children from 600 mothers. They showed that exercising regularly during pregnancy helps newborn children develop better lung function. This may benefit the long-term prospect of suffering from asthma.

A systematic review of managing postpartum depression gave support to the notion that exercise can be beneficial (Pritchett *et al.*, 2017). The authors accepted that the results should be treated with caution, as there was a risk of bias and substantial heterogeneity. None the less, it appeared that group exercise, participant-chosen exercise and exercise with co-interventions could all be effective in reducing postpartum depressive symptoms.

Erectile Dysfunction

Erectile dysfunction can result from physiological and psychological aspects, and it is not always easy to differentiate the two. The penile artery is fairly narrow and any blockage, even minor, will impact on erection. The state of the penile artery may be an indication of the status of the overall cardiovascular system. A study by Hodges *et al.* (2007) demonstrated that the median time between evidence of erectile dysfunction and subsequent CVD was 5 years. The important message is that anyone suffering from erectile dysfunction should take all possible action, including exercise, to prevent further development of CVD (see Chapter 15, this volume).

Premenstrual and Menstrual Symptoms

Research suggests that aerobic exercise can help improve symptoms of premenstrual syndrome (PMS) such as depression and fatigue (Yesildere

DOI: 10.1079/9781800621855.0024

Saglam and Orsal, 2020). One study found that women who did 60-minute aerobic sessions three times weekly for 8 weeks felt much improved physically, mentally, and emotionally (Samadi *et al.*, 2013). Researchers have found that some women have fewer painful cramps during menstruation if they exercise regularly (Office on Women's Health, 2022).

The Cochrane database summarizes:

> The current low-quality evidence suggests that exercise, performed for about 45 to 60 minutes each time, three times per week or more, regardless of intensity, may provide a clinically significant reduction in menstrual pain intensity of around 25 mm on a 100 mm visual analogue scale (VAS).
>
> (Armour *et al.*, 2019)

All studies used exercise regularly throughout the month, with some studies asking women not to exercise during menstruation. Given the overall health benefits of exercise, and the relatively low risk of side effects reported in the general population, women may consider using exercise, either alone or in conjunction with other modalities, such as non-steroidal anti-inflammatory drugs (NSAIDs), to manage menstrual pain.

Menopause

Many women are left feeling tired and listless following the menopause. Hot flushes are also a common symptom, and it has been shown that regular exercise is highly beneficial (Moilanen *et al.*, 2012). Researchers from Liverpool John Moores University found that women who used the gym suffered fewer hot flushes than those with a more sedentary lifestyle. The flushes they did experience were also less severe. Moderate-intensity, supervised exercise was offered to postmenopausal women by Bailey *et al.* (2016). The results showed that exercise training led to a parallel reduction in the severity of hot flushes. Women with worse hot flushes and night sweats have been found to be at greater risk of heart problems and strokes (Huang *et al.*, 2018). This provides another justification for exercise in women who suffer from severe hot flushes. A team from the University of Copenhagen has argued that the menopause may be the ideal time to take up exercise (Olsen *et al.*, 2020). As oestrogen levels drop, the take-up of oxygen to the muscles may improve. This could lead to the ideal environment for exercise.

The amount of exercise to take to reduce menopausal symptoms is uncertain, although regular aerobic exercise is considered preferable to infrequent bursts of high-impact exercise. Researchers in Australia have found that even those women who do less than the recommended 30 minutes five times per week can experience benefits (Stojanovska *et al.*, 2014).

Joint Disease

It is generally believed that regular exercise, particularly running, is damaging to lower-limb joints. However, the opposite may be true. Regular physical activity may reduce the risk of developing painful osteoarthritis by improving cartilage resilience and increasing the strength of muscles that support the joints (Heesch *et al.*, 2007). Cycling and regular walking seem to reduce the need for hip-replacement surgery (Ageberg *et al.*, 2012). Activities like jogging which create impact for leg joints appear to be more protective than lower-impact activities (Hootman *et al.*, 2003).

A study at Southampton University, UK, found no link between the amount of exercise people do and the development of osteoarthritis in their knees (Gates *et al.*, 2022). The study combined 5000 people from six investigations and recorded the average time spent exercising. The analysis over 5 to 12 years showed that the chance of developing arthritis did not correlate with activity. High-impact activities are unwise for people suffering from arthritis, but low-impact exercises can strengthen knee joint muscles, thus reducing pain and slowing degeneration. Those with damaged knee joints who wish to continue running are well advised to switch to off-road running to reduce the impact.

Once osteoarthritis of the knees has developed, walking can both relieve pain and slow the rate of progression of joint damage (Lo *et al.*, 2022). NICE guidelines for the management of osteoarthritis have advised that muscle-strengthening and general aerobic exercise should replace the use of analgesics for this condition (NICE, 2022).

Prehabilitation has been considered with reference to cancer (see Chapter 22, this volume) and pregnancy (earlier in this chapter). In addition, it has been shown that exercise prior to many orthopaedic procedures, especially those of the lower limbs, is of value (Ditmyer *et al.*, 2002). The aim is to strengthen the quadriceps muscles and the muscles around the hip joint. This can prevent or delay the need for knee or hip replacement and certainly aid in recovery.

Driving for long distances can cause pain and stiffness and common sense would suggest that taking a regular break is beneficial. This was tested scientifically by researchers from Nottingham Trent, Imperial College and Loughborough universities (Varela *et al.*, 2016). Participants took part in a driving simulator for 2 hours with a 10-minute break after an hour. Those who exercised during this break prevented any feeling of discomfort for a further hour compared with those who remained seated.

Back pain was the topic of a study at the University of Sydney with over 30,000 people. Over a period of 6 months, it was found that patients with back pain who carried out a range of exercises reduced the risk of painful twinges by 35% (Ayre *et al.*, 2022).

Attention Deficit Hyperactivity Disorder

ADHD is a huge problem in most Westernized countries. In the UK, about 8% of children and 2% of adults are affected. The typical characteristics are inability to concentrate or apply oneself together with restlessness and impulsive behaviour. It is usually diagnosed in childhood but sometimes is first recognized in adult life. The usually recommended treatments are medication, counselling, CBT and educational support. Recently the place of exercise has been recognized. A systematic review of studies of exercise for ADHD involved 1723 sufferers (Villa-González *et al.*, 2020). Children with the condition undertaking exercise experienced improvements in their characteristic symptoms, mainly attention deficit and hyperactivity, in comparison to other sedentary tasks such as watching a video. Five minutes of jumping or 30 minutes on a treadmill or static bicycle were enough to produce appreciable improvements in inhibitory control or in cognitive and executive functions.

Inflammation

Inflammation is becoming an issue in medicine for a number of reasons and its association with exercise is now established. A full review of this topic can be found in Gleeson *et al.* (2011). A 2014 study by researchers from Loughborough and Leicester, UK, found that a brisk 30-minute walk five days a week led to a drop in inflammatory markers within 6 months (Viana *et al.*, 2014). This study did apply to kidney patients, but other studies have shown a similar effect on other people with higher levels of inflammation.

Inflammation is associated with oxidative stress and regular exercise can curb the oxidative stress which damages sperm. A study that examined sperm in exercising versus non-exercising groups (Maleki *et al.*, 2022) found that the exercisers increased their sperm volume by 8.3%, their cell motility by 12.4% and the quality of their cell shape by 17.1%.

Others

There are a number of other conditions worthy of mention with respect to exercise, although the extent of the research is far less.

Eyesight has been studied by a group from the universities of Iowa State and South Carolina in the USA (Meier *et al.*, 2018). This group looked at 9500 people and found that the most active had only half the risk of developing glaucoma compared with the least active group. Even creativity has been shown to improve following a brisk walk. A test of creativity called the Guilford Alternate Uses Test was used at Stanford University to compare those who had walked with those who had sat down for the test (Oppezzo and Schwartz, 2014). The walking group came up with 60% more ideas than the stationary group.

There has recently been considerable interest in vaccinations. Evidence from Sydney University concerning the flu vaccination indicates that the side effects after the jab are less for those who exercised beforehand (Edwards and Booy, 2013). It is not known yet whether this would translate to other forms of vaccination, but the prospect of an improved immune response cannot be dismissed.

Fertility, too, is affected by physical activity – greater levels of exercise reduce problems with conception among normal-weight women (Mena *et al.*, 2020).

The list of conditions that are helped by increasing levels of exercise seems inexhaustible: chronic kidney disease (Slomski, 2022), fatty liver (Hoene *et al.*, 2021), insomnia (Li *et al.*, 2021), chronic pain (Geneen *et al.*, 2017), fibromyalgia (Lazaridou *et al.*, 2020), polycystic ovary syndrome (Dos Santos *et al.*, 2020), migraine (Barber and Pace, 2020), schizophrenia (Firth *et al.*, 2015) and even psoriasis (Yeroushalmi *et al.*, 2022). Perhaps exercise is truly a panacea.

Summary

Some of the conditions whose outcomes are improved by regular exercise and high levels of physical fitness include pregnancy, the menopause, infertility, erectile dysfunction, osteoarthritis and ADHD. The common factor which mediates these effects in such a disparate group may be reduction in inflammation.

References

Ageberg, E., Engström, G., Gerhardsson de Verdier, M., Rollof, J., Roos, E.M. and Lohmander, L.S. (2012) Effect of leisure time physical activity on severe knee or hip osteoarthritis leading to total joint replacement: a population-based prospective cohort study. *BMC Musculoskeletal Disorders* 13, 73. https://doi.org/10.1186/1471-2474-13-73

Armour, M., Ee, C.C., Naidoo, D., Ayati, Z., Chalmers, K.J., *et al.* (2019) Exercise for dysmenorrhoea. *Cochrane Database of Systematic Reviews* 9(9), CD004142. https://doi.org/10.1002/14651858.CD004142.pub4

Ayre, J., Jenkins, H., McCaffery, K.J., Maher, C.G. and Hancock, M.J. (2022) Unique considerations for exercise programs to prevent future low back pain: the patient perspective. *Pain* 163(8), e953–e962. https://doi.org/10.1097/j.pain.0000000000002540

Baena-García, L., Coll-Risco, I., Ocón-Hernádez, O., Romero-Gallardo, L., Acosta-Manzano, P., *et al.* (2020) Association of objectively measured physical fitness during pregnancy with maternal and neonatal outcomes. The GESTAFIT Project. *PLoS One* 15(2), e0229079. https://doi.org/10.1371/journal.pone.0229079. Erratum in: *PLoS One* 15(4), e0231230. https://doi.org/10.1371/journal.pone.0231230

Bailey, T.G., Cable, N.T., Aziz, N., Atkinson, G., Cuthbertson, D.J., *et al.* (2016) Exercise training reduces the acute physiological severity of postmenopausal hot flushes *Journal of Physiology* 594(3), 657–667.

Barakat, R., Franco, E., Perales, M., López, C. and Mottola, M.F. (2018) Exercise during pregnancy is associated with a shorter duration of labor. A randomized clinical trial. *European Journal of Obstetrics & Gynecology and Reproductive Biology* 224, 33–40.

Barber, M. and Pace, A. (2020) Exercise and migraine prevention: a review of the literature. *Current Pain and Headache Reports* 24(8), 39. https://doi.org/10.1007/s11916-020-00868-6

Ditmyer, M.M., Topp, R. and Pifer, M. (2002) Prehabilitation in preparation for orthopaedic surgery. *Orthopaedic Nursing* 21(5), 43–51. https://doi.org/10.1097/00006416-200209000-00008

Dos Santos, I.K., Ashe, M.C., Cobucci, R.N., Soares, G.M., de Oliveira Maranhão, T.M. and Dantas, P.M.S. (2020) The effect of exercise as an intervention for women with polycystic ovary syndrome: a systematic review and meta-analysis. *Medicine* 99(16), e19644. https://doi.org/10.1097/MD.0000000000019644

Edwards, K.M. and Booy, R. (2013) Effects of exercise on vaccine-induced immune responses. *Human Vaccines & Immunotherapeutics* 9(4), 907–910. https://doi.org/10.4161/hv.23365

Firth, J., Cotter, J., Elliott, R., French, P. and Yung, A.R. (2015) A systematic review and meta-analysis of exercise interventions in schizophrenia patients. *Psychological Medicine* 45(7), 1343–1361. https://doi.org/10.1017/S0033291714003110

Gates, L.S., Perry, T.A., Golightly, Y.M., Nelson, A.E., Callahan, L.F., *et al.* (2022) Recreational physical activity and risk of incident knee osteoarthritis: an international meta-analysis of individual participant-level data. *Arthritis & Rheumatology* 74(4), 612–622. https://doi.org/10.1002/art.42001

Geneen, L.J., Moore, R.A., Clark, C., Martin D., Colvin, L.A. and Smith, B.H. (2017) Physical activity and exercise for chronic pain in adults: an overview of Cochrane Reviews. *Cochrane Database of Systematic Reviews* 1(1), CD011279. https://doi.org/10.1002/14651858.CD011279.pub3

Gleeson, M., Bishop, N.C., Stensel, D.J., Lindley, M.R., Mastana, S.S. and Nimmo, M.A. (2011) The anti-inflammatory effects of exercise: mechanisms and implications for the prevention and treatment of disease. *Nature Reviews Immunology* 11(9), 607–615.

Gudmundsdóttir, H.F., Carlsen, O.C.L., Bains, K.E.S., Färdig, M., Carlsen, K.-H., *et al.* (2021) Infant lung function and maternal physical activity in the first half of pregnancy. Presented at *ERS International Congress*, 5 September 2021, OA1294.

Heesch, K.C., Miller, Y.D. and Brown, W.J. (2007). Relationship between physical activity and stiff or painful joints in mid-aged women and older women: a 3-year prospective study. *Arthritis Research & Therapy* 9, R34. https://doi.org/10.1186/ar2154

Hodges, L.D., Kirby, M., Solanki, J., O'Donnell, J. and Brodie, D.A. (2007) The temporal relationship between erectile dysfunction and cardiovascular disease. *International Journal of Clinical Practice* 61(12), 2019–2025.

Hoene, M., Kappler, L., Kollipara, L., Hu, C., Irmler, M., *et al.* (2021) Exercise prevents fatty liver by modifying the compensatory response of mitochondrial metabolism to excess substrate availability. *Molecular Metabolism* 54, 101359. https://doi.org/10.1016/j.molmet.2021.101359

Hootman, J.M., Macera, C.A., Helmick, C.G. and Blair, S.N. (2003) Influence of physical activity-related joint stress on the risk of self-reported hip/knee osteoarthritis: a new method to quantify physical activity. *Preventive Medicine* 36(5), 636–644. https://doi.org/10.1016/s0091-7435(03)00018-5

Huang, C.H., Li, C.L., Kor, C.T. and Chang, C.C. (2018) Menopausal symptoms and risk of coronary heart disease in middle-aged women: a nationwide population-based cohort study. *PLoS One* 13(10), e0206036. https://doi.org/10.1371/journal.pone.0206036

International Weight Management in Pregnancy (i-WIP) Collaborative Group (2017) Effect of diet and physical activity based interventions in pregnancy on gestational weight gain and pregnancy outcomes: meta-analysis of individual participant data from randomised trials. *BMJ* 358, j3119. https://doi.org/10.1136/bmj.j3119. Erratum in: *BMJ* 2017, 358, j3991. https://doi.org/10.1136/bmj.j3991

Lazaridou, A., Paschali, M., Schreiber, K., Galenkamp, L., Berry, M., et al. (2020) The association between daily physical exercise and pain among women with fibromyalgia: the moderating role of pain catastrophizing. *Pain Reports* 5(4), e832. https://doi.org/10.1097/PR9.0000000000000832

Li, S., Li, Z., Wu, Q., Liu, C., Zhou, Y., et al. (2021) Effect of exercise intervention on primary insomnia: a meta-analysis. *Journal of Sports Medicine and Physical Fitness* 61(6), 857–866. https://doi.org/10.23736/S0022-4707.21.11443-4

Lo, G.H., Vinod, S., Richard, M.J., Harkey, M.S., McAlindon, T.E., et al. (2022) Association between walking for exercise and symptomatic and structural progression in individuals with knee osteoarthritis: data from the Osteoarthritis Initiative Cohort. *Arthritis & Rheumatology* 74(10), 1660–1667. https://doi.org/10.1002/art.42241

Maleki, B.H., Tartibian, B. and Chehrazi, M. (2022) Effectiveness of exercise training on male factor infertility: a systematic review and network meta-analysis. *Sports Health* 14(4), 508–517. https://doi.org/10.1177/19417381211055399

Meier, N.F., Lee, D.C., Sui, X. and Blair, S.N. (2018) Physical activity, cardiorespiratory fitness, and incident glaucoma. *Medicine and Science in Sports and Exercise* 50(11), 2253–2258. https://doi.org/10.1249/MSS.0000000000001692

Mena, G.P., Mielke, G.I. and Brown, W.J. (2020) Do physical activity, sitting time and body mass index affect fertility over a 15-year period in women? Data from a large population-based cohort study. *Human Reproduction* 35(3), 676–683. https://doi.org/10.1093/humrep/dez300

Moilanen, J.M., Mikkola, T.S., Raitanen, J.A., Heinonen, R.H., Tomas, E.I., et al. (2012) Effect of aerobic training on menopausal symptoms – a randomized controlled trial. *Menopause* 19(6), 691–696.

NICE (2022) Osteoarthritis in over 16s: diagnosis and management. NICE guideline. Available at: https://www.nice.org.uk/guidance/ng226 (accessed 22 January 2023).

Office on Women's Health (2022) Period problems. Available at: https://www.womenshealth.gov/menstrual-cycle/period-problems (accessed 22 January 2023).

Olsen, L.N., Hoier, B., Hansen, C.V., Leinum, M., Carter, H.H., et al. (2020) Angiogenic potential is reduced in skeletal muscle of aged women. *Journal of Physiology* 598, 5149–5164. https://doi.org/10.1113/JP280189

Oppezzo, M. and Schwartz, D. (2014) Give your ideas some legs: the positive effect of walking on creative thinking. *Journal of Experimental Psychology: Learning, Memory, and Cognition* 40(4), 1142–1152. https://doi.org/10.1037/a0036577

Pritchett, R.A., Daley, A.J. and Jolly, K. (2017) Does aerobic exercise reduce postpartum depressive symptoms? A systematic review and meta-analysis. *British Journal of General Practice* 67(663), e684–e691.

RCOG (2022) Physical activity and pregnancy. Available at: https://www.rcog.org.uk/for-the-public/browse-all-patient-information-leaflets/physical-activity-and-pregnancy/ (accessed 31 January 2023).

Samadi, Z., Taghian, F. and Valiani, M. (2013) The effects of 8 weeks of regular aerobic exercise on the symptoms of premenstrual syndrome in non-athlete girls. *Iranian Journal of Nursing and Midwifery Research* 18(1), 14–19.

Sanda, B., Vistad, I., Sagedal, L.R., Haakstad, L.A.H., Lohne-Seiler, H. and Torstveit, M.K. (2018) What is the effect of physical activity on duration and mode of delivery? Secondary analysis from the Norwegian Fit for Delivery trial. *Acta Obstetrica et Gynecologica Scandinavica* 97(7), 86–-871.

Schulkey, C.E., Regmi, S.K., Magnan, R.A., Danzo, M.T., Luther, H., et al. (2015) The maternal age-associated risk of congenital heart disease is modifiable. *Nature* 520, 230–233.

Slomski, A. (2022) Physical activity benefits older adults' kidney function. *JAMA* 328(1), 10. https://doi.org/10.1001/jama.2022.11059

Stojanovska, L., Apostolopoulos, V., Polman, R. and Borkoles, E. (2014) To exercise, or, not to exercise, during menopause and beyond. *Maturitas* 77(4), 318–323. https://doi.org/10.1016/j.maturitas.2014.01.006

Varela, M., Gyi, D. and Mansfield, M. (2016) Predicting the onset of driver musculoskeletal fatigue. In: Waterson, P., Sims, R. and Hubbard, E.-M. (eds) *Contemporary Ergonomics and Human Factors 2016,* Daventry, 19–21 April. Chartered Institute of Ergonomics and Human Factors, Loughborough, UK, pp. 1–2.

Viana, J.L., Kosmadakis, G.C., Watson, E.L., Bevington, A., Feehally, J., et al. (2014) Evidence for anti-inflammatory effects of exercise in CKD. *Journal of the American Society of Nephrology* 25(9), 2121–2130. https://doi.org/10.1681/ASN.2013070702

Villa-González, R., Villalba-Heredia, L., Crespo, I., Del Valle, M. and Olmedillas, H. (2020) A systematic review of acute exercise as a coadjuvant treatment of ADHD in young people. *Psicothema* 32(1), 67–74. https://doi.org/10.7334/psicothema2019.211

Yeroushalmi, S., Hakimi, M., Chung, M., Bartholomew, E., Bhutani, T. and Liao, W. (2022) Psoriasis and exercise: a review. *Psoriasis: Targets and Therapy* 12, 189–197. https://doi.org/10.2147/PTT.S349791

Yesildere Saglam, H. and Orsal, O. (2020) Effect of exercise on premenstrual symptoms: a systematic review. *Complementary Therapies in Medicine* 48, 102272. https://doi.org/10.1016/j.ctim.2019.102272

25 Frailty

Frailty in old age is a huge and growing problem and the role of exercise in the prevention and treatment of frailty is extremely important. This affects everyone and has the potential to decide the pattern not only of the future of individuals but also of the social and financial health of the nation. And frailty is *not* inevitable.

The Definition of Frailty

Frailty has been lengthily defined as a 'clinically recognizable state of increased vulnerability resulting from aging-associated decline in reserve and function across multiple physiologic systems such that the ability to cope with everyday or acute stressors is compromised' (Xue, 2011). In brief, old and feeble. Frailty is the condition of general weakness and debility which is often seen as an inevitable consequence of the ageing process. Some of the essential features include low grip strength, low energy, slowed walking speed, low physical activity and/or unintentional weight loss (Fried *et al.*, 2001). The term *pre-frailty* is used for those with lesser degrees of debility.

There are several scales which can be used to assess frailty. A good example is the FRAIL scale (Morley *et al.*, 2012). This includes five components: Fatigue, Resistance, Ambulation, Illness and Loss of weight. Frail scale scores range from 0 to 5 (i.e. 1 point for each component; 0 = best to 5 = worst) and represent frail (3–5), pre-frail (1–2) and robust (0) health status. A rapid clinical test is the get-up-and-go test: the subject sits in an upright chair, gets up and walks 3 yards, turns round, returns to the chair and sits down. A time of less than 10 seconds is normal, between 10 and 20 seconds is an indicator of encroaching frailty and more than 20 seconds is characteristic of frailty. Walking speed is also an indicator of frailty. To be capable of more than 1¾ mph (2.8 kph) excludes frailty. However, below 1½ mph (2.4 kph), the slower a person walks the frailer that individual is likely to be. Among older people, those with a slow pace are three times as likely to need care as those who walk at faster speeds (Srithumsuk *et al.*, 2020).

The Causes of Frailty

Frailty is closely allied to loss of muscle tissue. As people age, they all lose muscle mass and strength, a condition called *sarcopenia*. A degree of age-related sarcopenia is unavoidable but the rate at which muscle is lost is largely dependent on how much exercise is taken. By the seventh and eighth decades of life, maximal voluntary muscle contractile strength is decreased, on average, by 20 to 40% for both men and women. Most of this loss of strength is caused by decreased muscle mass. Underlying processes include programmed cell death, oxidative stress, inflammation, hormonal changes and mitochondrial dysfunction (Lanza and Nair, 2009). The resulting progressive loss of neuromuscular function leads to increasing disability and loss of independence. The prevalence of sarcopenia increases with each 5-year age group from about 15% among the 65- to 70-year-olds to as much as 50% in the over-85s and probably becoming increasingly common thereafter. It accelerates with the passing of the years. As the age of the population grows so will the numbers with sarcopenia (Doherty, 2003).

Sarcopenia and the resulting frailty are usually the result of the accumulation of all the chronic diseases discussed earlier – obesity, diabetes, heart disease, osteoporosis, osteoarthritis and general unfitness. As the British Diabetic Association informs its members: 'Evidence is emerging that frailty has a significant impact on inpatients in terms of increased adverse outcomes and reduced survival' (Joint British Diabetes Societies, 2022). Other contributory factors include excessive sedentary behaviour (Webster *et al.*, 2021), obesity and a variety of lifestyle factors including smoking, poor diet (Gil-Salcedo *et al.*, 2020), socio-economic inequalities (Zaninotto *et al.*, 2020) and genetic influences (Romero-Blanco *et al.*, 2021).

Fleg *et al.* summarize the problem thus:

> The accelerated loss of aerobic capacity with advancing age has important clinical ramifications. The ability of older persons to function independently in the community depends largely on maintenance of sufficient aerobic capacity and muscle strength to perform daily activities. The perceived degree of effort and breathlessness of a given activity is determined by its oxygen cost relative to a person's peak. Tasks perceived as requiring substantial effort in deconditioned individuals tend to be avoided, setting off a vicious circle of further reduction in aerobic capacity, causing further avoidance of physical activity and further loss of muscle mass and strength.
>
> (Fleg *et al.*, 2005)

This is precisely the essence of frailty. It is ***not*** an inevitable consequence of ageing but, at least in part, a lifestyle choice (English and Paddon-Jones, 2010).

The ADNFS (Fentem *et al.*, 1994) highlighted the low level of fitness in the general population and the progressive further reduction with increasing age. Physical capacity becomes increasingly important as age increases. For 50-year-olds, not being as fit as they should be for that age will not make a substantial difference to their daily living (unless they are extremely unfit). But for an 80- or 90-year-old, poor fitness levels (relative to that age group) may mean that the individual is unable to maintain an independent life. The difference between being fit or unfit at this age means the difference between being able to get out of bed and dress unaided or relying on carers. Another example would be the difference between people being able to get up from a chair and put the kettle on or being dependent on others to do it for them. The level of VO_{2max} (physical fitness) that predicts loss of independence has been calculated at about 18 ml/min/kg for men and 15 ml/kg/min for women (Shephard, 2009). These figures appear unreasonably high as there are plenty of people with much lower fitness levels who can continue to look after themselves. However, the point is well made that the lower people's VO_{2max}, the less able they are to look after themselves. Old people are particularly liable to become dependent on others if they develop another age-related disease (e.g. osteoarthritis or atrial fibrillation) (Richard *et al.*, 2022).

The Consequences of Frailty

The social and financial consequences of frailty are enormous and growing. When frail people become ill, they have poorer outcomes for mortality, morbidity and institutionalization than the non-frail. If frail people are discharged from hospital, they have a high rate of readmission – as much as 40% over 6 months. If they need surgery, frail people are much more likely to suffer complications or die. Our hospitals are full of 'bed blockers' who only needed admission because they were frail and who are unable to go home because of lack of carers and lack of money to pay for them. The frail elderly occupy increasing numbers of beds in residential homes and nursing homes for dependent people. If able to stay at home, they require regular visits from informal or formal carers to allow them to keep a semblance of normal life. Frail elderly people are major users of emergency medical services, presenting with such problems as falls, immobility, incontinence and confusion. They are at particular risk of falling. Fifty per cent of people over 80 years old fall at least once a year and about 5% of these falls result in a fracture, most seriously of the neck of the femur. Falls are a major threat to older adults' quality of life, often causing a decline in self-care ability and in participation in physical and social activities. Fear of falling can lead to further limiting of activity, independent of injury. Current estimates are that falls cost the NHS more than £2.3 billion per year (Age UK, 2021).

There is a growing number of dependent elderly people, with increasing social care costs, increasing difficulty in finding enough younger carers and an inability to afford them. The trajectory of this problem is inexorably upwards with the proportion of the population aged over 80 set to double over the next 40 years. The number of over-85s requiring 24-hour care is also expected to double to 446,000 during the same time period, a staggering number. The media frequently publicizes the crisis in social care funding, predicting it to rise to over £2.6 billion annually. There is a dose-response increase in healthcare costs from good health through pre-frailty to full-blown frailty (Kojima, 2019). The Institute for Fiscal Studies has predicted that, unless they are supported financially by the Government, local councils will have to spend up to 60% of their revenues on social care by 2034. The problems of caring for our ageing population will be compounded by cuts in funding and by the restriction of immigration on which staffing depends.

The Association of Directors of Adult Social Services (ADASS) has published figures on the numbers of those needing care, and the inability of our current systems to meet this need. The numbers are shocking. At the end of April 2022 nearly 300,000 people were waiting for assessments for social care. Of these, 74,000 had been waiting for more than half a year, up by 80% from the previous estimate. The total of those waiting had increased by over 90,000 over the previous 6 months – an increase of 600 more people every day. If those who had been assessed but were still waiting for care to start are added in, more than half a million people need, but are not receiving, care (ADASS, 2022).

For those who have had assessments and been found to qualify, the battle is not over. There is a nationwide lack of carers. Pay for carers is miserly, discouraging new recruits and leading to many quitting this highly pressured and vital service. Even if care can be identified, the allowance given to the clients often fails to reach the real cost, low though this is. The results include:

- People are suffering at home without the right support in place, with some dying alone.

- Family members have to give up their jobs to care for their relative with a completely inadequate carer's allowance. Many are at risk of being pushed into poverty.
- Unsupported older people are more likely to need hospital treatment for any inter-current illness.
- After treatment in hospital there are lengthy waits before adequate care at home is available.
- Hospital beds are full of patients ready for discharge but nowhere to go – so admission of new patients becomes increasingly difficult.
- Patients are stacked up on trolleys in accident and emergency (A&E) departments.
- The queues of ambulances outside A&E departments grow ever longer.

The Role of Unfitness in Frailty

Frailty goes hand in hand with end-of-life dependence. Figure 25.1 illustrates the range of differences in strength and balance with increasing age.

Everyone deteriorates in ability as they age, but the fitter they keep, the slower is that rate of decline, and the flatter is the trajectory of reducing function (Tidy and Knott, 2016). Individuals can only maintain independence if their ability is maintained

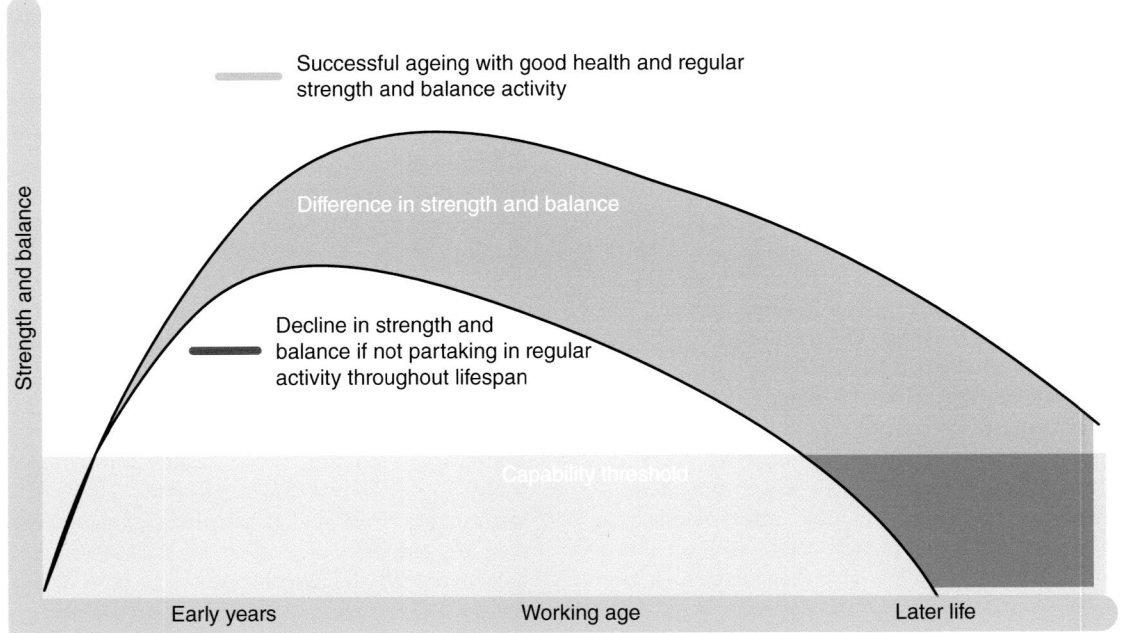

Fig. 25.1. The effect of regular exercise on strength, balance and capability throughout life. (From Department of Health and Social Care, 2019).

above a certain level. The less able people become, the earlier in life they reach that level, labelled the *capability threshold*.

The problem may be exacerbated because the frail elderly are particularly vulnerable to acute deterioration in health mainly due to falls, fractures and infections. Such events lead to a sudden steepening of the curve of loss of function so that the line of dependency is reached much earlier.

This becomes even worse if hospital admission is needed. In hospital immobility is the rule, a result both of the reason for admission and of the usual hospital culture of bed rest for poorly patients. Unfortunately the frail elderly not only start with reduced muscle mass and strength but also, when bed-rested, suffer a more rapid further loss than younger subjects. For many this means that their goal of maintaining independence is finally made impossible. They become confined in hospital awaiting long-term care where it can be found. This disastrous progression of disability can partly be ameliorated by planned inpatient exercise programmes and these are now being implemented in many geriatric departments, with some success (Martínez-Velilla *et al.*, 2019).

Healthspan

The desirability of decreasing the period of dependency at the end of life cannot be overstated. Average lifespan is increasing but as lives extend so also do the years of end-of-life dependency. What is needed is not just more years of life but also more years of healthy and active life. This is sometimes referred to as 'healthspan' and is a much better measure of the health of the nation than lifespan. Shortening the proportion of life spent in end-of-life debility is often called 'compression of morbidity'. This is what is needed – to live well until as near to death as possible (Fig. 25.2).

Unfortunately the most recent evidence indicates that individuals' lives, far from improving, are worsening in this respect. The Office of National Statistics (2014) report showed that a 65-year-old man could expect to be free from disability and long-term illness for a further 10.6 years in 2012, but by 2014 this had decreased to 10.3 years. For women the figures were 11.2 years falling to 10.9 years. The life expectancy of someone born today gives another perspective. A boy born now can expect to live to age 78.5 years but only have a healthy life expectancy (healthspan) of 62.7 years, i.e. 20% of his life will be with some form of disability or chronic illness. The picture for women is even worse. They may have a life expectancy 82.5 years, but a healthy life expectancy of only 63.9 years. This gives a total of 23% of life expectancy being lived with a chronic illness or disability. Socio-economic inequalities magnify these figures. One study of older people in England and the USA suggested that disability-free life expectancy was largest for the wealthy. In both countries, 50-year-olds in the poorest group could expect to live 7 to 9 years fewer without disability than those in the richest group (Zaninotto *et al.*, 2020).

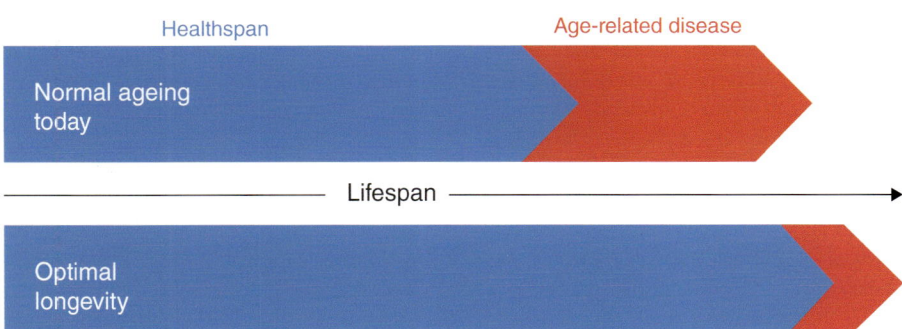

Fig. 25.2. Healthspan and lifespan – today's normal compared with what can be achieved by regular exercise. (From Seals and Melov, 2014. Article available under the terms of the Creative Commons Attribution 3.0 Unported (CC BY 3.0) licence; https://creativecommons.org/licenses/by/3.0/.)

The harm done by premature frailty is even observed in the workplace:

If state pension age rises but the gains in HWLE [healthy working life expectancy] do not keep pace, then individuals (especially those with chronic health problems) may increasingly face challenges. These challenges could include securing suitable employment or engaging productively and healthily at work, to the detriment of their health and well-being and that of their families.

(Lynch *et al.*, 2022)

Exercise for Prevention of Frailty

Frailty is mainly the long-term result of an accumulation of one or more of the degenerative diseases described above. They are all promoted by lack of exercise and thus the main risk factor for the development of frailty is insufficient physical activity, usually over a very long period. The inactive and the sedentary are those at risk. The key may be found in the difference between chronological age and physiological age. It is common to be aware of people who seem much younger than their real age would suggest. Increasingly the reverse is true, and people are seen who appear much older than their real age. This difference between chronological age and physiological age is measurable and enormous differences are apparent. In the FIT study in the USA, nearly 60,000 subjects of all ages were assessed (Blaha *et al.*, 2016). Fitness levels were used to assess physiological age and varied enormously at each chronological age. There were variations of between 18 and 38 years between chronological and physiological age. Physical fitness is a product of a number of factors including age, hormonal changes, heredity, socio-economic status, etc. Among all these there is only one risk factor which is easily influenced by the individual – the level of physical activity. A study of active, non-elite, cyclists aged 55 to 79 found very high levels of fitness. For those aged 55 the fitness was equivalent to the average for 20-year-olds, for those aged 65 it was equivalent to the average for 25-year-olds and for those aged 75 it was equivalent to 35-year-olds (Pollock *et al.*, 2015). Similar findings were found by the Stanford Arthritis Center study of runners aged over 50 compared with non-exercising controls, with both groups being followed up for 8 years. There were striking differences between the two groups for development of disability, more marked in women than

men (Fries, 1996). Over 500 members of a running club, aged 50 or more, were followed up over 9 years and compared to a similar number of non-running members of the same community. The disability scores were low in both groups at the start of the study and remained so in the runners over the whole period of follow-up. However, the disability scores in the non-runners rose steadily throughout the 9 years. When this group was followed up for a total of 19 years, the benefits sustained by the runners continued to accumulate (Chakravarty *et al.*, 2008). The average time until the onset of measurable disability was 16 years later for the runners compared with the controls. The health gap between the groups increased through the period of study and was still widening into the tenth decade of life.

Lower-level exercise than cycling and running is also preventive of frailty and can produce biological evidence of benefit. Regular walking improves aerobic fitness, lower-body strength, balance and agility in older adults (Sithichoksakulchai *et al.*, 2022). A study of over 400,000 UK Biobank subjects compared the walking pace of middle-aged people with their leucocyte telomere length (LTL) (Dempsey *et al.*, 2022). LTL is considered a strong marker of biological age – and this study found that a faster walking pace was associated with longer telomeres.

The improved health status of elderly people who have exercised regularly has been emphasized by one study (Ferrucci *et al.*, 1999) which found that the average 65-year-old can expect an additional 12.7 years of healthy life – meaning that they will live disability-free until age 77.7. Highly active 65-year-olds, however, have an additional 5.7 years of healthy life expectancy – they will remain disability-free until age 83.4.

Many other studies have confirmed that regular exercise reduces dependency in older people (Singh, 2002; Young and Dinan, 2005). As with so many exercise benefits, an early start is important. The Whitehall Study, initiated by Gerry Morris, tracked 6357 civil servants for 20 years. Physical activity at age 50 predicted frailty at the age of 70. Those who were exercising for 150 minutes weekly at the start had the risk of future frailty reduced by a third (Simoes *et al.*, 2006). Intervention later in life, before the onset of frailty, can also be very effective. The Buck study (Melov *et al.*, 2007) compared the effects of 6 months of weight training in 25 healthy old people (average age 70) with 26 younger (average age 30). The older individuals increased their strength by about 50%. Before exercise training, the older adults were 59% weaker than the younger, but strength improved significantly in the older adults so that they were only 38% weaker than the young adults after 6 months of training. Before-and-after muscle biopsies indicated that the healthy older adults showed evidence of mitochondrial impairment and muscle weakness but that this was partially reversed by the training programme.

Frailty leads to 'terminal dependence', which is the interval between total independence and death. It is the sedentary and inactive who not only die earlier but also suffer a longer period of dependence at the end of life. Regular exercisers keep themselves fit, flexible and strong and also reduce their chances of developing other diseases which contribute to frailty – heart disease, obesity, lower-limb arthritis, diabetes and dementia.

Exercise in the Treatment of Frailty

Advanced age is no barrier to the benefits of tailored exercise (Izquierdo *et al.*, 2020; Hayashi *et al.*, 2021). Although improvements in function may result from exercise interventions to treat the elderly infirm, once frailty has become established it may be too late to make major differences to performance. Treatment should start before debility is apparent. A 2008 meta-analysis of exercise interventions in frail elderly showed improvements in both functional and physical performance in the treated groups but no increase in ability to perform ADL (Gu and Conn, 2008). A further review in 2011 confirmed a limited benefit from applying exercise programmes to frail older adults (Theou *et al.*, 2011) and found that only more prolonged and vigorous exercise programmes were effective in improving functional ability. They state that 'multicomponent training interventions, of long duration (≥5 months), performed three times per week, for 30–45 minutes per session, generally had superior outcomes than other exercise programs.' This view was reinforced by the SPRINTT project, which studied the effect of multicomponent intervention in preventing mobility disability in frail older adults (Bernabei *et al.*, 2022).

A Cochrane Review in 2021 involving 29 studies compared the effect of high-intensity intermittent training versus moderate-intensity exercise. It showed that high-intensity intermittent training induces favourable adaptions in CRF, physical fitness, muscle power, cardiac contractile function and mitochondrial citrate synthase activity in older individuals. It also reduced blood triglyceride and glucose levels. All of these may help to maintain aerobic fitness and slow down the progress of sarcopenia.

The effect of physical training on muscle structure and function has indicated that it has a larger effect on physical performance, a medium effect on muscle strength but little or no effect on muscle mass (Escriche-Escuder *et al.*, 2021).

There is some evidence that the effectiveness of exercise in controlling sarcopenia is enhanced by increasing protein intake (Tieland *et al.*, 2012), but protein alone has no such effect (Oktaviana *et al.*, 2020).

For elderly patients who already have some functional limitations, further decline in physical functioning can be slowed by maintaining even a low level of physical activity. The LIFE study in the USA randomized a volunteer sample of 1635 mildly impaired sedentary men and women aged between 70 and 89 years into a programme of physical training or no intervention. The treated group showed a significantly better mobility after 2.6 years of training (Theou *et al.*, 2011). This effect is seen in 'younger' old people and the less disabled, but exercise may not help those who are very disabled, particularly those with severely limited mobility. Once again, exercise intervention is needed before debility has advanced too far.

If it is to be of any value at all, exercise must be maintained. It is recognized that this is something that becomes increasingly difficult for the elderly. A trial that investigated weight training in nursing-home residents, aged 90 years or older, showed the training to be clearly beneficial in terms of strength and self-care scores. Unfortunately the scores soon fell back to their pre-trial levels after the study ended (Pahor *et al.*, 2014).

Balance and Risk of Falling

A particular role for exercise as a treatment for frailty is in the prevention of falls in those who have or have not already suffered accidental falls. Around one-third of over-65s and half of over-80s fall at least once a year. Frailty predicts both falls and fractures (Faber *et al.*, 2006; Kojima *et al.*, 2015). Falls are the leading cause of death from injury in the over-70s. Falls lead to fractures, including 80,000 hip fractures per annum in the

UK. About 40% of people over the age of 75 who break their hips are no longer able to care for themselves. Ten per cent die within 30 days and nearly 30% die within 12 months. Moreover, poor balance predicts excess mortality (Araujo *et al.*, 2022). People with balance disorder are at a higher risk of death from all causes, CVD and cancer. After adjusting for sociodemographic characteristics, lifestyle factors and chronic conditions, the HRs among people with balance disorder compared with those without balance disorder are 1.44 for all-cause mortality, 1.65 for CVD mortality and 1.37 for cancer mortality (Cao *et al.*, 2021).

To lessen these risks, some of the types of beneficial exercises include improving balance and regular stretching. These can maintain joint flexibility, reduce fibrosis in the tissues and maintain mobility. Exercises involving balance can also prevent falls. Yoga, tai chi, Pilates and table tennis are excellent examples of these as they will help develop core strength without being too demanding.

The provision of exercise and education programmes to reduce the risk of falling is growing. One example is those established by ambulance stations for the patients whom staff have retrieved after a fall. A large meta-analysis of such programmes involved more than 4000 elderly fallers. The study has shown a subsequent reduction in falls by 30% and of falls leading to fractures by 60%, clearly of substantial benefit (de Vries *et al.*, 2013). The 2018 Cochrane Review of the use of exercise to prevent recurrent falls in the elderly concluded that a combination of balance and functional training with strength training is the most effective (Sherrington *et al.*, 2019). The review included 108 RCTs, involving 23,407 participants in exercise versus control groups. It found a reduction of 23% in the rate of falls in the treated groups and a significant reduction in falls-related fractures. Functional training aimed at improving the strength and movements of daily tasks are shown to be more effective than general muscle-strengthening exercises (Resende-Neto *et al.*, 2021).

If such training regimes were widely applied, they should reduce by a quarter the overall number of falls per year. This would amount to about 140 fewer falls per 1000 older people over 1 year in the general population and twice as many in older people at high risk of falls (El-Khoury *et al.*, 2013). Aquatic exercise may be particularly suitable (Moreira *et al.*, 2020).

Conclusion

Frailty, a devastating condition of later life, is not inevitable and everyone has the opportunity to reduce or prevent it for themselves. It is never too late to take up exercise, but if it is left too long it may be too late to reduce dependency on others. As individuals age, it becomes increasingly important to maintain a physically active lifestyle. Lapsing into a lazy old age is a recipe for detraining and the onset of inevitable dependency.

Summary

The prevention and treatment of frailty in old age is now recognized as very important as the population ages and the issues of care become paramount. As people age, they lose certain abilities and independence, but the fitter they are, the slower is the rate of decline. The aim is to increase the proportion of 'healthspan' throughout life and exercise is the main method of achieving this. For elderly people who are already frail, even a low level of exercise is beneficial. Improved balance training is particularly helpful to reduce the prospect of falls, with consequent fractures.

References

ADASS (2022) ADASS Survey: People waiting for assessments, care or reviews. Available at: https://www.adass.org.uk/surveys/waiting-for-care-july-22 (accessed 30 January 2023).

Age UK (2021) Falls in the over 65s cost NHS £4.6 million a day. Available at: https://www.ageuk.org.uk/latest-press/archive/falls-over-65s-costnhs/#:~:text=Up%20to%20one%20in%20three,Concern%20and%20Help%20the%20Aged (accessed 22 January 2023).

Araujo, C.G., de Souza e Silva, C.G., Laukkanen, J.A., Singh, M.F., Kunutsor, S.K., et al. (2022) Successful 10-second one-legged stance performance predicts survival in middle-aged and older individuals. *British Journal of Sports Medicine* 56, 975–980. https://doi.org/10.1136/bjsports-2021-105360

Bernabei, R., Landi, F., Calvani, R., Cesari, M., Del Signore, S., et al. (2022) Multicomponent intervention to prevent mobility disability in frail older adults: randomised controlled trial (SPRINTT project). *BMJ* 377, e068788. https://doi.org/10.1136/bmj-2021-068788

Blaha, M.J., Hung, R.K., Dardari, Z., Feldman, D.I., Whelton, S.P., et al. (2016) Age-dependent prognostic value of exercise capacity and derivation of fitness-associated biologic age. *Heart* 102(6), 431–437. https://doi.org/10.1136/heartjnl-2015-308537

Cao, C., Cade, W.T., Li, S., McMillan, J., Friedenreich, C. and Yang, L. (2021) Association of balance function with all-cause and cause-specific mortality among US adults. *JAMA Otolaryngology – Head & Neck Surgery* 147(5), 460–468. https://doi.org/10.1001/jamaoto.2021.0057

Chakravarty, E.F., Hubert, H.B., Lingala, V.B. and Fries, J.F. (2008) Reduced disability and mortality among aging runners: a 21-year longitudinal study. *Archives of Internal Medicine* 168, 1638–1646.

Dempsey, P.C., Musicha, C., Rowlands, A.V., Davies, M., Khunti, K., et al. (2022) Investigation of a UK biobank cohort reveals causal associations of self-reported walking pace with telomere length. *Community Biology* 5, 381. https://doi.org/10.1038/s42003-022-03323-x

Department of Health and Social Care (2019) *UK Chief Medical Officers' Physical Activity Guidelines*. Department of Health and Social Care, London.

de Vries, O.J., Peters, G.M., Lips, P. and Deeg, D.J. (2013) Does frailty predict increased risk of falls and fractures? *Osteoporosis International* 24(9), 2397–2403.

Doherty, T.J. (2003) Ageing and sarcopenia. *Journal of Applied Physiology* 95, 1717–1727.

El-Khoury, F., Cassou, B., Charles, M.-A. and Dargent-Molina, P. (2013) The effect of fall prevention exercise programmes on fall induced injuries in community dwelling older adults: systematic review and meta-analysis of randomised controlled trials. *BMJ* 347, f6234.

English, K. and Paddon-Jones, D. (2010) Protecting muscle mass and function in older adults during bed rest. *Current Opinion in Clinical Nutrition and Metabolic Care* 13, 34–39. https://doi.org/10.1097/MCO.0b013e328333aa66

Escriche-Escuder, A., Fuentes-Abolafio, I.J., Roldán-Jiménez, C. and Cuesta-Vargas, A.I. (2021) Effects of exercise on muscle mass, strength, and physical performance in older adults with sarcopenia: a systematic review and meta-analysis according to the EWGSOP criteria. *Experimental Gerontology* 151, 111420. https://doi.org/10.1016/j.exger.2021.111420

Faber, M.J., Bosscher, R.J., Paw, M.J.C.A. and van Wieringen, P.C. (2006) Effects of exercise programs on falls and mobility in frail and pre-frail older adults: a multicenter randomized controlled trial. *Archives of Physical Medicine and Rehabilitation* 87, 885–896.

Fentem, P.H., Collins, M.F., Tuxworth, W., Walker, A., Hoinville, E., et al. (1994) *Allied Dunbar National Fitness Survey. Technical Report.* Allied Dunbar, Health Education Authority and Sports Council, London.

Ferrucci, L., Izmirlian, G., Leveille, S., Phillips, C.L., Corti, M.-C., et al. (1999) Smoking, physical activity and active life expectancy. *American Journal of Epidemiology* 149(7), 645–653.

Fleg, J.L., Morrell, C.H., Bos, A.G., Brant, L.J., Talbot, L.A., et al. (2005) Accelerated longitudinal decline of aerobic capacity in healthy older adults. *Circulation* 112, 674–682.

Fried, L.P., Tangen, C.M., Walston, J., Newman, A.B., Hirsch, C., et al. (2001) Frailty in older adults: evidence for a phenotype. *Journal of Gerontology* 56(3), M146–M156.

Fries, J.F. (1996) Physical activity, the compression of morbidity, and the health of the elderly *Journal of the Royal Society of Medicine* 89(2), 64–68.

Gil-Salcedo, A., Dugravot, A., Fayosse, A., Dumurgier, J., Bouillon, K., et al. (2020) Healthy behaviors at age 50 years and frailty at older ages in a 20-year follow-up of the UK Whitehall II cohort: a longitudinal study. *PLoS Medicine* 17(7), e1003147. https://doi.org/10.1371/journal.pmed.1003147

Gu, M.O. and Conn, V.S. (2008) Meta-analysis of the effects of exercise interventions on functional status in older adults. *Research in Nursing and Health* 31, 594–603.

Hayashi, C., Ogata, S., Okano, T., Toyoda, H. and Mashino, S. (2021) Long-term participation in community group exercise improves lower extremity muscle strength and delays age-related declines in walking speed and physical function in older adults. *European Review of Aging and Physical Activity* 18(1), 6. https://doi.org/10.1186/s11556-021-00260-2

Izquierdo, M., Morley, J. and Lucia, A. (2020) Exercise in people over 85: advanced age is no barrier to the benefits of tailored exercise. *BMJ* 368, m402. https://doi.org/10.1136/bmj.m402

Joint British Diabetes Societies (2022) Inpatient care of the frail older adult with diabetes. Available at: https://www.diabetes.org.uk/resources-s3/2019-10/frailty-jbds-ipfinal-28-10-19.pdf (accessed 30 January 2023).

Kojima, G. (2019) Increased healthcare costs associated with frailty among community-dwelling older people: a systematic review and meta-analysis. *Archives of Gerontology and Geriatrics* 84, 103898. https://doi.org/10.1016/j.archger.2019.06.003

26 Longevity

There is no answer to the question 'What is normal life expectancy?' but it is certain that our population is nowhere near reaching it. Indeed, it has been suggested that humans have evolved not only to live longer but also to exercise into old age (Lieberman *et al.*, 2021). That this can happen is illustrated by the 'Blue Zone' phenomenon. These optimal wellness enclaves are found around the globe from Okinawa in Japan to Ikaria in Greece. They are home to an extraordinarily high number of people who live far longer than average, into their nineties and hundreds. What these healthy nonagenarians and centenarians all seem to share is that they exercise moderately as part of their daily lives. This kind of natural daily movement is known as NEAT, which stands for non-exercise activity thermogenesis (Levine, 2002). NEAT is all the non-planned physical activity we do each day, like climbing stairs, walking, cooking and brushing our teeth. These types of movement may seem insignificant, but when added up, NEAT may account for as many as 2000 Calories of energy output per day.

Until very recently, despite our thoroughly unhealthy lifestyles, we have seen a gradual increase in lifespan. In the years between 1991 and 2014 average life expectancy for men rose from 73.6 years in 1991 to 79.4 years in 2014. For women the figures were from 79.0 to 83.1 years (Office for National Statistics, 2014). This unexpectedly good news has recently 'hit the buffers' with figures produced by Public Health England (2017) suggesting that the trend has now flattened. Indeed, before the Covid-19 pandemic, the Institute and Faculty of Actuaries (2018) calculated that at the age of 65, the life expectancy of a man has fallen by 4 months and that of a woman has fallen by a whole year. This will be good news for the pensions industry, which will reap a reward of £27 billion in liabilities from company balance sheets. The same is true in the USA (Woolf and Schoomaker, 2019), where life expectancy fell in 2017 from 78.7 to 78.6 years, after rising from 69.9 years over the previous six decades. More importantly, the duration of healthy life – healthspan (see Chapter 25, this volume) – has been falling for several years, while the years spent in poor health have increased. One reason given for this decline in lifespan has been socio-economic disadvantage aggravated by austerity measures (Hawkes, 2019). Low income is linked to most of the non-communicable diseases that contribute to premature death and a possible link is provided by the lower levels of exercise and fitness among the less well-off (Matsuo and So, 2021).

Effect of Exercise on Lifespan

As discussed in Chapter 7 (this volume), there are two ways of judging how much and how effectively a person exercises:

1. *Assessing physical activity by either questionnaire or direct observation.* The former is biased by the individual's tendency to exaggerate, driven by so-called 'social desirability bias', and almost always gives a much greater exercise estimate than the latter. Direct observation gives the most accurate measure of physical activity but has a number of problems – it is difficult to do, difficult to compare between exercise types, takes special equipment and is expensive, and it only gives a result which applies to the period of observation. Most people will 'up their game' when they know they are being observed.

2. *Measuring physical fitness.* There is a direct relationship between amount of exercise taken and physical fitness level, but with wide variations (Stofan *et al.*, 2008). There are other variables which affect the relationship such as inherited characteristics. However, this method has the strength of giving a measurement which does not depend upon the unreliable witness of the participant.

© H.J.N. Bethell and D. Brodie 2023. *Exercise: A Scientific and Clinical Overview*
(H.J.N. Bethell and D. Brodie)
DOI: 10.1079/9781800621855.0026

Araujo, C.G., de Souza e Silva, C.G., Laukkanen, J.A., Singh, M.F., Kunutsor, S.K., *et al.* (2022) Successful 10-second one-legged stance performance predicts survival in middle-aged and older individuals. *British Journal of Sports Medicine* 56, 975–980. https://doi.org/10.1136/bjsports-2021-105360

Bernabei, R., Landi, F., Calvani, R., Cesari, M., Del Signore, S., *et al.* (2022) Multicomponent intervention to prevent mobility disability in frail older adults: randomised controlled trial (SPRINTT project). *BMJ* 377, e068788. https://doi.org/10.1136/bmj-2021-068788

Blaha, M.J., Hung, R.K., Dardari, Z., Feldman, D.I., Whelton, S.P., *et al.* (2016) Age-dependent prognostic value of exercise capacity and derivation of fitness-associated biologic age. *Heart* 102(6), 431–437. https://doi.org/10.1136/heartjnl-2015-308537

Cao, C., Cade, W.T., Li, S., McMillan, J., Friedenreich, C. and Yang, L. (2021) Association of balance function with all-cause and cause-specific mortality among US adults. *JAMA Otolaryngology – Head & Neck Surgery* 147(5), 460–468. https://doi.org/10.1001/jamaoto.2021.0057

Chakravarty, E.F., Hubert, H.B., Lingala, V.B. and Fries, J.F. (2008) Reduced disability and mortality among aging runners: a 21-year longitudinal study. *Archives of Internal Medicine* 168, 1638–1646.

Dempsey, P.C., Musicha, C., Rowlands, A.V., Davies, M., Khunti, K., *et al.* (2022) Investigation of a UK biobank cohort reveals causal associations of self-reported walking pace with telomere length. *Community Biology* 5, 381. https://doi.org/10.1038/s42003-022-03323-x

Department of Health and Social Care (2019) *UK Chief Medical Officers' Physical Activity Guidelines.* Department of Health and Social Care, London.

de Vries, O.J., Peters, G.M., Lips, P. and Deeg, D.J. (2013) Does frailty predict increased risk of falls and fractures? *Osteoporosis International* 24(9), 2397–2403.

Doherty, T.J. (2003) Ageing and sarcopenia. *Journal of Applied Physiology* 95, 1717–1727.

El-Khoury, F., Cassou, B., Charles, M.-A. and Dargent-Molina, P. (2013) The effect of fall prevention exercise programmes on fall induced injuries in community dwelling older adults: systematic review and meta-analysis of randomised controlled trials. *BMJ* 347, f6234.

English, K. and Paddon-Jones, D. (2010) Protecting muscle mass and function in older adults during bed rest. *Current Opinion in Clinical Nutrition and Metabolic Care* 13, 34–39. https://doi.org/10.1097/MCO.0b013e328333aa66

Escriche-Escuder, A., Fuentes-Abolafio, I.J., Roldán-Jiménez, C. and Cuesta-Vargas, A.I. (2021) Effects of exercise on muscle mass, strength, and physical performance in older adults with sarcopenia: a systematic review and meta-analysis according to the EWGSOP criteria. *Experimental Gerontology* 151, 111420. https://doi.org/10.1016/j.exger.2021.111420

Faber, M.J., Bosscher, R.J., Paw, M.J.C.A. and van Wieringen, P.C. (2006) Effects of exercise programs on falls and mobility in frail and pre-frail older adults: a multicenter randomized controlled trial. *Archives of Physical Medicine and Rehabilitation* 87, 885–896.

Fentem, P.H., Collins, M.F., Tuxworth, W., Walker, A., Hoinville, E., *et al.* (1994) *Allied Dunbar National Fitness Survey. Technical Report.* Allied Dunbar, Health Education Authority and Sports Council, London.

Ferrucci, L., Izmirlian, G., Leveille, S., Phillips, C.L., Corti, M.-C., *et al.* (1999) Smoking, physical activity and active life expectancy. *American Journal of Epidemiology* 149(7), 645–653.

Fleg, J.L., Morrell, C.H., Bos, A.G., Brant, L.J., Talbot, L.A., *et al.* (2005) Accelerated longitudinal decline of aerobic capacity in healthy older adults. *Circulation* 112, 674–682.

Fried, L.P., Tangen, C.M., Walston, J., Newman, A.B., Hirsch, C., *et al.* (2001) Frailty in older adults: evidence for a phenotype. *Journal of Gerontology* 56(3), M146–M156.

Fries, J.F. (1996) Physical activity, the compression of morbidity, and the health of the elderly *Journal of the Royal Society of Medicine* 89(2), 64–68.

Gil-Salcedo, A., Dugravot, A., Fayosse, A., Dumurgier, J., Bouillon, K., *et al.* (2020) Healthy behaviors at age 50 years and frailty at older ages in a 20-year follow-up of the UK Whitehall II cohort: a longitudinal study. *PLoS Medicine* 17(7), e1003147. https://doi.org/10.1371/journal.pmed.1003147

Gu, M.O. and Conn, V.S. (2008) Meta-analysis of the effects of exercise interventions on functional status in older adults. *Research in Nursing and Health* 31, 594–603.

Hayashi, C., Ogata, S., Okano, T., Toyoda, H. and Mashino, S. (2021) Long-term participation in community group exercise improves lower extremity muscle strength and delays age-related declines in walking speed and physical function in older adults. *European Review of Aging and Physical Activity* 18(1), 6. https://doi.org/10.1186/s11556-021-00260-2

Izquierdo, M., Morley, J. and Lucia, A. (2020) Exercise in people over 85: advanced age is no barrier to the benefits of tailored exercise. *BMJ* 368, m402. https://doi.org/10.1136/bmj.m402

Joint British Diabetes Societies (2022) Inpatient care of the frail older adult with diabetes. Available at: https://www.diabetes.org.uk/resources-s3/2019-10/frailty-jbds-ipfinal-28-10-19.pdf (accessed 30 January 2023).

Kojima, G. (2019) Increased healthcare costs associated with frailty among community-dwelling older people: a systematic review and meta-analysis. *Archives of Gerontology and Geriatrics* 84, 103898. https://doi.org/10.1016/j.archger.2019.06.003

Kojima, G., Kendrick, D., Skelton, D.A., Morris, R.W., Gawler, S. and Iliffe, S. (2015) Frailty predicts short-term incidence of future falls among British community-dwelling older people: a prospective cohort study nested within a randomised controlled trial. *BMC Geriatrics* 15, 155.

Lanza, I.R. and Nair, K.S. (2009) Muscle mitochondrial changes with aging and exercise. *American Journal of Clinical Nutrition* 89(1), 467S–471S. https://doi.org/10.3945/ajcn.2008.26717D

Lynch, M., Bucknall, M., Jagger, C. and Wilkie, R. (2022) Projections of healthy working life expectancy in England to the year 2035. *Nature Aging* 2, 13–18. https://doi.org/10.1038/s43587-021-00161-0

Martínez-Velilla, N., Casas-Herrero, A., Zambom-Ferraresi, F., Sáez de Asteasu, M.L., Lucia, A., *et al.* (2019) Effect of exercise intervention on functional decline in very elderly patients during acute hospitalization: A randomized clinical trial. *JAMA Internal Medicine* 179(1), 28–36. https://doi.org/10.1001/jamainternmed.2018.4869

Melov, S., Tarnopolsky, M.A., Beckman, K., Felkey, K. and Hubbard, A. (2007) Resistance exercise reverses aging in human skeletal muscle. *PLoS One* 2(5), e465. https://doi.org/10.1371/journal.pone.0000465

Moreira, N.B., da Silva, L.P. and Rodacki, A.L.F. (2020) Aquatic exercise improves functional capacity, perceptual aspects, and quality of life in older adults with musculoskeletal disorders and risk of falling: a randomized controlled trial. *Experimental Gerontology* 142, 111135. https://doi.org/10.1016/j.exger.2020.111135

Morley, J.E., Malmstrom, T.K. and Miller, D.K. (2012) A simple frailty questionnaire (FRAIL) predicts outcomes in middle aged African Americans. *Journal of Nutrition, Health & Aging* 16(7), 601–608. https://doi.org/10.1007/s12603-012-0084-2

Office of National Statistics (2014) *Life Expectancy at Birth and at Age 65 by Local Areas in England and Wales: 2012 to 2014.* Office for National Statistics, London. Available at: https://www.ons.gov.uk/peoplepopulationandcommunity/birthsdeathsandmarriages/lifeexpectancies/bulletins/lifeexpectancyatbirthandatage65bylocalareasinenglandandwales/2015-11-04 (accessed 31 January 2023).

Oktaviana, J., Zanker, J., Vogrin, S. and Duque, G. (2020) The effect of protein supplements on functional frailty in older persons: a systematic review and meta-analysis. *Archives of Gerontology and Geriatrics* 86, 103938. https://doi.org/10.1016/j.archger.2019.103938

Pahor, M., Guralnik, J.M., Ambrosius, W.T., Blair, S., Bonds, D.E., *et al.* (2014) Effect of structured physical activity on prevention of major mobility disability in older adults: the LIFE study randomized clinical trial. *JAMA* 311, 2387–2396.

Pollock, R.D., Carter, S., Velloso, C.P., Duggal, N.A., *et al.* (2015) An investigation into the relationship between age and physiological function in highly active older adults. *Journal of Physiology* 593(3), 657–680. https://doi.org/10.1113/jphysiol.2014.282863

Resende-Neto, A.G., Silva Resende, M., Oliveira-Andrade, B.C., da Silva Chaves, L.M., Brandão, L.H.A., *et al.* (2021) Functional training in comparison to traditional training on physical fitness and quality of movement in older women. *Sport Sciences for Health* 17, 213–222. https://doi.org/10.1007/s11332-020-00675-x

Richard, G., O'Halloran, A.M., Doody, P., Harbison, J., Kenny, R.A. and Romero-Ortuno, R. (2022) Atrial fibrillation and acceleration of frailty: findings from the Irish Longitudinal Study on Ageing. *Age and Ageing* 51(2), afab273. https://doi.org/10.1093/ageing/afab273

Romero-Blanco, C., Artiga González, M.J., Gómez-Cabello, A., Vila-Maldonado, S., Casajús, J.A., *et al.* (2021) ACTN3 R577X polymorphism related to sarcopenia and physical fitness in active older women. *Climacteric* 24(1), 89–94. https://doi.org/10.1080/13697137.2020.1776248

Seals, D.R. and Melov, S. (2014) Translational geroscience: emphasizing function to achieve optimal longevity. *Aging* 6(9), 718–730.

Shephard, R.J. (2009) Maximal oxygen intake and independence in old age. *British Journal of Sports Medicine* 43, 342–346.

Sherrington, C., Fairhall, N.J., Wallbank, G.K., Tiedemann, A., Michaleff, Z.A., *et al.* (2019) Exercise for preventing falls in older people living in the community. *Cochrane Database of Systematic Reviews* 1(1), CD012424. https://doi.org/10.1002/14651858.CD012424.pub2

Simoes, E.J., Kobau, R., Kapp, J., Waterman, B., Mokdad, A. and Anderson, L. (2006) Associations of physical activity and body mass index with activities of daily living in older adults. *Journal of Community Health* 31, 45–67.

Singh, M.A. (2002) Exercise comes of age: rationale and recommendations for a geriatric exercise prescription. *Journal of Gerontology* 57, M262–M282.

Sithichoksakulchai, S., Chen, M.-C. and Chen, K.-M. (2022) Walking promotes physical fitness of community-dwelling older adults: a systematic review and meta-analysis. *Topics in Geriatric Rehabilitation* 38(2), 101–109. https://doi.org/10.1097/TGR.0000000000000351

Srithumsuk, W., Kabayama, M., Godai, K., Klinpudtan, N., Sugimoto, K., *et al.* (2020) Association between physical function and long-term care in community-dwelling older and oldest people: the SONIC study. *Environmental Health and Preventive Medicine* 25, 46. https://doi.org/10.1186/s12199-020-00884-3

Theou, O., Stathokostas, L., Roland, K.P., Jakobi, J.M., Patterson, C., *et al.* (2011) The effectiveness of exercise interventions for the management of frailty: a systematic review. *Journal of Aging Research* 2011, 569194. https://doi.org/10.4061/2011/569194

Tidy, C. and Knott, K. (2016) Prevention of falls in the elderly. Available at: https://patient.info/doctor/prevention-of-falls-in-the-elderly-pro (accessed 12 December 2022).

Tieland, M., van de Rest, O., Dirks, M.L., van der Zwaluw, N., Mensink, M., *et al.* (2012) Protein supplementation improves physical performance in frail elderly people: a randomized, double-blind, placebo-controlled trial. *Journal of the American Medical Directors Association* 13(8), 720–726. https://doi.org/10.1016/j.jamda.2012.07.005

Webster, K.E., Zhou, W., Gallagher, N.A., Smith, E.M.L., Gothe, N.P., *et al.* (2021) Device-measured sedentary behavior in oldest old adults: a systematic review and meta-analysis. *Preventive Medicine Reports* 23, 101405. https://doi.org/10.1016/j.pmedr.2021.101405

Xue, Q.-L. (2011) The frailty syndrome: definition and natural history. *Clinics in Geriatric Medicine* 27(1), 1–15.

Young, A. and Dinan, S. (2005) ABC of sports and exercise medicine. Activity in later life. *BMJ* 330, 189–191.

Zaninotto, P., Batty, G., Stenholm, S., Kawachi, I., Hyde, M., *et al.* (2020) Socioeconomic inequalities in disability-free life expectancy in older people from England and the United States: a cross-national population-based study. *The Journals of Gerontology: Series A* 75(5), 906–913. https://doi.org/10.1093/gerona/glz266

26 Longevity

There is no answer to the question 'What is normal life expectancy?' but it is certain that our population is nowhere near reaching it. Indeed, it has been suggested that humans have evolved not only to live longer but also to exercise into old age (Lieberman *et al.*, 2021). That this can happen is illustrated by the 'Blue Zone' phenomenon. These optimal wellness enclaves are found around the globe from Okinawa in Japan to Ikaria in Greece. They are home to an extraordinarily high number of people who live far longer than average, into their nineties and hundreds. What these healthy nonagenarians and centenarians all seem to share is that they exercise moderately as part of their daily lives. This kind of natural daily movement is known as NEAT, which stands for non-exercise activity thermogenesis (Levine, 2002). NEAT is all the non-planned physical activity we do each day, like climbing stairs, walking, cooking and brushing our teeth. These types of movement may seem insignificant, but when added up, NEAT may account for as many as 2000 Calories of energy output per day.

Until very recently, despite our thoroughly unhealthy lifestyles, we have seen a gradual increase in lifespan. In the years between 1991 and 2014 average life expectancy for men rose from 73.6 years in 1991 to 79.4 years in 2014. For women the figures were from 79.0 to 83.1 years (Office for National Statistics, 2014). This unexpectedly good news has recently 'hit the buffers' with figures produced by Public Health England (2017) suggesting that the trend has now flattened. Indeed, before the Covid-19 pandemic, the Institute and Faculty of Actuaries (2018) calculated that at the age of 65, the life expectancy of a man has fallen by 4 months and that of a woman has fallen by a whole year. This will be good news for the pensions industry, which will reap a reward of £27 billion in liabilities from company balance sheets. The same is true in the USA (Woolf and Schoomaker, 2019), where life expectancy fell in 2017 from 78.7 to 78.6 years, after rising from 69.9 years over the previous six decades. More importantly, the duration of healthy life – healthspan (see Chapter 25, this volume) – has been falling for several years, while the years spent in poor health have increased. One reason given for this decline in lifespan has been socio-economic disadvantage aggravated by austerity measures (Hawkes, 2019). Low income is linked to most of the non-communicable diseases that contribute to premature death and a possible link is provided by the lower levels of exercise and fitness among the less well-off (Matsuo and So, 2021).

Effect of Exercise on Lifespan

As discussed in Chapter 7 (this volume), there are two ways of judging how much and how effectively a person exercises:

1. *Assessing physical activity by either questionnaire or direct observation.* The former is biased by the individual's tendency to exaggerate, driven by so-called 'social desirability bias', and almost always gives a much greater exercise estimate than the latter. Direct observation gives the most accurate measure of physical activity but has a number of problems – it is difficult to do, difficult to compare between exercise types, takes special equipment and is expensive, and it only gives a result which applies to the period of observation. Most people will 'up their game' when they know they are being observed.

2. *Measuring physical fitness.* There is a direct relationship between amount of exercise taken and physical fitness level, but with wide variations (Stofan *et al.*, 2008). There are other variables which affect the relationship such as inherited characteristics. However, this method has the strength of giving a measurement which does not depend upon the unreliable witness of the participant.

DOI: 10.1079/9781800621855.0026

Exercise Volume and Longevity

Volume of exercise

The original observations on the relationship between physical activity and disease came from the comparison between London bus drivers and bus conductors. Professor Jerry Morris's 1950s study looked at heart attack rates and mortality of the two groups. The drivers represented inactivity, sitting behind the wheel, unable to exercise while suffering all the frustration of steering a bus around the city. The conductors on the other hand personified physical activity, on their feet all day, running up and down the stairs and taking plenty of exercise. As was anticipated, the drivers had a higher mortality, largely due to a greater risk of coronary disease (Morris *et al.*, 1953).

In those days the number of physically active workers was considerably greater than is the case nowadays. Mechanization has greatly reduced the role of work in making the working man take exercise. Morris repeated his findings in a comparison of the leisure-time activities of civil servants. Those who exercised vigorously as part of their leisure activity fared much better than their sedentary colleagues (Morris *et al.*, 1990). One of his findings was the presence of a threshold for the effect of exercise. It was only those taking vigorous exercise in their leisure time who benefited. Lower levels of exercise did not prolong life. An approximate level

for this threshold was 40 minutes' exercise to a state of breathlessness three to four times per week. However there is a paradox. More recent studies have indicated that leisure-time exercise does reduce mortality, but work-related exercise may actually increase premature death (Holtermann *et al.*, 2021).

The threshold effect has not been confirmed by subsequent studies, nearly all of which have found a graded effect of increasing activity on mortality starting with very modest levels of exercise. The Framingham study followed a large group of middle-aged and older citizens in the USA. For this cohort, moderate activity increased the length of life by 1.3 years in men and 1.5 years in women. High levels of physical activity further increased these figures to 3.7 and 3.5 years, respectively (Franco *et al.*, 2005).

Wen *et al.* (2011) performed an 8-year follow-up of more than 400,000 adults who had been questioned about their physical activity at baseline. They found a steady increase in longevity from the lowest to the highest activity, levelling off at very high exercise rates. They concluded that optimal results were achieved by exercising for 90 to 100 minutes per day, which is far more than is recommended by health guidelines and achieved only by very few dedicated individuals (Fig. 26.1).

These findings have been replicated by a number of subsequent studies (Moore *et al.*, 2012; Zhao *et al.*, 2019) which have concluded that those who

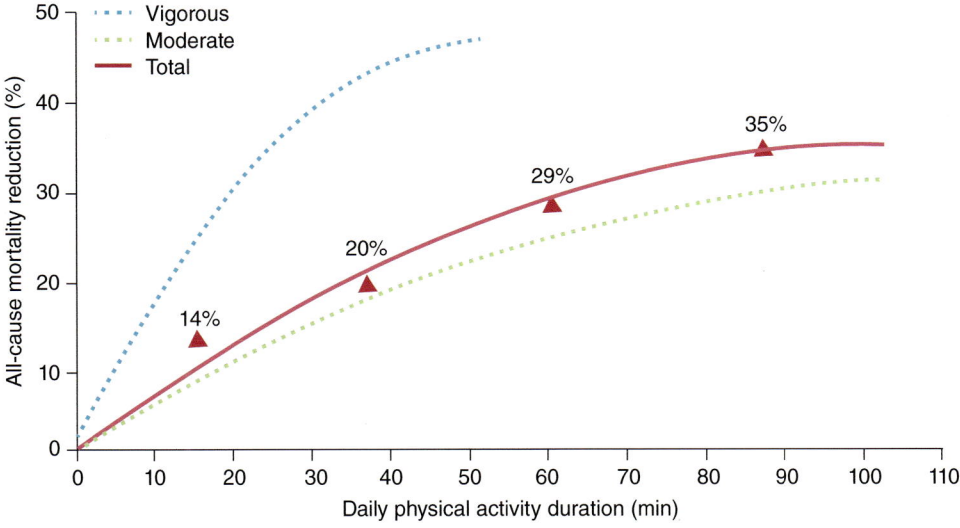

Fig. 26.1. Effects of duration and intensity of exercise on reduction of all-cause mortality. (From Wen *et al.*, 2011, used with permission.)

satisfy the widely used recommendation of 150 minutes of moderate-to-vigorous exercise per week gain between 3.4 and 4.5 life years (Wen *et al.* 2011). Other follow-up studies have reported similar findings, with step counting (Lee *et al.*, 2019; Paluch *et al.*, 2021) showing a dose response increase in benefit from less than 2700 steps to more than 7500 steps.

Not all studies have agreed on the optimal amount of exercise for prolonging life. Some have found a ceiling effect (Schnohr *et al.*, 2015), but the majority have shown a clear association with increasing duration, intensity and frequency of exercise at least up to 300 minutes of vigorous exercise per week (Samitz *et al.*, 2011; Moore *et al.*, 2012; Lear *et al.*, 2017). Aerobic exercise is more effective for prolonging life than muscle strengthening but a combination of the two has the greatest effect (Zhao *et al.*, 2020). There is some evidence that regular swimming may be even more effective in postponing mortality (Chase *et al.*, 2008).

Commuting to work can have an effect. A study of more than half a million adults aged 40 to 69, followed up for 5 years, found that those who cycled to work had about half the risk of dying during this time as those who used public transport (Celis-Morales *et al.*, 2017).

Intensity of exercise

Exercise intensity is also a factor. A systematic review and meta-analysis showed a 10% survival advantage of moderate-to-vigorous exercise compared with light exercise (Ramakrishnan *et al.*, 2021). When the ratio of vigorous to moderately vigorous exercise was compared in 403,000 US adults, the higher the proportion of vigorous exercise, the greater the reduction in all-cause mortality (Wang *et al.*, 2021).

Aerobic versus muscle-strengthening exercise

The type of exercise also influences reduction in mortality. The US National Health Interview Survey of nearly half a million subjects comparing their patterns of exercise showed a mortality reduction of 11% for muscle-strengthening exercise, 29% for aerobic and 40% for a combination of the two (Zhao *et al.*, 2020). In ex-Olympic champions a greater benefit is found for those involved in aerobic sport than in power events and the effect is also enhanced in those who maintained regular exercise after their days of Olympic glory, with an increase in life expectancy of up to 5 years (Bauman and Blair, 2012). Others have confirmed that, compared with the general population, endurance athletes live longer than members of the general public but power athletes do not share this benefit (Lemez and Baker, 2015).

Recreational and competitive sport

Examples of the life-prolonging effect of regular exercise have also looked at those who take regular vigorous exercise as part of their sporting activities such as runners, cyclists and swimmers. One study reviewed 500 runners aged 50–59 and compared them with age-matched and sex-matched controls. After 19 years, 15% of the runners but 34% of controls had died (Chakravarty *et al.*, 2008). A review of all the available evidence indicates that runners have a 30–50% reduced risk of mortality during follow-up and live approximately 3 years longer than non-runners (Lee *et al.*, 2017). Increasing the time spent running and increasing the intensity are both related to benefit up to about 4 hours per week and a total dose of 50 MET hours per week. Above this dose of exercise, further benefit is doubtful and there might be a small reduction. A much-quoted criticism of the benefit of exercise is the cynical suggestion that the amount of time spent exercising is about the same as the increase in lifespan. Such cynicism is convincingly debunked in Lee *et al.*'s (2017) study. The authors calculate that every hour spent in exercise increases lifespan by 7 hours.

A study of 15,000 Olympic Medal winners gives another perspective – a survival of about 3 years longer than the general population – irrespective of the colour of the medal (Clarke *et al.*, 2012). When it comes to specific sports, an analysis of longevity of 'sporting legends' found that Wimbledon finalists lived longest, followed by rugby captains, cricket captains and British Open champions (Mayhew, 2021). Boxing champions, however, had shorter lives.

Starting later

Is it ever too late to start exercising? The answer is a qualified no, but the effect on longevity takes a while to become established. It probably takes about 10 years of high levels of activity to increase longevity (Byberg *et al.*, 2009). A cohort of more than 315,000 Americans aged 50 to 71 had their exercise habits tracked and were followed up for 20 years. Unsurprisingly the mortality during follow-up was about 35% lower in the habitually active group than in those who took little exercise. Surprising, however, was the finding that those who took up exercise later in life and then maintained it had a similar reduction in mortality to that of the active group (Mok *et al.*, 2019; Saint-Maurice *et al.*, 2019).

Regular exercise reduces the risk of a number of non-communicable diseases, and this must largely explain its effect on life expectancy. However, there other intriguing contributors including an effect on cellular ageing. DNA is the genetic chromosome-carrying material, which is found in all the cells in our bodies. Telomeres are the caps on the end of each strand of DNA and they protect the DNA from damage each time a cell reproduces itself. With time and repeated cell division the telomeres become shortened and may indeed become so short that they cannot protect the DNA, with subsequent cellular disruption. Telomere length (LTL) is thus allied to cellular age and represents our biological age rather than our chronological age. Regular exercise has an effect on telomere length. There is a positive and significant relationship between both physical activity and CRF and telomere length, most marked in middle-aged and older people, which emphasizes the importance of CRF for healthy ageing (Tucker, 2017; Marques *et al.*, 2020). A study at Leicester University looked at the relationship between walking speed and LTL. The researchers found that steady/average and brisk walkers had significantly longer LTL compared with slow walkers, with accelerometer-assessed measures of physical activity further supporting this through an association between LTL and habitual activity intensity, but not with total amount of activity (Dempsey *et al.*, 2022). Bidirectional Mendelian randomization analyses suggest a causal link between walking pace and LTL, but not the other way around.

The reduction in cellular ageing has been found to be about 9 years in very active older people (Tucker, 2017). This effect may be enhanced by the ability of exercise to influence mitochondrial structure and protein production (Robinson *et al.*, 2017).

Physical Fitness and Longevity

There is a clear relationship between increasing habitual exercise and increasing physical fitness (Public Health England, 2017). Take running, for instance: every 30 minutes of running per week is associated with 0.5 MET higher fitness level. Numerous studies have confirmed the relationship between physical fitness and life expectancy. Indeed physical fitness in middle age is the best predictor bar none of what age you will achieve, and that includes blood cholesterol level, presence of obesity, high BP or diabetes or even pre-existent heart disease, and cigarette smoking (Blair, 2009). Only increasing age is a better predictor of how many years are left to you. The reduction in mortality in the fit compared with the unfit is largely due to lower rates of CVD and cancer (Sandvik *et al.*, 1993).

A summary of the results of 33 studies which compared physical fitness and mortality was published in 2009 (Kodama *et al.*, 2009). The population included over 100,000 people without heart disease, diabetes, high BP or high blood cholesterol. The subjects had all had an initial exercise test to measure their fitness and were then followed for a mean of 11 years. Fitness was expressed in metabolic equivalents, METs. It was divided into three categories – low fitness being less than 7.9 METs (VO_2 = 27.6 ml/min/kg), intermediate fitness between 7.9 and 10.6 METs (27.6–37.1 ml/min/kg) and high fitness above 10.7 METs (37.4 ml/min/kg). There was a clear correlation between low fitness level and mortality, with the risk of dying being 70% higher in the low-fitness group than in the high-fitness group. Moreover, for every 1-MET increase in fitness (equivalent to an increase in walk/jog speed of 1 kph) there was a 13% decrease in risk of dying. A similar study in 2015 found that the effect of fitness was even greater than this for younger age groups, with an 18% lower mortality rate per 1-MET increase in fitness for those aged under 40 compared with the 12% figure for those aged over 70 (Blaha *et al.*, 2016). A study from Cleveland, Ohio, tested the relationship between physical fitness and mortality in 122,000 people followed up for an average of 8 years following a treadmill test. The relationship was stark, with CRF being inversely related to mortality over the period of study. This was most obvious in those with the very highest levels of fitness. These individuals had just one-fifth the risk of dying than the least fit. The greatest benefit between being fit and being very fit was found in the over-70s, confirming the effectiveness and importance of exercise in older people (Mandsanger *et al.*, 2018).

Walking pace can be used as an indication of CRF (Yates *et al.*, 2017) and the UK Biobank study recorded a lifespan advantage for higher walking speeds (Laukkanen and Kunutsor, 2019). That study of walking pace in nearly half a million participants found a fast pace to be associated with increased lifespan across a wide range of BMI. The fast walkers lived about 5 years longer than the slower. There is a clear relationship between CRF and age-related mortality – the fitter the individual, the lower the mortality (Fig. 26.2).

The Copenhagen study of middle-aged men also put figures to the expected years of life gained at different levels of fitness (Clausen *et al.*, 2018). More than 5000 men aged around 50 had formal exercise testing. They were then followed up for 46 years. Compared with those in the bottom 5% for CRF, those with low normal fitness lived an extra 2.1 years, those with high normal fitness lived an extra 2.9 years and the top 5% lived an extra 4.9 years. They calculated that for each unit increase in VO_{2max} there was an increase in life expectancy of 45 days (Fig. 26.3).

As with taking up exercise later in life, older individuals who improve their fitness also improve their life expectancy (Kokkinos *et al.*, 2010). In a large epidemiological study involving older male veterans (age 65–92 years) with an 8-year median follow-up, an inverse and graded association between impaired exercise capacity (in METs) and all-cause mortality was noted. Mortality risk was 12% lower for every 1-MET increase in exercise capacity, regardless of age, remarkably similar to the finding above. The biggest relative benefit was found for the higher fitness groups.

Special Situations

- Obese individuals gain as much as those of normal weight but the life shortening of a combination of fatness and unfitness can be disastrous. These individuals die on average more than 7 years sooner than those of normal weight and physical activity (Clausen *et al.*, 2018).
- The lifespan of diabetics can be increased by regular cycling, and the more the better. Compared with no cycling, any cycling reduced 5-year mortality by 24% in one group of diabetics with the greatest reduction for those who

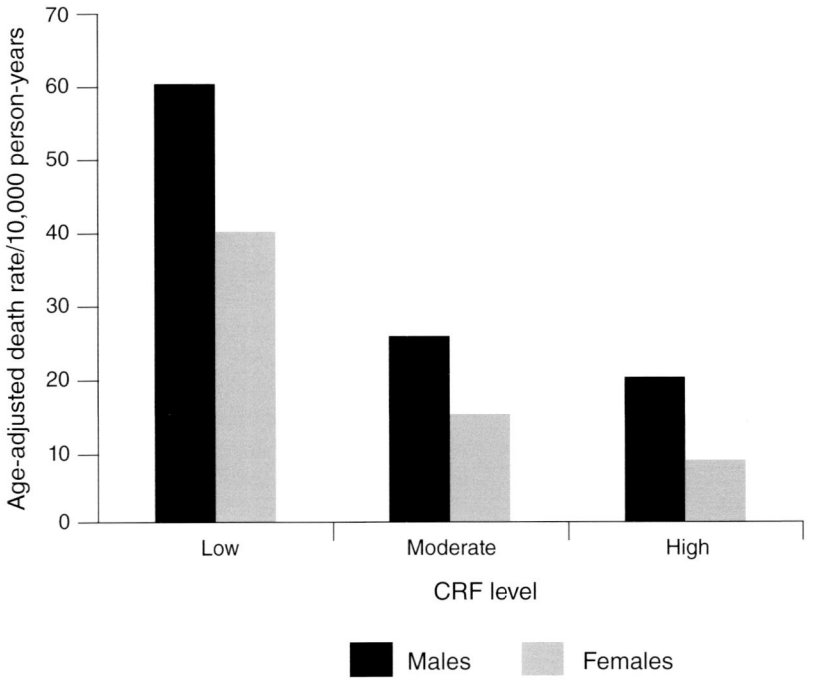

Fig. 26.2. Effect of different levels of CRF on age-adjusted mortality.

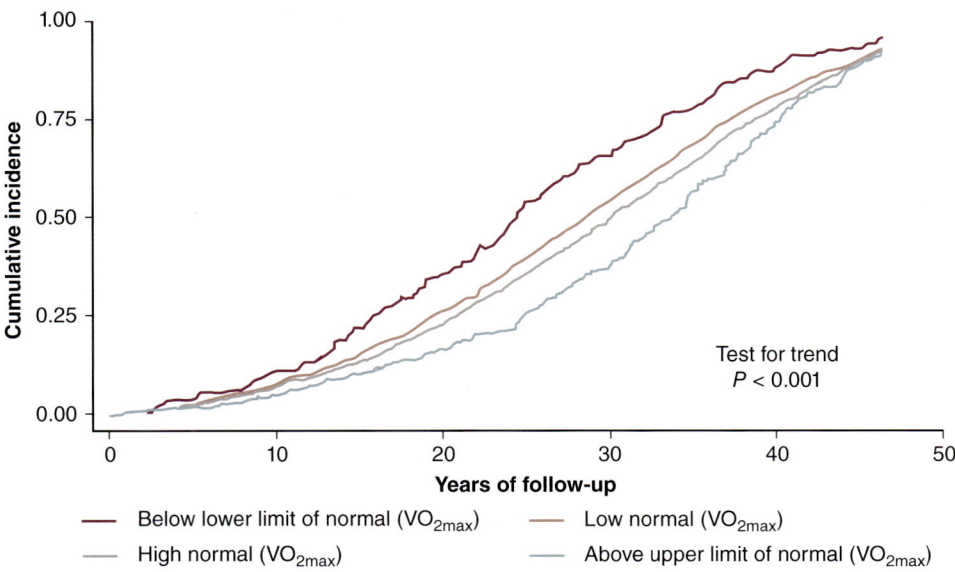

Fig. 26.3. Mortality rates over time for different levels of physical fitness. (From Clausen *et al.*, 2018, used with permission.)

cycled for between 150 and 299 minutes per week (Ried-Larsen *et al.*, 2021).

- In hypertensive patients there is a dose-response effect of exercise on mortality at all levels of BP (Joseph *et al.*, 2019).
- Running has been shown to be highly protective against cancer mortality – any amount of running reduces death rates. One meta-analysis showed that running participation is associated with 27, 30 and 23% lower risk of all-cause, cardiovascular and cancer mortality, respectively, compared with no running (Pedisic *et al.*, 2020).
- Regular exercise and high levels of CRF protect against sudden cardiac death. One meta-analysis found the relative risk of sudden death to be 0.52 for the highest versus the lowest levels of physical activity and 0.58 for the highest versus the lowest CRF (Aune *et al.*, 2020). There is a dose-response relationship between physical activity and the risk of sudden death – compared with inactive people the HR is 0.79 for low levels, 0.67 for moderate levels and 0.55 for high levels of activity (Hansen *et al.*, 2021).

The facts are clear. Low levels of exercise and low physical fitness are both predictors of premature mortality and shortening of total lifespan. Low fitness levels have been calculated to account for 16% of premature deaths, substantially more than any other risk factor including cigarette smoking, diabetes, obesity, raised blood cholesterol or hypertension. And we should not be surprised that other measures of physical performance are also associated with longer life, including grip strength and balance (Cooper *et al.*, 2010) as well as leg-muscle strength (Ruiz *et al.*, 2008).

- The possible impact of an increase in the level of physical activity of the population at large would be considerable. A study of nearly 5000 adults between the ages of 40 and 85 suggested that an increase in average moderate intensity physical activity by 10, 20 and 30% could reduce premature mortality by 6.9, 13.0 and 16.9%, respectively (Saint-Maurice *et al.*, 2022). Moreover, the effects of increasing physical activity compare well with the effects of a number of different medications (Naci and Ioannidis, 2015) and of other healthy behaviours (Maron *et al.*, 2018).

Summary

Regular exercise and high levels of physical fitness are associated with an increase in life expectancy of between 3 and 10 years. For similar doses of exercise, vigorous activity is more effective than moderate activity. The increase in longevity is mediated by lower rates of the common degenerative diseases of later life. The steady increase in life expectancy seen over the past half century has stalled recently, which is probably due to higher rates of obesity, diabetes, cancers, etc. – all more prevalent in sedentary populations.

References

Aune, D., Schlesinger, S., Hamer, M., Norat, T. and Riboli, E. (2020) Physical activity and the risk of sudden cardiac death: a systematic review and meta-analysis of prospective studies. *BMC Cardiovascular Disorders* 20(1), 318. https://doi.org/10.1186/s12872-020-01531-z

Bauman, A.E. and Blair, S.N. (2012) Elite athletes' survival advantage. *BMJ* 345, e8338.

Blaha, M.J., Hung, R.K., Dardarl, Z., Feldman, D.I., Whelton, S.P., et al. (2016) Age-dependent value of exercise capacity and derivation of fitness-associated biologic age. *Heart* 102, 431–437.

Blair, S.N. (2009) Physical inactivity: the biggest public health problem of the 21st century. *British Journal of Sports Medicine* 43, 1–2.

Byberg, L., Melhus, H., Gedeborg, R., Sundström, J., Ahlbom, A., et al. (2009) Total mortality after changes in leisure time physical activity in 50 year old men: 35 year follow-up of population based cohort. *British Journal of Sports Medicine* 43, 482.

Celis-Morales, C.A., Lyall, D.M., Welsh, P., Anderson, J., Steell, L., et al. (2017) Association between active commuting and incident cardiovascular disease, cancer and mortality. *BMJ* 357, j1456.

Chakravarty, E.F., Hubert, H.B., Lingala, V.B. and Fries, J.F. (2008) Reduced disability and mortality among aging runners: a 21-year longitudinal study. *Archives of Internal Medicine* 168, 1638–1646.

Chase, N.L., Sui, X. and Blair, S.N. (2008) Swimming and all-cause mortality risk compared with running, walking, and sedentary habits in men. *International Journal of Aquatic Research and Education* 2(3), 3.

Clarke, P.M., Walter, S.J., Hayen, A., Mallon, W.J., Heijmans, J. and Studdert, D.M. (2012) Survival of the fittest: retrospective cohort study of the longevity of Olympic medallists in the modern era. *BMJ* 345, e8308. https://doi.org/10.1136/bmj.e8308

Clausen, J.S.R., Marott, J.L., Holtermann, A., Gyntelberg, F. and Jensen, M.T. (2018) Midlife cardiorespiratory fitness and the long-term risk of mortality: 46 years of follow-up. *Journal of the American College of Cardiology* 72(9), 987–995. https://doi.org/10.1016/j.jacc.2018.06.045

Cooper, R., Kuh, D. and Hardy, R. (2010) Objectively measured physical capability levels and mortality: systematic review and meta-analysis. *BMJ* 341, c4467.

Dempsey, P.C., Musicha, C., Rowlands, A.V., Davies, M., Khunti, K., et al. (2022) Investigation of a UK biobank cohort reveals causal associations of self-reported walking pace with telomere length. *Communications Biology* 5, 381.

Franco, O.H., de Laet, C., Peeters, A., Jonker, J., Mackenbach, J. and Nusselder, W. (2005) Effects of physical activity on life expectancy with cardiovascular disease. *Archives of Internal Medicine* 165, 2355–2360.

Hansen, K.W., Peytz, N., Blokstra, A., Bojesen, S.E., Celis-Morales, C., et al. (2021) Association of fatal myocardial infarction with past level of physical activity: a pooled analysis of cohort studies. *European Journal of Preventive Cardiology* 28(14), 1590–1598. https://doi.org/10.1093/eurjpc/zwaa146

Hawkes, N. (2019) The 2010s: a decade of disappointment in UK healthcare. *BMJ* 367, l6895. https://doi.org/10.1136/bmj.l6895

Holtermann, A., Schnohr, P., Nordestgaard, B.G. and Marott, J.L. (2021) The physical activity paradox in cardiovascular disease and all-cause mortality: the contemporary Copenhagen General Population Study with 104 046 adults. *European Heart Journal* 42(15), 1499–1511. https://doi.org/10.1093/eurheartj/ehab087

Institute and Faculty of Actuaries (2018) CMI_2018: the latest version of the CMI Mortality Projections Model. Available at: https://www.actuaries.org.uk/system/files/field/document/CMI%20WP119%20v01%202019-03-07%20-%20CMI%20Mortality%20Projections%20Model%20CMI_2018%20Briefing%20Note.pdf (accessed 31 January 2023).

Joseph, G., Marott, J.L., Torp-Pedersen, C., Biering-Sørensen, T., Nielsen, G., et al. (2019) Dose-response association between level of physical activity and mortality in normal, elevated, and high blood pressure. *Hypertension* 74(6), 1307–1315. https://doi.org/10.1161/HYPERTENSIONAHA.119.13786

Kodama, S., Saito, K., Tanaka, S., Maki, M., Yachi, Y., et al. (2009) Cardiorespiratory fitness as a quantitative predictor of all-cause mortality and cardiovascular

Chapter 26

events in healthy men and women: a meta-analysis. *JAMA* 301, 202–2035.

Kokkinos, P., Myers, J., Faselis, C., Panagiotakos, D.B., Doumas, M., et al. (2010) Exercise capacity and mortality in older men: a 20-year follow-up study. *Circulation* 122, 790–797.

Laukkanen, J.A. and Kunutsor, S.K. (2019) Fitness equals longer life expectancy regardless of adiposity levels. *Mayo Clinic Proceedings* 94(6), 942–945. https://doi.org/10.1016/j.mayocp.2019.04.016

Lear, S.A., Hu, W., Rangarajan, S., Gasevic, D., Leong, D., et al. (2017) The effect of physical activity on mortality and cardiovascular disease in 130 000 people from 17 high-income, middle-income, and low-income countries: the PURE study. *Lancet* 390, 2643–2654.

Lee, D., Brellenthin, A.G., Thompson, P.D., Sui, X., Lee, I.-M. and Lavie, C.J. (2017) Running as a key lifestyle medicine for longevity. *Progress in Cardiovascular Diseases* 60(1), 45–55. https://doi.org/10.1016/j.pcad.2017.03.005

Lee, I.-M., Shiroma, E.J., Kamada, M., Bassett, D.R., Matthews, C.E. and Buring, J.E. (2019) Association of step volume and intensity with all-cause mortality in older women. *JAMA Internal Medicine* 179(8), 1105–1112. https://doi.org/10.1001/jamainternmed.2019.0899

Lemez, S. and Baker, J. (2015) Do elite athletes live longer? A systematic review of mortality and longevity in elite athletes. *Sports Medicine Open* 1(1), 16. https://doi.org/10.1186/s40798-015-0024-x

Levine, J.A. (2002) Non-exercise activity thermogenesis (NEAT). *Best Practice & Research Clinical Endocrinology & Metabolism* 16(4), 679–702. https://doi.org/10.1053/beem.2002.0227

Lieberman, D.E., Kistner, T.M., Richard, D., Lee, I.-M. and Baggish, A.L. (2021) The active grandparent hypothesis: physical activity and the evolution of extended human healthspans and lifespans. *Proceedings of the National Academy of Sciences USA* 118(50), e2107621118. https://doi.org/10.1073/pnas.2107621118

Mandsanger, K., Harb, S., Cremer, P., Phelan, D., Nissen, S.E. and Jaber, W. (2018) Association of cardiorespiratory fitness with long-term mortality among adults undergoing exercise treadmill testing. *JAMA Network Open* 1(6), e183605. https://doi.org/10.1001/jamanetworkopen.2018.3605

Maron, D.J., Mancini, G.B.J., Hartigan, P.M., Spertus, J.A., Sedlis, S.P., et al. (2018) Healthy behavior, risk factor control, and survival in the COURAGE trial. *Journal of the American College of Cardiology* 72(19), 2297–2305. https://doi.org/10.1016/j.jacc.2018.08.2163

Marques, A., Gouveira, É.R., Peralta, M., Martins, J., Venturini, J., et al. (2020) Cardiorespiratory fitness and telomere length: a systematic review. *Journal of Sports Sciences* 38(14), 1690–1697. https://doi.org/10.1080/02640414.2020.1754739

Matsuo, T. and So, R. (2021) Socioeconomic status relates to exercise habits and cardiorespiratory fitness among workers in the Tokyo area. *Journal of Occupational Health* 63(1), e12187. https://doi.org/10.1002/1348-9585.12187

Mayhew, L. (2021) The longevity of sporting legends. Available at: https://www.researchgate.net/publication/352379982_The_longevity_of_sporting_legends (accessed 24 January 2023).

Mok, A., Khaw, K.-T., Luben, R., Wareham, N. and Brage, S. (2019) Physical activity trajectories and mortality: population based cohort study. *BMJ* 365, l2323. https://doi.org/10.1136/bmj.l2323

Moore, S.C., Patel, A.V., Matthews, C.E., Berrington de Gonzalez, A., Park, Y., et al. (2012) Leisure time physical activity of moderate to vigorous intensity and mortality: a large pooled cohort analysis. *PLoS Medicine* 9(11), e1001335. https://doi.org/10.1371/journal.pmed.1001335

Morris, J.N., Heady, J.A., Raffle, P.A., Roberts, C.G. and Parks, J.W. (1953) Coronary heart disease and physical activity of work. *Lancet* 262, 1053–1057.

Morris, J.N., Clayton, D.G., Everitt, M.G., Semmence, A.M. and Burgess, E.H. (1990) Exercise in leisure time: coronary attack and death rates. *British Heart Journal* 63, 325–334.

Naci, H. and Ioannidis, J.P. (2015) Comparative effectiveness of exercise and drug interventions on mortality outcomes: metaepidemiological study. *British Journal of Sports Medicine* 49(21), 1414–1422. https://doi.org/10.1136/bjsports-2015-f5577rep

Office for National Statistics (2014) Life expectancy at birth and at age 65 by local areas in England and Wales: 2012 to 2014. Available at: https://www.ons.gov.uk/peoplepopulationandcommunity/birthsdeathsandmarriages/lifeexpectancies/bulletins/lifeexpectancyatbirthandatage65bylocalareasinenglandandwales/2015-11-04 (accessed 31 January 2023).

Paluch, A.E., Gabriel, K.P., Fulton, J.E., Lewis, C.E., Schreiner, P.J., et al. (2021) Steps per day and all-cause mortality in middle-aged adults in the Coronary Artery Risk Development in Young Adults study. *JAMA Network Open* 4(9), e2124516. https://doi.org/10.1001/jamanetworkopen.2021.24516

Pedisic, Z., Shrestha, N., Kovalchik, S., Stamatakis, E., Liangruenrom, N., et al. (2020) Is running associated with a lower risk of all-cause, cardiovascular and cancer mortality, and is the more the better? A systematic review and meta-analysis. *British Journal of Sports Medicine* 54, 898–905.

Public Health England (2017) Health profile for England: 2017. Chapter 1: Life expectancy and healthy life expectancy. Available at: https://www.gov.uk/government/publications/health-profile-for-england/chapter-1-life-expectancy-and-healthy-life-expectancy (accessed 31 January 2023).

Ramakrishnan, R., He, J.R., Ponsonby, A.L., Woodward, M., Rahimi, K., et al. (2021) Objectively measured physical activity and all-cause mortality: a systematic review and meta-analysis. *Preventive Medicine* 143, 106356. https://doi.org/10.1016/j.ypmed.2020.106356

Ried-Larsen, M., Rasmussen, M.G., Blond, K., Overvad, T.F., Overvad, K., *et al.* (2021) Association of cycling with all-cause and cardiovascular disease mortality among persons with diabetes: the European Prospective Investigation into Cancer and Nutrition (EPIC) study. *JAMA Internal Medicine* 181(9), 1196–1205. https://doi.org/10.1001/jamainternmed.2021.3836

Robinson, M.M., Dasari, S., Konopka, A.R., Johnson, M.L., Manjunatha, S., *et al.* (2017) Enhanced protein translation underlies improved metabolic and physical adaptations to different exercise training modes in young and old humans. *Cell Metabolism* 25(3), 581–592. https://doi.org/10.1016/j.cmet.2017.02.009

Ruiz, J.R., Sui, X., Lobelo, F., Morrow, J.R. Jr, Jackson, A.W., *et al.* (2008) Association between muscular strength and mortality in men: prospective cohort study. *BMJ* 337, a439.

Saint-Maurice, P., Coughlan, D., Kelly, S.P., Keadle, S.K., Cook, M.B., *et al.* (2019) Association of leisure time physical activity across the adult life course with all-cause and cause-specific mortality. *JAMA Network Open* 2(3), e190355. https://doi.org/10.1001/jamanetworkopen.2019.0355

Saint-Maurice, P.F., Graubard, B.I., Troiano, R.P., Berrigan, D., Galuska, D.A., *et al.* (2022) Estimated number of deaths prevented through increased physical activity among US adults. *JAMA Internal Medicine* 182(3), 349–352. https://doi.org/10.1001/jamainternmed.2021.7755

Samitz, G., Egger, M. and Zwahlen, M. (2011) Domains of physical activity and all-cause mortality: systematic review and dose–response meta-analysis of cohort studies. *International Journal of Epidemiology* 40(5), 1382–1400.

Sandvik, L., Erikssen, J., Thaulow, E., Mundal, R. and Rodahl, K. (1993) Physical fitness as a predictor of mortality among healthy, middle-aged Norwegian men. *New England Journal of Medicine* 328, 533–537.

Schnohr, P., O'Keefe, J.H., Marott, J.L., Lange, P. and Jensen, G.B. (2015) Dose of jogging and long-term mortality: the Copenhagen City Heart Study. *Journal of the American College of Cardiology* 65(5), 411–419. https://doi.org/10.1016/j.jacc.2014.11.023

Stofan, J.R., DiPietro, L., Davis, D., Kohl, H.W. 3rd and Blair, S.N. (2008) Physical activity patterns associated with cardiorespiratory fitness and reduced mortality: the Aerobics Centre Longitudinal Study. *American Journal of Public Health* 88, 1807–1813.

Tucker, L.A. (2017) Physical activity and telomere length in US men and women: an NHANES investigation. *Preventive Medicine* 100, 145–151. https://doi.org/10.1016/j.ypmed.2017.04.027

Wang, Y., Nie, J., Ferrari, G., Rey-Lopez, J.P. and Rezende, L.F.M. (2021) Association of physical activity intensity with mortality: a national cohort study of 403 681 US adults. *JAMA Internal Medicine* 181(2), 203–211. https://doi.org/10.1001/jamainternmed.2020.6331

Wen, C.P., Wai, J.P., Tsai, M.K., Yang, Y.C., Cheng, T.Y., *et al.* (2011) Minimum amount of physical activity for reduced mortality and extended life expectancy: a prospective cohort study. *Lancet* 378(9798), 1244–1253. https://doi.org/10.1016/S0140-6736(11)60749-6

Woolf, S.H. and Schoomaker, H. (2019) Life expectancy and mortality rates in the United States, 1959–2017. *JAMA* 322(20), 1996–2016. https://doi.org/10.1001/jama.2019.16932

Yates, T., Zaccardi, F., Dhalwani, N.N., Davies, M.J., Bakrania, K., *et al.* (2017) Association of walking pace and handgrip strength with all-cause, cardiovascular, and cancer mortality: a UK Biobank observational study. *European Heart Journal* 38(43), 3232–3240. https://doi.org/10.1093/eurheartj/ehx449

Zhao, M., Veeranki, S.P., Li, S., Steffen, L.M. and Xi, B. (2019) Beneficial associations of low and large doses of leisure time physical activity with all-cause, cardiovascular disease and cancer mortality: a national cohort study of 88,140 US adults. *British Journal of Sports Medicine* 53, 1405–1411.

Zhao, M., Veeranki, S.P., Magnussen, C.G. and Xi, B. (2020) Recommended physical activity and all cause and cause specific mortality in US adults: prospective cohort study. *BMJ* 370, m2031. https://doi.org/10.1136/bmj.m2031

27 The Social and Economic Costs of Inactivity

Maintaining good health and fighting disease and other health problems are enormously expensive. The UK NHS annual budget was set to be £212.1 billion in 2020/21, which is 9.9% of GDP and 30% of the spending on public services. The social-care budget is even higher. NHS spending is planned to increase by 4% per annum for the foreseeable future, but the demands are set to rise even more steeply. Currently about 18% of the population is over 65 and this will have risen to 25% by 2046. None of this takes account of the astronomical costs of managing the Covid-19 pandemic.

Increasing age brings increasing debility and medical advances compound this. These advances, while helping with the treatment of individual diseases, also result in longer survival and ultimately more cost to the NHS. Any effective treatment for the management of disease increases costs in the long term, because more people live longer with all the chronic diseases and dependency which old age brings. Exercise is the only treatment that does not increase NHS and social expenses. By improving health overall and reducing old-age dependency, it actually reduces the bill.

The Cost of Sedentary Behaviour

Inactivity, or sedentary behaviour, is associated with poor health at all ages. The social and economic costs of this are virtually impossible to calculate. The various estimates made by different bodies using assorted methods differ wildly, but they are all very large! One example calculated some of the associated costs in five common conditions, which are in part caused by inactivity. These were CVD, type 2 diabetes, cancer of the colon, cancer of the breast and cancer of the uterus (Heron *et al.*, 2019). They chose these conditions because they had well-validated measures of the 'population attributable fractions' for physical inactivity. This refers to what proportion of the cause of each disease could be blamed on a lack of exercise. For this small number of diseases – out of 20 possible conditions – their conclusion was that the cost to NHS-funding bodies was £800 million per annum. This may be a considerable underestimate. They also calculated that if excessive sedentary behaviour were eliminated, about 70,000 premature deaths annually in the UK could be avoided.

The medical costs of disease are only a very small part of the overall cost to the nation. For instance, the British Heart Foundation and Oxford University used the same diseases to calculate the direct cost to the NHS (Allender *et al.*, 2007). They believed that in 2003/4, over 35,000 deaths could have been avoided if the population were physically active at the levels recommended by the UK government. Physical inactivity was directly responsible for 3.1% of morbidity and mortality in the UK. Preventable sickness absence from work costs about £5 billion and premature death about £1 billion.

Again, this estimate vastly understates the overall costs to all those involved. These include the NHS, the national economy, the individual's finances and their employers' productivity and expenses. Some idea of the extent of these costs was given by another British Heart Foundation publication, *Physical Inactivity and Sedentary Behaviour Report* (BHF, 2017), based on 2010/11 figures. Table 27.1 illustrates the overall costs and the costs to the NHS of those conditions to which inactivity is a substantial contributor.

For CVD, there were almost 180,000 deaths and over 1.6 million hospital episodes (including consultant visits, ordinary admissions and day cases). The direct healthcare cost of all CVD was £8.7 billion, and the total economic cost (including healthcare cost, informal care and loss of productivity) was £18.9 billion. The average cost of a hospital admission for a CVD event is estimated to be £4614.

For colorectal cancer, annual treatment costs were approximately £1.1 billion, 18% of which

© H.J.N. Bethell and D. Brodie 2023. *Exercise: A Scientific and Clinical Overview*
(H.J.N. Bethell and D. Brodie)
DOI: 10.1079/9781800621855.0027

Table 27.1. The costs of inactivity – 2011 figures. (From BHF, 2017.)

Condition	Cost to NHS (£, billions)	Contribution of inactivity (%)	Cost of inactivity (£, millions)
CHD	5.0	10.5	543
Type 2 diabetes	1.2	13.0	158
Breast cancer	0.3	17.9	54
Colon cancer	3.5	18.7	65

could be prevented by regular exercise. The figures for breast cancer were a cost of £300 million, of which 18% could be prevented.

For diabetes, the cost of direct NHS patient care (which includes treatment, intervention and complications) for those living with type 2 diabetes was estimated at £8.8 billion, and the indirect costs (such as loss of productivity) were estimated to be £13 billion, 13% of which is preventable.

For obesity, the total annual cost to the NHS (including treatment and its consequences) was estimated to be £2 billion, with a total economic impact to the nation of around £10 billion. In the USA there is a large effect of obesity on healthcare costs, with an average increase in cost of US$2505 for the obese compared with those of normal weight (Cawley *et al.*, 2021). There is a 'dose-response' relationship with the figure being US$1703 for Class 1 obesity rising to US$5852 for Class 3. The total annual cost to the US healthcare system is in the region of US$260 billion.

Physical Activity and Costs

A number of studies have examined the relationship between CRF and costs to society. In the USA, a sample of nearly 10,000 subjects from the Veterans Exercising Testing Study (Myers *et al.*, 2018) showed a relationship between CRF and healthcare costs. The least-fit quartile had higher costs by US$14,662 per annum compared with the fittest quartile. There was a dose-response relationship with each MET increment in fitness being associated with a reduced cost per patient per annum of US$1592.

There has been an inverse relationship between CRF and likelihood of being admitted to hospital for those infected by Covid-19. The Mayo Clinic group (Brawner *et al.*, 2021) identified 246 patients with Covid-19 who had received a recent exercise

test. Among these, 89 (36%) were hospitalized. CRF was significantly lower among patients who were hospitalized (mean 6.7 METs) compared with those not hospitalized (mean 8.0 METs). Each unit higher of peak METs was independently associated with 13% lower odds of hospitalization. If these figures were generalized, the implication for the costs of the pandemic to the NHS would be huge.

Simple community initiatives to increase exercise levels have been shown to reduce healthcare costs. One practice which has organized a walking programme for 10 years analysed its hospital costs and compared them with those of a comparable local practice. The 'walking' practice had hospital costs of about £8000 per 1000 patients per annum compared with £12,000–13,000 for the other practice (Cracknell, 2014).

A European Perspective

A 2015 report from the Centre for Economic and Business Research and the International Sport and Culture Association calculated that physical inactivity was the fourth leading risk factor for global deaths and the cause of 500,000 deaths in the European Union, with a cost of £84 billion per year to the European economy (ISCA Report, 2015). The report considered that physical inactivity was a bigger risk to public health than smoking. The study also showed that being physically inactive goes beyond physical disorders. One in four Europeans (or 83 million people) is affected by mental ill health. The research estimates the indirect cost of inactivity-related mood and anxiety disorders to be over €23 billion per year.

The Costs of Care for the Elderly

A report from the All-Party Commission on Physical Activity (2014) estimates that inactivity is costing the UK £20 billion per year and causing 37,000 premature deaths. This financial estimate includes the costs of treating all those conditions that are caused by a sedentary lifestyle. These conditions include obesity, high BP, diabetes and all the others discussed above. It also considers lost working days due to sickness and lack of productivity of unfit workers. It must be a vast underestimate, since it does not take account of the huge costs of caring for elderly dependent people. A current estimate of the cost to the public purse of care of the elderly is about £22 billion – and the notional cost of informal care is an incredible £68 billion. Despite this, in the past 5 years £900 million has been cut from the UK Public Health grants given to local councils, who bear the brunt of the social-care expenses. Moreover, our current social-services provision is underfunded and totally inadequate. More than 500,000 adults in the UK are awaiting social-care assessments and if these deficiencies are to be met the costs will escalate further (BMJ News, 2022).

Inactivity also brings all the social costs discussed in previous chapters of this book. The most important of these is the progressive loss of physical ability in later life. This includes the difficulty in carrying out ADL, the loss of well-being, the loss of independence and the consequent financial burden of needing care. The overall benefits of good health are incalculable, but these benefits are quite transparent and easily recognizable.

Political action is urgently needed to prioritize the promotion and encouragement of physical activity for the whole population, particularly in later life.

Summary

The economic and social costs of inactivity and subsequent health issues are huge. Over 37,000 deaths could be avoided annually if people were more physically active. Simple community activities, such as walking, can reduce healthcare costs significantly. Physical inactivity is considered to be the fourth leading risk factor in global deaths. Inactivity is costing the UK over £20 billion per year.

References

Allender, S., Foster, C., Scarborough, P. and Rayner, M. (2007) The burden of physical activity-related ill health in the UK. *Journal of Epidemiology and Community Health* 61(4), 344–348.

All-Party Commission on Physical Activity (2014) Tackling physical inactivity – a coordinated approach. Available at: https://parliamentarycommissiononphysicalactivity. files.wordpress.com/2014/04/apcopa-final.pdf (accessed 30 January 2023).

BHF (2017) *Physical Inactivity and Sedentary Behaviour Report 2017*. British Heart Foundation, London. Available at: https://www.bhf.org.uk/informationsupport/publications/statistics/physical-inactivity-report-2017 (accessed 30 January 2023).

BMJ News (2022) Seven days in medicine: 11–17 May 2022. *BMJ* 377, o1227.

Brawner, C.A., Ehrman, J.K., Bole, S., Kerrigan, D.J., Parikh, S.S., *et al.* (2021) Inverse relationship of maximal exercise capacity to hospitalization secondary to coronavirus disease 2019. *Mayo Clinic Proceedings* 96(1), 32–39. https://doi.org/10.1016/j.mayocp.2020. 10.003

Cawley, J., Biener, A., Meyerhoefer, C., Ding, Y., Zvenyach, T., *et al.* (2021) Direct medical costs of obesity in the United States and the most populous states. *Journal of Managed Care and Speciality Pharmacy* 27(3), 354–366. https://doi.org/10.18553/ jmcp.2021.20410

Cracknell, K. (2014) Interview – Dr John Morgan. *Health Club Management*, November/December 2014. Available at: https://www.healthclubmanagement.co. uk/health-club-management-people/Dr-John-Morgan/ 29483 (accessed 24 January 2023).

Heron, L., O'Neill, C., McAneney, H., Kee, F. and Tully, M.A. (2019) Direct healthcare costs of sedentary behaviour in the UK. *Journal of Epidemiology and Community Health* 73, 625–793.

ISCA Report (2015) *The Economic Cost of Physical Inactivity in Europe*. An ISCA/Cebr Report. International Sport and Culture Association (ISCA), Copenhagen/Centre for Economics and Business Research (Cebr), London

Myers, J., Doom, R., King, R., Fonda, H., Chan, K., *et al.* (2018) Association between cardiorespiratory fitness and health care costs: the Veterans Exercise Testing Study. *Mayo Clinic Proceedings* 93(1), 48–55. https:// doi.org/10.1016/j.mayocp.2017.09.019

28 Encouraging Exercise

Every study of exercise behaviour confirms that the level of physical activity in the population is lamentably low. The only question is just how low. When exercise performance is estimated from questionnaires, the level looks reasonably encouraging. About 50% of the adult population believe that they achieve the current government recommendation for physical activity. Later in life, the exercise volume reduces significantly. By the age of 75 the level is 8% for men and 3% for women. As was seen in Chapter 7 (this volume), however, when exercise level is actually *measured*, the figures are startlingly different. The HSE 2008 report, which did undertake measurements, found that just 6% of men and 4% of women achieved the government's recommended physical activity level (Health and Social Care Information Centre, 2009). This was only one-sixth of the level of compliance indicated by the individuals' own questionnaire response. Society needs to invest a great deal more finance and effort into promoting exercise to a reluctant general public (Hillsdon *et al*., 2005b). The National Institute for Health Research (2019) has published a substantial document entitled *Moving Matters – Interventions to Increase Physical Activity* and this can be read in parallel with the section on 'Other Ideas' below.

Starting Young

The main beneficiaries of regular exercise are adults, but a national culture of exercise must begin in childhood. Unfortunately, children are as reluctant as adults in their attitude to exercise. The Chief Medical Officers' guidelines recommend that all children and young people aged 5–17 should engage in at least 60 minutes of physical activity per day, of which 30 minutes should be in school (Department of Health and Social Care, 2019). In reality, less than 20% of children meet this target and as they reach adolescence even this low figure plummets. Schemes to reverse the trend have nearly always been unsuccessful. A fun exercise programme aimed at maintaining physical activity into adolescence, *GoActive*, was trialled with over 1500 youngsters in eight schools. At the end of the study, there was no difference in activity between the children in the *GoActive* arm compared with the controls (Corder *et al*., 2020).

Government policy does not help. The figures on school sports grounds are shocking. Since the London Olympics in 2012, the equivalent of almost one school playing field per fortnight has been sold off and that rate has recently risen. In 2016, 21 schools sold all their playing fields to developers, the highest number since 2013. Permission to sell was often denied by local authorities, who were then overruled by the Department of Education.

Schoolteachers, even if lacking their own sports grounds, can play a major part in encouraging children to exercise outside school hours. One recent initiative has been the *Daily Mile*. Participating primary schools – and at the time of writing there are more than 3500 in the UK, with many more in other countries – ensure their charges run for 15 minutes each morning before the start of lessons. Teachers at one of the schools involved, St Ninian's Primary School in Stirling, UK, report that none of the children who have been engaged in the scheme for 3 years is overweight. Another promising area is the recruitment of Internet technology. Over recent years there has been a surge of new online apps, blogs and videos specifically targeting young people with messages about personal improvement in their health and lifestyle. These technologies offer opportunities for young people, including collecting, tracking and sharing data, e.g. about how far they walk or run. Despite their proliferation, there is currently no official assessment nor recommendation for their use, but there are exciting opportunities for applying information technology (IT) and social media in this area.

© H.J.N. Bethell and D. Brodie 2023. *Exercise: A Scientific and Clinical Overview*
(H.J.N. Bethell and D. Brodie)
DOI: 10.1079/9781800621855.0028

The most important people in promoting children's exercise, however, must be their parents. The country is amazingly well endowed with altruistic adults, mostly parents, who supervise children's sporting activities such as football, rugby, tennis and athletics. Parents may be helped by members of community groups or professional coaches, who, in return, are allowed to use school playing fields (where these have been retained) in the holidays.

Adults

In adult life the main reason given for not engaging in exercise is the lack of time resulting from full-time employment and/or bringing up children. A short chapter is devoted to this issue later (see Chapter 31, this volume). For working people, either in or outside the home, the most important incentive to exercise must be an understanding of just how vital it is to future health, happiness and longevity. This is the fundamental theme of this book, and the scientific and clinical evidence is legion.

Motivation is a huge issue at any age, and this has been considered extensively by Dr Jennifer Heisz in her book *Move the Body, Heal the Mind* (Heisz, 2022). She includes in her book many suggestions including the following: making a bargain with yourself, focusing on breathing, choosing a time of day that suits you best and exercising with others.

The Role of the Medical Profession

Encouraging people to take more exercise is a difficult task. The NHS workforce 'could help change society's view of sedentary older people, passive care and distorted perceptions of risk' (McNally, 2020). Healthcare professionals *should* target appropriate patients, but seldom do so. Latest research suggests that half of Britons who are at risk of life-threatening heart disease are not being offered diet and exercise advice by their doctor. A US study of consultations for diabetes or hypertension showed that exercise was recommended on only one-sixth of all occasions (Kraschnewski et al., 2013). Even when advice is given it is largely ineffective (Lawlor and Hanratty, 2001). A meta-analysis of trials of physical activity promotion in primary care did find a slight increase in self-reported physical activity at 12 months, but those trials that also measured physical fitness showed no significant increase (Orrow et al., 2012). In the USA, a survey study showed that physicians did not prioritize lifestyle interventions despite large potential benefits (Zhang et al., 2020).

There are many schemes that encourage GPs to prescribe exercise and most local authorities have systems for 'exercise on prescription' at their local sports centres (Craig et al., 2000). Winchcombe Medical Centre in the Cotswolds, UK, for example, offers walks on prescription. A pilot scheme in the south-west of England may find a GP prescribing patients to go outdoors in Devon. The more conventional proposal is that the GP 'prescribes' a course of exercise and the individual has an initial assessment at the sports centre, followed by a course of exercise of around 10 weeks. The cost is somewhat lower than that charged to the general public. At the end of the course the individual is encouraged to continue to attend the sports centre at the usual rate.

Exercise training and physical activity are not part of the usual medical student's curriculum, however, and this may explain why the level of referral to such schemes is extremely low. The uptake and completion of prescribed exercise programmes are even lower. Analysis of a number of these schemes shows that they do not lead to an increase in physical fitness, health-related quality of life or exercise habit in the longer term (Hillsdon et al., 2005a; Pavey et al., 2011). The UK National Referral Database analysed 13 exercise referral schemes lasting between 6 weeks and 3 months involving 24,000 people. They found small improvements in the health and well-being of most participants, but these changes were too small to be clinically significant (Wade et al., 2020). A quality improvement study in the UK comprised internal system alerts, GP education using the 'Making Every Contact Count' framework and targeted patient group text alerts (Zayer et al., 2020). The interventions, specifically targeted at the obese, increased the number of attendees at exercise referral schemes by only 1%.

The idea of exercise on prescription is a sound one, but more attention needs to be paid to barriers to attendance and continued adherence. Some of the factors that have been identified include poor organization of the scheme, inconvenient opening hours, poor social support and exercise leaders lacking motivational skills (Williams et al., 2007). However, regular telephone support and follow-up of absences for those who have been prescribed exercise programmes can be both effective and cost-effective in increasing long-term compliance (Elley et al., 2011).

Prescribing exercise may not be a natural consideration and action for most GPs. However, financial incentives are known to be effective. This is the basis of the Quality Outcomes Framework (QOF) through which GPs are paid to achieve various clinical targets. GPs are rewarded for including their patients on the obesity register, for ensuring BPs or blood sugars are properly monitored and for prescribing a number of the drugs that the NHS recommends. They may be paid to refer a patient to various agencies for support and education, but there is no incentive at all to encourage the same patient to take exercise. Perhaps if referral to an exercise programme were included in the QOF, then both the individual and the nation as a whole would benefit.

Doctors could also benefit from understanding and applying the principles of *motivational interviewing*. This is a patient-centred counselling style to change behaviour by helping patients to explore and resolve ambivalence. Training courses are available online and this approach has been shown to be effective in exploring attitudes and reluctance to exercise (Brodie and Inoue, 2004; Gallé *et al.*, 2020). The quality of the motivational interviewing is very important, and this is emphasized in a study by Ismail *et al.* (2019) which demonstrates that weight loss and increased physical activity are dependent on the style of motivational interviewing.

Encouraging the population to take exercise needs the commitment of doctors. They should regard exercise as a medicine, as equally effective against disease as any drug. The time may be coming for an overarching lifestyle approach. As a feature article in the *BMJ* puts it, 'Is lifestyle medicine emerging as a new medical specialty?' (Sayburn, 2018). The British Society of Lifestyle Medicine was founded in 2016 and some medical schools are now adopting this approach, including Cambridge University. Ideally, lifestyle medicine should not need a label of its own but should become integral to the delivery of healthcare. In its delivery, the medical profession needs to be supported by political action to make physical activity promotion and facilitation key goals in public health strategy. It is also the duty of all health professionals to set a good example. Most doctors do not smoke. They should also be seen to take exercise.

Enhancing Exercise Schemes

Exercise schemes can be somewhat effective, but only if combined with considerable input to encourage the individual and nurture the changed attitudes and behaviour required. A New Zealand study enrolled 1089 women aged 40–74 into a controlled trial of exercise referral and achieved a modest increase in exercising rate in the treated groups at 2 years (Lawton *et al.*, 2008). The intervention included initial motivational interviewing, regular follow-up telephone calls (a total of 75 minutes per patient) and a home visit at 6 months. Even with this level of input, the apparent increased exercise was not associated with improved clinical outcomes but unfortunately was associated with an increased risk of falls and injuries. A study in Norway examined the impact of the country's Healthy Life Centres, which provided tailored support to change physical activity, diet and smoking. The results after 3 months found small positive impacts on participants' physical activity levels, aerobic fitness and obesity (Blom *et al.*, 2020). A combination of exercise instruction with telephone-based motivational interviewing has been found to increase total physical activity, vigorous physical activity and CRF in middle-aged and older adults. A study in Portugal showed that to increase exercise adherence, the interpersonal behaviour of the instructors was critical. The clients who perceived the instructors as supportive showed the best outcomes (Rodrigues *et al.*, 2019). The attractiveness of the exercise leader may be important (Soekmawati *et al.*, 2022). One of the major international programmes to enhance fitness was targeted at male soccer fans (EuroFIT). Over a 5-year period the intervention was not seen to be cost-effective compared with no intervention, but over 10 years it did become cost-effective (Kolovos *et al.*, 2020).

Most local, district or county authorities have schemes to promote healthy living, which includes exercise. Buckinghamshire Council, for example, has collaborated with the local NHS clinical commissioning group to produce *Livewell Stay Well* promotions (https://www.livewellstaywellbucks.co.uk (accessed 24 January 2023)) and provide free online workshops (https://directory.familyinfo.buckinghamshire.gov.uk/service/44 (accessed 30 January 2023)).

Other Ideas

The British Heart Foundation (2015) publication, *Physical Activity Statistics 2015*, provides a number of ideas for increasing physical activity in adults. These include the following.

Workplace interventions

Adults spend up to 60% of their waking hours in the workplace, which should therefore be a useful place to start. Such initiatives include creating workplace exercise facilities, providing one-to-one exercise advice, encouraging use of the stairs rather than lifts, and providing short breaks during the working day for employees to engage in physical activity. In Canada, the Alberta Centre for Active Living (2015) analysed some of the factors currently used to encourage increased physical activity in the workplace. They include challenges and competitions (pedometer challenges, physical activity and sedentary time), information and counselling (posters and handouts, individual and shared counselling), organizational changes (regular active breaks and moving about) and the physical environment (office layout, active workstations, secure bike racks). Again, the effects of these measures appear to be limited.

One multi-intervention health programme trial of 160 work sites did achieve an increase in self-reported physical activity at 18 months but produced no change in any clinical outcome such as BP, blood cholesterol or BMI (Song and Baicker, 2019). A much simpler scheme was operated in Arizona and Minneapolis, where multilevel sit-stand workstations meant that employees could sit or stand when working (Pereira et al., 2020). They resulted in large reductions in sitting time over 12 months.

Environmental interventions

Improving the environment in a number of ways can encourage exercise. This includes walking and biking trails, outdoor gyms, traffic calming, encouraging 'active travel' (walking or cycling rather than taking the bus or train) and notices promoting the use of stairs rather than lifts in public places.

Residents living in neighbourhoods where it is easy and pleasant to walk have less likelihood of developing some health problems, such as pre-diabetes (Fazli et al., 2020). Evidence from existing low-traffic neighbourhoods is encouraging. The London Borough of Waltham Forest has implemented growing numbers of these neighbourhoods since 2015. A survey found that after 3 years residents had increased their walking by 115 minutes and cycling by 20 minutes per week relative to people living elsewhere in Outer London (Aldred and Goodman, 2020).

In the USA, Active Living Research (2022) has expanded this theme by specifying some of the environmental improvements that can encourage greater physical activity. These include aesthetics of the area, plenty of vegetation, parks with open vistas, perceived safety from traffic and crime, general neatness, and play and exercise equipment. The importance of a good exercise environment was shown by the International Physical Activity and Environment Network (Sallis et al., 2016). Across 14 cities on five continents, the difference in physical activity between participants living in the most and the least activity-friendly neighbourhoods ranged from 68 minutes per week to 89 minutes per week. A similar result was found in Ontario, where the incidence of pre-diabetes was reduced in the highly walkable areas (Fazli et al., 2020). That study was confirmed by another one undertaken in Nova Scotia, where there was a reduction in the prevalence of some chronic diseases in more walkable communities (Keats et al., 2020). Canada seems to be the model for showing the benefits of 'neighbourhood walkability' as a further study has shown that adults living in less-walkable neighbourhoods had a higher predicted 10-year CVD risk than those living in highly walkable areas (Howell et al., 2019). Exactly the same conclusions applied to another Canadian study looking at walkable neighbourhoods and obesity and general health (Colley et al., 2019). The same results were found in Barcelona for the relationship between the quality of urban spaces and obesity (Knobel et al., 2021). There was also an improvement in health-related fitness levels in those people who frequented urban spaces (McCormack et al., 2020).

There are a number of recommendations for exercising in outside, green areas (Richardson et al., 2013). Scientists at the University of Queensland found visiting a park for just 30 minutes a week reduced the risk of developing heart disease, stress, anxiety and depression (Shanahan et al., 2016). Even hospital patients recovered more quickly by just being able to see trees and nature from their window. GPs in the Shetland Isles are prescribing a dose of nature alongside medication and therapy for anxiety and depression (Nutt, 2018). It is thought that phytoncides, oils from plants, can trigger the release of the 'happy hormone' serotonin. This encourages a drop in BP and cortisol levels. In Canada, doctors are allowed to write prescriptions for free annual passes to Canada's national parks. Exercising outdoors has considerable benefits including increased production of vitamin D, decreased levels of anger, boosting immunity, improved concentration and self-esteem. It has also been found that people who exercise outdoors work harder and longer than in the gym and avoid the numerous germs associated with the indoor environment. A study at the Oregon Research Institute found that walking outdoors on uneven surfaces significantly improved the balance in adults over the age of 60 (Li *et al.*, 2003). Proximity to green spaces appears to be sufficient to promote physical activity. A study on people who had received coronary artery bypass surgery showed that those who lived in greener areas were significantly more likely to increase their post-surgical physical activity than those who did not (Sadeh *et al.*, 2019). This particularly applied to those patients who did not engage in cardiac rehabilitation.

To improve overall health, there is a need to 'transition to healthier and more environmentally sustainable travel patterns, and low traffic neighbourhoods may substantially contribute to this goal' (Laverty *et al.*, 2021). Avoiding the health damage of a car-based society will require bravery and a commitment to evidence-based decisions from policy makers, supported by strong advocacy from civil society groups.

Active commuting

Defined as walking or cycling to work, active commuting has been shown to be positively associated with physical fitness and also with lower BMI, obesity, BP and insulin levels (Gordon-Larsen *et al.*, 2009). Active commuting reduces heart disease, cancer and age-related mortality, with cycling being more effective than walking (Celis-Morales *et al.*, 2017). The bicycle-hire system in major cities (e.g. 'Boris Bikes' in London) has increased active travel. Sustrans (https://www.sustrans.org (accessed 26 January 2023)) is a charity that aims to enable and increase public exercise by walking, cycling and using public transport (which involves walking to and from bus stops, stations, etc.), leading to healthier, cheaper journeys. Their flagship project is the National Cycle Network, which has created over 14,000 miles of signed cycle routes throughout the UK. About 70% of the network is on previously existing, mostly minor roads where motor traffic will be encountered. On the downside, it is to be deplored that some train companies prevent the transport of bicycles on commuter trains.

Financial reward

Paying people to take exercise has been discussed and a trial is currently underway (Heise *et al.*, 2021).

Community interventions

Social-support systems, group activities, buddy systems and 'Walking for Health' groups all promote more exercising, though to a limited degree. Telephone encouragement and mass-media campaigns are also recognized as providing social support.

Jogging and running

Another initiative has been the *parkrun* scheme. On every Saturday morning more than 700 parks around the UK host 5-kilometre runs without charge. About 50,000 runners, of all abilities, participate each weekend. An excellent introduction to this form of exercise is the *Couch to 5K* initiative, which helps anyone to get off the sofa and gradually increase their activity level to walking/walk-jogging/jogging 5 km. The programme is supported by a website, a phone app and plenty of available encouraging and motivating podcasts.

Internet-delivered interventions

A number of schemes to increase physical activity within various populations have been delivered via the Internet. This has the benefit of reaching a large number of people at a lower cost relative to other types of intervention, such as making physical environmental changes or having regular direct contact with individuals. Internet-delivered interventions have produced positive results, but there is still insufficient evidence of their ability to produce long-term change.

They have the particular advantages of providing easy self-monitoring and feedback information and enabling communication with health professionals or other users via email and chat lines. Many people find that feeding their accelerometer results on to a website allows them to monitor their performance over time. Comparing it to that of others can be an effective incentive.

Smartphone apps

For encouraging exercise, some smartphone apps concentrate on helping with behavioural change.

Others measure activity, like the pedometer apps and the Public Health England app *Active 10*. Results of exercise sessions, for instance runs, can be uploaded to a website which will track performance and compare it with previous performances or compare results with other participants. The idea is that competition is a stimulus and should encourage individuals to keep exercising or even increase their performance. So far, there is little evidence of their efficacy in increasing exercise in either the short or the long term. One block to their implementation is the need for the user to be motivated to take exercise in the first instance. One hopeful development has been an app which is also a game that demands physical activity. An RCT of use of the game for 24 weeks in 36 type 2 diabetics found an average increase in walking of 3128 daily steps and an increase in peak oxygen uptake of 1.9 ml/min/kg. Unfortunately, inadequate exercise and inadequate compliance led to no change in diabetic control (Höchsmann *et al.*, 2019). One study found that fitness apps emphasizing illness or death-related messaging were more likely to be effective in motivating participation than those with social stigma, obesity or financial-cost messaging (Oyibo, 2021).

There are numerous apps, websites and blogs available purporting to improve health and this book is not in a position to make comparisons. The NHS website is often a good starting point, but others include: https://www.myfitnesspal.com, https://www.fightingfifty.co.uk, https://dailycupo-fyoga.com, https://www.exi.life, https://patient.info, https://www.sustrans.org.uk, https://www.nerdfitness.com, https://www.ramblers.org.uk, https://www.lazygirlrunning.com, https://www.countryfile.com and https://www.mentalhealth.org.uk (all accessed 26 January 2023).

Pedometers

At an individual level, sedentary individuals can do much for themselves by just leaving the chair and walking about for a few minutes every hour, going out for short walks, or pacing about when answering the telephone. A pedometer or fitness tracker is an excellent addition to the armamentarium for encouraging increased exercise. Worn regularly, it provides the baseline and allows targets to be set that are easily monitored.

Such 'trackers' come in a variety of forms with a variety of characteristics. They can monitor movement, calories burned, heart rate and even sleep patterns. The Consumers' Association produces a listing of available devices ranging in price from £18 to £700 (Which?, 2023). Anyone deciding that this is the right approach should choose one that is appropriate for the sport or activity they wish to track. Sadly, one controlled trial of weight-loss strategies found that overweight people using exercise trackers lost less weight over 2 years than their controls who did not use trackers (Jakicic *et al.*, 2016). A systematic review has shown that interventions based upon physical activity monitors are safe and effectively increase physical activity and MVPA (Larsen *et al.*, 2022). The authors do warn that the results might be overestimated owing to publication bias.

Applying the concept of biological age

It has been suggested that telling patients their biological age, particularly if it is much greater than their chronological age (see Chapter 7, this volume), could be a tool for encouraging them to become more active and thus bring the two ages into harmony.

Food labelling

Including 'activity equivalent' values of the calories about to be consumed on food labels does not make very comfortable reading but may be all to the good, provided it does not induce a sense of despair in the consumer. For instance, it takes a person of average weight about 26 minutes to walk off the calories in a can of fizzy drink. It takes a run of about 43 minutes to burn off a quarter of a large pizza (Cramer, 2016). This information may be encouraging for some but disheartening for many.

Reducing exercise targets, particularly for older people

The thinking is that for some individuals even the rather modest goals set by the Department of Health and other national bodies may be too challenging. Setting lower targets may help older, sedentary people to move towards recommended activity levels over time. The fact remains that all exercise is good and a little is much better than none (Sparling *et al.*, 2015). As a review by the National Institute for Health Research (2019) said: 'older people are more likely to keep active through structured group activities than exercising on their own at home. The social aspects of exercise and activity are particularly important. Successful approaches include walking programmes tailored to older people'.

Walking

Natural England has established that for every £1 spent on healthy walking schemes, the NHS could save £7.18 in the cost of treating conditions such as heart disease, stroke and diabetes (Natural England, 2009). An analysis of the trials of physical-activity promotion in 1996 concluded that:

> interventions that encourage walking and do not require attendance at a facility are most likely to lead to sustainable increases in overall physical activity. Brisk walking has the greatest potential for increasing overall activity levels of a sedentary population and meeting current public health recommendations.
>
> (Hillsdon and Thorogood, 1996)

One example of this is the *Walking for Health* programme offered by many local authorities. For those who would promote exercise, persistent criticism seems not to be the answer. Alternatively, strategies involving gentle persuasion might be more successful. People need to be convinced of the pleasure of exercise. Activities should be chosen, above all, that will be enjoyed. The 'feel-good' effects will surprise the uninitiated and the post-exercise glow has been described by McCartney (2015) as 'on the orgasmic spectrum'.

Ultimately, it is necessary to 'nudge' people into exercise, remembering those motivating factors identified by the ADNFS (Fentem *et al.*, 1994). These were 'to feel in good shape physically', 'to improve or maintain health', 'to feel a sense of achievement' and 'to get outdoors'. Specifically for men the motivating factors were 'having fun' and 'relaxing', and for women 'looking good' and 'controlling body weight'. Remember also that many people reject exercise because they do not regard themselves as 'sporty' or because they are shy, feel overweight or lack energy.

One way to make walking more palatable is dog ownership. Dog walkers are known to be 20% more active and spend 20 minutes per day longer walking than dog non-owners (Dall *et al.*, 2017). Dog ownership may motivate older adults to engage in appropriate levels of physical activity. Those people who do not own a dog could connect with others in a dog-sharing scheme to improve their personal health. It appears that owning a large breed of dog is especially beneficial.

The Political Approach

The promotion of exercise in the community requires a politically led multidisciplinary approach, strongly supported by the medical profession. Unfortunately, it is not yet known how this may best be implemented. Sport England, which was set up in 1994 with National Lottery money to achieve this, has overseen a reduction rather than an increase in sports participation over the past few years. Sport England has now joined with the Faculty of Sport and Exercise Medicine and Public Health England to launch a new project, *Moving Medicine*. This aims to educate doctors and their patients to turn to exercise as the treatment of choice for many clinical problems. Its aim is to introduce a culture of physical activity into the lives of everyone. It is encouraging to see how many other organizations are involved in promoting exercise and producing policies to enable exercise to become the norm rather than the exception. These include the World Health Organization, the National Institute for Health and Care Excellence, the UK Health Forum, Sustrans, the Sport and Recreation Alliance, the Department of Transport, the Local Government Association and the Royal Society for Public Health. Political actions and public education should produce a cultural shift that will make inactivity as unacceptable as cigarette smoking. To be effective, this needs to be supported by the full weight of public opinion and public pressure. This statement is supported by a letter to the *BMJ* which argues for funded prevention programmes to end the cycle of preventable mortality (Van Duinen, 2020). It is sincerely hoped that this book will contribute to this cultural shift.

Summary

The levels of physical activity in the community are lamentably low. Some examples of attempts to increase exercise-taking have been successful but most have failed to show sustained benefit. Political action will be needed to introduce a culture of physical fitness. The aims should address the need to start young and also to convince older people of the importance of maintaining their activity levels.

References

Active Living Research (2022) Active Living resources for parks & recreation. Available at: https://activelivingresearch.org/taxonomy/parks-recreation (accessed 30 January 2023).

Alberta Centre for Active Living (2015) Alberta survey on physical activity: Executive summary. Available at: https://www.ualberta.ca/kinesiology-sport-recreation/media-library/research/centres-and-units/centre-for-active-living/alberta-survey-of-physical-activity/2015/2015-ab-survey-executive-summary.pdf (accessed 30 January 2023).

Aldred, R. and Goodman, A. (2020) Low traffic neighbourhoods, car use, and active travel: Evidence from the People and Places Survey of Outer London Active Travel Interventions. *Findings*, 11 September 2020. Available at: https://doi.org/10.32866/001c.17128 (accessed 26 January 2023).

Blom, E.E., Aadland, E., Solbraa, A.K. and Oldervoll, L.M. (2020) Healthy Life Centres: a 3-month behavior change programme's impact on participants' physical activity levels, aerobic fitness and obesity: an observational study. *BMJ Open* 10, e035888. https://doi.org/10.1136/bmjopen-2019-035888

British Heart Foundation (2015) *Physical Activity Statistics 2015*. British Heart Foundation, London. Available at: https://www.bhf.org.uk/what-we-do/our-research/heart-statistics/heart-statistics-publications/physical-activity-statistics-2015 (accessed 26 January 2023).

Brodie, D.A. and Inoue, A. (2004) Motivational interviewing to promote physical activity for people with chronic heart failure. *Journal of Advanced Nursing* 50(5), 518–527.

Celis-Morales, C.A., Lyall, D.M., Welsh, P., Anderson, J., Steell, L., *et al.* (2017) Association between active commuting and incident cardiovascular disease, cancer, and mortality: prospective cohort study. *BMJ* 357, j1456.

Colley, R.C., Christidis, T., Tjepkema, M., Michaud, I. and Ross, N.A. (2019) An examination of the associations between walkable neighbourhoods and obesity and self-rated health in Canadians. *Health Reports* 30(9), 14–24.

Corder, K., Sharp, S.J., Jong, S.T., Foubister, C., Brown, H.E., *et al.* (2020) Effectiveness and cost-effectiveness of the GoActive intervention to increase physical activity among UK adolescents: a cluster randomised controlled trial. *PLoS Medicine* 17(7), e1003210. https://doi.org/10.1371/journal.pmed.1003210

Craig, A., Dinan, S., Smith, A., Taylor, A. and Webborn, N. (2000) *NHS Exercise Referral Systems: A National Quality Assurance Framework*. The Stationery Office, London.

Cramer, S. (2016) Label food with equivalent exercise to counter obesity. *BMJ* 353, i1856.

Dall, P.M., Ellis, S.L.H., Ellis, B.M., Grant, P.M., Colyer, A., *et al.* (2017) The influence of dog ownership on objective measures of free-living physical activity and sedentary behaviour in community-dwelling older adults: a longitudinal case-controlled study. *BMC Public Health* 17, 496. https://doi.org/10.1186/s12889-017-4422-5

Department of Health and Social Care (2019) *UK Chief Medical Officers' Physical Activity Guidelines*. Department of Health and Social Care, London.

Elley, C.R., Garrett, S., Rose, S.B., O'Dea, D., Lawton, B.A., *et al.* (2011) Cost-effectiveness of exercise on prescription with telephone support among women in general practice over 2 years. *British Journal of Sports Medicine* 45(15), 1223–1229. https://doi.org/10.1136/bjsm.2010.072439

Fazli, G.S., Moineddin, R., Chu, A., Bierman, A.S. and Booth, G.L. (2020) Neighborhood walkability and prediabetes incidence in a multiethnic population. *BMJ Open Diabetes Research & Care* 8, e000908. https://doi.org/10.1136/bmjdrc-2019-000908

Fentem, P.H., Collins, M.F., Tuxworth, W., Walker, A., Hoinville, E., *et al.* (1994) *Allied Dunbar National Fitness Survey. Technical Report*. Allied Dunbar, Health Education Authority and Sports Council, London.

Gallé, F., Marte, G., Cirella, A., Di Dio, M., Miele, A., *et al.* (2020) An exercise-based educational and motivational intervention after surgery can improve behaviors, physical fitness and quality of life in bariatric patients. *PLoS One* 15(10), e0241336. https://doi.org/10.1371/journal.pone.0241336

Gordon-Larsen, P., Boone-Heinonen, P., Sidney, S., Sternfeld, B., Jacobs, D.R. Jr and Lewis, C.E. (2009)

Active commuting and cardiovascular disease risk the CARDIA study. *Archives of Internal Medicine* 169, 1216–1223.

Health and Social Care Information Centre (2009) Health survey for England – 2008: Physical activity and fitness. Available at: https://digital.nhs.uk/data-and-information/publications/statistical/health-survey-for-england/health-survey-for-england-2008-physical-activity-and-fitness (accessed 13 January 2023).

Heise, T.L., Frense, J., Christianson, L. and Seuring, T. (2021) Using financial incentives to increase physical activity among employees as a strategy of workplace health promotion: protocol for a systematic review. *BMJ Open* 11, e042888. https://doi.org/10.1136/bmjopen-2020-042888

Heisz, J. (2022) *Move the Body, Heal the Mind: Overcome Anxiety, Depression, and Dementia and Improve Focus, Creativity, and Sleep*. Mariner Books, Boston, Massachusetts.

Hillsdon, M. and Thorogood, M. (1996) A systematic review of physical activity promotion strategies. *British Journal of Sports Medicine* 30, 84–89.

Hillsdon, M., Foster, C., Cavill, N., Crombie, H. and Naidoo, B. (2005a) *The Effectiveness of Public Health Interventions for Increasing Physical Activity among Adults: A Review of Reviews. Evidence Briefing*, 2nd edn. Health Development Agency, London.

Hillsdon, M., Foster, C. and Thorogood, M. (2005b) Interventions for promoting physical activity. *Cochrane Database of Systematic Reviews* (1), CD003180.

Höchsmann, C., Müller, O., Ambühl, M., Klenk, C., Königstein, K., *et al.* (2019) Novel smartphone game improves physical activity behavior in type 2 diabetes. *American Journal of Preventive Medicine* 57(1), 41–50.

Howell, N.A., Tu, J.V., Moineddin, R., Chu, A. and Booth G.L. (2019) Association between neighborhood walkability and predicted 10-year cardiovascular disease risk: the CANHEART (Cardiovascular Health in Ambulatory Care Research Team) cohort. *Journal of the American Heart Association* 8(21), e013146.

Ismail, K., Bailey, A., Twist, K., Stewart, K., Ridge, K., *et al.* (2019) Reducing weight and increasing physical activity in people at high risk of cardiovascular disease: a randomised controlled trial comparing the effectiveness of enhanced motivational interviewing intervention with usual care. *Heart* 106(6), 447–454.

Jakicic, J.M., Davis, K.K., King, W.C., Marcus, M.D., Helsel, D., *et al.* (2016) Effect of wearable technology combined with a lifestyle intervention on long-term weight loss. The IDEA randomized clinical trial. *JAMA* 316(11), 1161–1171. https://doi.org/10.1001/jama.2016.12858

Keats, M.R., Cui, Y., DeClercq, V., Grandy, S.A., Sweeney, E. and Dummer, T.J.B. (2020) Associations between neighborhood walkability, physical activity, and chronic disease in Nova Scotian adults: an Atlantic PATH Cohort Study. *International Journal of Environmental Research and Public Health* 17, 8643.

Knobel, P., Maneja, R., Bartoll, X., Borrell, C., Alonso, L., *et al.* (2021) Quality of urban green spaces influences residents' use of these spaces, physical activity, and overweight/obesity. *Environmental Pollution* 271, 116393.

Kolovos, S., Finch, A.P., van der Ploeg, H.P., van Nassau, F. and Broulikova, H.M. (2020) Five-year cost-effectiveness of the European fans in training (EuroFIT) physical activity intervention for men versus no intervention. *International Journal of Behavioral Nutrition and Physical Activity* 17, 30. https://doi.org/10.1186/s12966-020-00934-7

Kraschnewski, J.L., Sciamanna, C.N., Stuckey, H.L., Chuang, C.H., Lehman, E.B., *et al.* (2013) A silent response to the obesity epidemic: decline in US physician weight counseling. *Medical Care* 51, 186–192.

Larsen, R.T., Wagner, V., Korfitsen, C.B., Keller, C., Juhl, C.B., *et al.* (2022) Effectiveness of physical activity monitors in adults: systematic review and meta-analysis. *BMJ* 376, e068047. https://doi.org/10.1136/bmj-2021-068047

Laverty, A.A., Goodman, A. and Aldred, R. (2021) Low traffic neighbourhoods and population health. *BMJ* 372, n443. https://doi.org/10.1136/bmj.n443

Lawlor, D. and Hanratty, B. (2001) The effectiveness of physical activity advice given in routine primary care consultations: a systematic review. *Journal of Public Health Medicine* 23, 219–226.

Lawton, B.A., Rose, S.B., Elley, C.R., Dowell, A.C., Fenton, A. and Moyes, S.A. (2008) Exercise on prescription for women aged 40–74 recruited through primary care: two year randomised controlled trial. *BMJ* 337, a2509.

Li, F., Harmer, P., Wilson, N.L. and Fisher, K.J. (2003) Health benefits of cobblestone-mat walking: preliminary findings. *Journal of Aging and Physical Activity* 11(4), 487–501. https://doi.org/10.1123/japa.11.4.487

McCartney, M. (2015) Margaret McCartney: Nagging people is a futile exercise. *BMJ* 351, h4515.

McCormack, G.R., Frehlich, L., Blackstaffe, A., Turin, T.C. and Doyle-Baker, P.K. (2020) Active and fit communities. Associations between neighborhood walkability and health-related fitness in adults. *International Journal of Environmental Research and Public Health* 17, 1131. https://doi.org/10.3390/ijerph17041131

McNally, S.A. (2020) Exercise: the miracle cure for surgeons to fix the NHS and social care. *Royal College of Surgeons Bulletin* 102(1), 28–33.

National Institute for Health Research (2019) *Moving Matters – Interventions to Increase Physical Activity*. National Institute for Health and Care Research, London. https://doi.org/10.3310/themedreview-03898

Natural England (2009) *An Estimate of the Economic and Health Value and Cost Effectiveness of the*

Expanded WHI Scheme 2009. Natural England Technical Information Note TIN055. Natural England, York, UK.

Nutt, K. (2018) Nature to be prescribed to help health and wellbeing. Available at: https://www.rspb.org.uk/about-the-rspb/about-us/media-centre/press-releases/nature-prescribed-to-help-health/ (accessed 26 January 2023).

Orrow, G., Kinmonth, A.-L., Sanderson, S. and Sutton, S. (2012) Effectiveness of physical activity promotion based in primary care: systematic review and meta-analysis of randomised controlled trials. *BMJ* 344, e1389.

Oyibo, K. (2021) The relationship between perceived health message motivation and social cognitive beliefs in persuasive health communication. *Information* 12(9), 350. https://doi.org/10.3390/info12090350

Pavey, T.G., Taylor, A.H., Fox, K.R., Hillsdon, M., Anokye, N., *et al.* (2011) Effect of exercise referral schemes in primary care on physical activity and improving health outcomes: systematic review and meta-analysis. *BMJ* 343, d6462.

Pereira, M.A., Mullane, S.L., Toledo, M.J.L., Larouche, M.L., Rydell, S.A., *et al.* (2020) Efficacy of the '*Stand and Move at Work*' multicomponent workplace intervention to reduce sedentary time and improve cardiometabolic risk: a group randomized clinical trial. *International Journal of Behavioral Nutrition and Physical Activity* 17, 133. https://doi.org/10.1186/s12966-020-01033-3

Richardson, E., Pearce, J., Mitchell, R. and Kingham, S. (2013) Role of physical activity in the relationship between urban green space and health. *Public Health* 127(4), 1318–1324. https://doi.org/10.1016/j.puhe.2013.01.004

Rodrigues, F., Teixeira, D.S., Cid, L. and Monteiro, D. (2019) Promoting physical exercise participation: the role of interpersonal behaviors for practical implications. *Journal of Functional Morphology and Kinesiology* 4, 40. https://doi.org/10.3390/jfmk4020040

Sadeh, M., Brauer, M., Chudnovsky, A., Ziv, A. and Dankner, R. (2019) Residential greenness and increased physical activity in patients after coronary artery bypass graft surgery. *European Journal of Preventive Cardiology* 28(11), 1184–1191. https://doi.org/10.1177/2047487319886017

Sallis, J.F., Cerin, E., Conway, T.L., *et al.* (2016) Physical activity in relation to urban environment in 14 cities worldwide: a cross-sectional study. *Lancet* 387, 2207–2217. https://doi.org/10.1016/S0140-6736(15)01284-2

Sayburn, A. (2018) Is lifestyle medicine emerging as a new medical specialty? *BMJ* 363, 138–139.

Shanahan, D.F., Bush, R., Gaston, K.J., Lin, B.B., Dean, J., *et al.* (2016) Health benefits from nature experiences depend on dose. *Scientific Reports* 6, 22551. https://doi.org/10.1038/srep28551

Soekmawati, Nathan, R.J., Tan, P.-K. and Vijay, V. (2022) Fitness trainers' physical attractiveness and gym goers' exercise intention. *International Journal of Business and Society* 23(1), 496–517.

Song, Z. and Baicker, K. (2019) Effect of a workplace wellness program on employee health and economic outcomes: a randomized clinical trial. *JAMA* 321(15), 1491–1501. https://doi.org/10.1001/jama.2019.3307. Erratum in: *JAMA* 2019, 321(18), 1830. https://doi.org/10.1001/jama.2019.5197

Sparling, P.B., Howard, B.J., Dunstan, D.W. and Owen, N. (2015) Recommendations for physical activity in older adults. *BMJ* 350, h100.

Van Duinen, G.L. (2020) Healthy lifestyle and life expectancy: fund prevention programmes to end the cycle of preventable morbidity. *BMJ* 368, m427. https://doi.org/10.1136/bmj.m427

Wade, M., Mann, S., Copeland, R.J. and Steele, J. (2020) Effect of exercise referral schemes upon health and well-being: initial observational insights using individual patient data meta-analysis from the National Referral Database. *Journal of Epidemiology and Community Health* 74(1), 32–41. https://doi.org/10.1136/jech-2019-212674

Which? (2023) Best fitness trackers 2023: Which? Best Buys and expert advice, Available at: https://www.which.co.uk/reviews/fitness-trackers/article/how-to-buy-the-best-fitness-or-activity-tracker-aCTU90C40v8E (accessed 1 February 2023).

Williams, N.H., Hendry, M., France, B., Lewis, R. and Wilkinson, C. (2007) Effectiveness of exercise-referral schemes to promote physical activity in adults: systematic review. *British Journal of General Practice* 57, 979–986.

Zayer, V., Wormall, S., Prasad, V. and Perera, K. (2020) How can referrals of patients who are obese to the local exercise referral scheme be increased? A UK based primary care quality improvement study. *British Journal of General Practice* 70(Suppl. 1), bjgp20X711221.

Zhang, J.J., Rothberg, M.B., Misra-Hebert, A.D., Gupta, N.M. and Taksler, G.B. (2020) Assessment of physician priorities in delivery of preventive care. *JAMA Network Open* 3(7), e2011677. https://doi.org/10.1001/jamanetworkopen.2020.11677

29 Sedentary Behaviour

Sedentary behaviour is any waking time spent primarily sitting or lying down and which involves expenditure of 1.5 METs or less. Examples are sitting, watching TV, playing video games and using a computer (Katzmarzyk *et al.*, 2019). Too much sitting, however, is distinct from too little exercise (Owen, 2012). Just sitting is dangerous in its own right even if you do take enough exercise. Many adults may meet the minimal public health recommendations on physical activity on most days each week. However, the 9–10 hours of sitting that can occupy their remaining, 'non-exercise', time can still have a damaging effect on their health (Healy *et al.*, 2008). A new physical-activity grouping known as 'active couch potatoes' has emerged: those who apparently take the recommended amount of exercise but spend excess time just sitting around. Activity, even at low levels, has been shown to control the blood-sugar response to food, to sustain mental health and even to help new brain cells to grow. Avoiding sedentary behaviour should be complementary to the benefits of sustained physical activity associated with more demanding exercise.

How Much Sitting is Taking Place?

The HSE 2008 reported that around 40% of adults spend 6 hours or more per day sitting down at weekends and slightly fewer on weekdays (Health and Social Care Information Centre, 2009). A more recent assessment of sedentary behaviour comes from the HSE 2016 (Health and Social Care Information Centre, 2017). The self-reported average daily sitting time was 5.3 hours for men and 4.9 hours for women at weekends. On weekdays the figure was 4.8 hours for men and 4.6 hours for women. In each case, about 3 hours per day was spent watching TV. The trend was for more sedentary behaviour among the young (16–24 years), with an average sedentary time of 7 hours per day, and the elderly (70–79), at 9 hours per day. This is the characteristic U-shaped curve, with the lowest incidence of sitting occurring in the age range 25–69, usually associated with employment. The figures from the USA are similar. A national study of nearly 6000 adults in 2015/16 found that 26% sat for more than 8 hours per day, with 45% not getting any moderate or vigorous exercise. About 11% were sitting for more than 8 hours daily and being completely physically inactive (Ussery *et al.*, 2018). Things may have become worse for young people with the huge growth in smartphone use. Among university students, there is a direct relationship between time spent on the phone and decreasing levels of physical fitness (Yoo *et al.*, 2020). US researchers examined the habits of 3500 people and compared it with their health. They found that those who watched more than 4 hours of TV per day had a 50% higher risk of heart disease and early death (Garcia *et al.*, 2019).

Older people were also considered by the SITLESS study, which examined the sedentary behaviour of 1360 community-dwelling elderly adults, average age 75. It reported that 79% of waking time was spent sitting, 18.6% in light activity and just 2.6% in moderately vigorous activity. Watching TV and reading accounted for 47% of waking time (Gine-Garriga *et al.*, 2020). There are clear occupational variations in sedentary behaviour, with office workers, as expected, spending more time sitting than blue-collar workers (Prince *et al.*, 2019). Office workers do partly compensate for this risk by taking more moderate and vigorous exercise in their leisure time than manual workers.

The Harmful Effects of Too Much Sitting

The risk of premature death increases for any sedentary time greater than 7 hours per day. Both total sedentary time per day and length of sedentary bouts are predictors of premature death and the combination of the two triples the risk of premature

DOI: 10.1079/9781800621855.0029

mortality (Diaz *et al.*, 2017). A further study involving almost 110,000 participants (Li *et al.*, 2022) showed that high amounts of sitting time were associated with an increased risk of both all-cause mortality and CVD. This has even received a label – 'the sedentary death syndrome'. The news is not all bad. Though regular exercise does not eliminate the perils induced by too much TV watching, it does reduce the impact. A meta-analysis involving more than 1 million people found that it is necessary to watch TV for more than 5 hours per day to reduce the benefits of a regular exercise habit (Ekelund *et al.*, 2016). About an hour's exercise daily offsets the ill effects of sitting at work for 8 hours.

A Canadian research team, based in Ottawa, followed 278 patients who had been through a cardiac rehabilitation programme (Prince *et al.*, 2015). They found that the less time the patients spent sedentary, the better their markers of health. They recommended that patients with cardiovascular symptoms should get up and move every 30 minutes throughout the day.

The more that people sit about, the higher the risk of developing CVD and diabetes (Oggioni *et al.*, 2014). A recent study by Hooker *et al.* (2022) used accelerometry to measure sedentary time. They found that greater time being sedentary and longer bouts of sedentary time were associated with a higher risk of stroke. They calculated that for sedentary people, every extra hour spent on the sofa was linked to a 14% greater likelihood of stroke.

The PURE study tracked 105,677 adults aged 35 to 70 years with a median follow-up of 11 years. Compared to those who sat for fewer than 4 hours per day, those who sat for 8 hours or more per day had a 20% higher risk for all-cause death. Sitting for 6 to 8 hours per day was associated with a 12% increased risk. The conditions involved included cardiovascular death, myocardial infarction, stroke and heart failure. The risks caused by too much sitting were partly offset by physical activity.

The extent of the damage from sedentary behaviour has been quantified by a study conducted in Dallas, Texas, of the coronary calcium scores in heart patients (Kulinski *et al.*, 2015). This score indicates the amount of calcium detectable in coronary arteries and is a good indicator of the presence of coronary narrowing, with its attendant risks of heart attacks and sudden death. For this group of over 2000 patients, each hour of sedentary time per day on average was associated with a 14% increase in coronary-artery calcification. TV viewing time

has also been studied extensively. For every additional hour per day watching TV, there is an increase in the risk of CVD of 3% and an increase in BMI of 0.54 kg/m^2 (Patterson *et al.*, 2020). Other conditions that have been shown to be aggravated or even caused by too much sitting about include obesity and some cancers, while the death rate from all causes is increased (Biswas *et al.*, 2015; Gilchrist *et al.*, 2020). In one study, 435 adults at risk for developing diabetes wore activity monitors to see how much time they spent in various activities. Findings from the study provided further evidence that simply substituting standing for sitting throughout the day improved markers of type 2 diabetes, with a 5% drop in fasting insulin levels (Henson *et al.*, 2016).

The global burden associated with inactivity is substantial according to a study based at the Pennington Biomedical Research Centre in Louisiana (Katzmarzyk *et al.*, 2019). Their report states that one out of every 11 deaths in rich countries is linked to inactivity and 8.1% of dementia cases are similarly related to sedentary behaviour. Reducing sedentary behaviour by as little as 1 hour per day lowers the risk of CVD by 12%. There is a view that idleness 'will kill as many people as smoking' (Doyle, 2015).

The Cost of Sedentary Behaviour

Sedentary behaviour brings a substantial cost to the national economy. A Queen's University Belfast study for the year 2016/17 estimated that the cost of sedentary behaviour to the NHS was £700 million per annum, with up to 70,000 deaths per year. Most of this is due to the increased prevalence of CVD, type 2 diabetes, colon cancer, lung cancer and cancer of the uterus (Heron *et al.*, 2018).

Reducing Sedentary Behaviour

What is the best strategy to reduce sedentary behaviour? Perhaps surprisingly, even fidgeting appears to be very effective (Hagger-Johnson *et al.*, 2016). There is no shortage of ideas given by the authors of the Dallas Heart Study paper (Kulinski *et al.*, 2015). These include taking a walk at lunchtime, pacing about when on the phone, taking the stairs not the lift and using a pedometer as a prompt to keep moving. Other suggestions are using more 'active travel', such as cycling to work, getting off the bus a stop or two early and walking rather than driving for short trips, as well as getting up and moving about during TV commercial breaks.

There is a move in some companies to introduce standing workstations in place of the traditional desk and chair. The Stand More AT (SMArT) Work intervention is an approach adopted by one NHS trust (Edwardson *et al.*, 2018). A special workstation has been invented to make the user become more active. The Stir Kinetic MI is a computerized desk which detects when its owner has been sitting for too long and moves up and down a few centimetres to force them to stand up. It can be programmed to account for the height of the user and the frequency of movement required. The price of £2000 is a costly incentive to move more frequently! Professor Alan Hedge, from Cornell University, suggests that for every half an hour working in an office, people should sit for 20 minutes, stand for 8 minutes, and then move around and stretch for 2 minutes (Hedge, 2019). Standing up to answer the phone would be a start. The Privy Council of the UK traditionally stands for all meetings. This was originally a way of keeping the meetings short, but perhaps all should follow this model of good practice.

Summary

Sedentary behaviour is defined as energy expenditure of 1.5 METs or less. Examples include sitting, watching TV or using a computer. Studies suggest that 40% of adults spend at least 6 hours sitting per day. As the use of screens starts to dominate life, this figure is likely to be an underestimate. The risk of premature death increases for any sedentary time more than 7 hours per day. Sedentary behaviour is costly, with one study suggesting that the cost to the NHS is £700 million annually. Any strategy to reduce sedentary behaviour is beneficial, with a few companies encouraging employees to be more active, even by using telephone prompts to move.

References

Biswas, A., Oh, P.I., Faulkner, G.E., Bajaj, R.R., Silver, M.A., *et al.* (2015) Sedentary time and its association with risk for disease incidence, mortality, and hospitalisation in adults: a systematic review and meta-analysis. *Annals of Internal Medicine* 162, 123–132. Erratum in: *Annals of Internal Medicine* 2015, 163, 400.

Diaz, K.M., Howard, V.J., Hutto, B., Colabianchi, N., Vena, J.E., *et al.* (2017) Patterns of sedentary behavior and mortality in US middle-aged and older adults: a national cohort study. *Annals of Internal Medicine* 167, 465–475.

Doyle, J. (2015) Idleness 'will end up killing as many people as smoking'. *Mail Online*, 4 August 2015. Available at: https://www.dailymail.co.uk/health/article-3184468/idleness-end-killing-people-smoking-Study-finds-quarter-adults-don-t-mamge-30-minutes-exercise-week.html (accessed 31 January 2023).

Edwardson, C.L., Yates, T., Biddle, S.J.H., Davies, M.J., Dunstan, D.W., *et al.* (2018) Effectiveness of the Stand More AT (SMArT) Work intervention: cluster randomised controlled trial. *BMJ* 363, k3870. https://doi.org/10.1136/bmj.k3870

Ekelund, U., Steene-Johannessen, J., Brown, W.J., Fagerland, M.W., Owen, N., *et al.* (2016) Does physical activity attenuate, or even eliminate, the detrimental association of sitting time with mortality? A harmonised meta-analysis of data from more than 1 million men and women. *Lancet* 388, 1302–1310.

Garcia, J.M., Duran, A.T., Schwartz, J.E., Booth, J.N. 3rd, Hooker, S.P., *et al.* (2019) Types of sedentary behavior and risk of cardiovascular events and mortality in blacks: the Jackson Heart Study. *Journal of the American Heart Association* 8(13), e010406. https://doi.org/10.1161/JAHA.118.010406

Gilchrist, S.C., Howard, V.J., Akinyemiju, T., Judd, S.E., Cushman, M., *et al.* (2020) Association of sedentary behavior with cancer mortality in middle-aged and older US adults. *JAMA Oncology* 6(8), 1210–1217. https://doi.org/10.1001/jamaoncol.2020.2045

Gine-Garriga, M., Sansano-Nadal, O., Tully, M.A., Caserotti, P., Coll-Planas, L., *et al.* (2020) Accelerometer-measured sedentary and physical activity time and their correlates in European older adults: the SITLESS study. *The Journals of Gerontology, Series A* 75(9), 1754–1762. https://doi.org/10.1093/gerona/glaa016

Hagger-Johnson, G., Gow, A.J., Burley, V., Greenwood, D. and Cade, J.E. (2016) Sitting time, fidgeting, and all-cause mortality in the UK Women's Cohort Study. *American Journal of Preventive Medicine* 50(2), 154–160. https://doi.org/10.1016/j.amepre.2015.06.025

Health and Social Care Information Centre (2009) Health Survey for England – 2008: Physical activity and fitness. Available at: https://digital.nhs.uk/data-and-information/publications/statistical/health-survey-for-england/

health-survey-for-england-2008-physical-activity-and-fitness (accessed 13 January 2023).

Health and Social Care Information Centre (2017) Health Survey for England, 2016: Physical activity in adults. Available at: http://healthsurvey.hscic.gov.uk/support-guidance/public-health/health-survey-for-england-2016/physical-activity-in-adults.aspx (accessed 12 January 2023).

Healy, G.N., Dunstan, D.W., Salmon, J., Shaw, J.E., Zimmet, P.Z. and Owen, N. (2008) Television time and continuous metabolic risk in physically active adults. *Medicine and Science in Sports and Exercise* 40, 639–645.

Hedge, A. (2019) Ergonomic tips: Computer use by senior citizens. Available at: https://www.spineuniverse.com/wellness/ergonomics/ergonomic-tips-computer-use-senior-citizens (accessed 29 January 2023).

Henson, J., Dunstan, D.W., Davies, M.J. and Yates, T. (2016) Sedentary behaviour as a new behavioural target in the prevention and treatment of type 2 diabetes. *Diabetes Metabolism Research and Reviews* 32(Suppl. 1), 213–220. https://doi.org/10.1002/dmrr.2759

Heron, L., O'Neill, C., McAneney, H., Kee, F. and Tully, M.A. (2018) Direct healthcare costs of sedentary behaviour in the UK. *Journal of Epidemiology and Community Health* 73(7), 625–629. https://doi.org/10.1136/jech-2018-211758

Hooker, P.S., Diaz, K.M., Blair, S.N., Colabianchi, N., Hutto, B., *et al.* (2022) Association of accelerometer-measured sedentary time and physical activity with risk of stroke among US adults. *JAMA Network Open* 5(6), e2215385.

Katzmarzyk, P.T., Powell, K.E., Jakicic, J.M., Troiano, R.P., Piercy, K., *et al.* (2019) Sedentary behavior and health: update from the 2018 Physical Activity Guidelines Advisory Committee. *Medicine and Science in Sports and Exercise* 51, 1227–1241. https://doi.org/10.1249/MSS.0000000000001935

Kulinski, J., Kozlitina, J., Berry, J., de Lemos, J. and Khera, A. (2015) Sedentary behavior is associated with coronary artery calcification in the Dallas Heart Study. *Journal of the American College of Cardiology* 65(10), A1446. https://doi.org/10.1016/S0735-1097(15)61446-2

Li, S., Lear, S.A., Rangarajan, S., Hu, B., Yin, L., *et al.* (2022) Association of sitting time with mortality and cardiovascular events in high-income, middle-income, and low-income countries. *JAMA Cardiology* 7(8), 796–807. https://doi.org/10.1001/jamacardio.2022.1581

Oggioni, C., Lara, J., Wells, J.C.K., Soroka, K. and Siervo, M. (2014) Shifts in population dietary patterns and physical inactivity as determinants of global trends in the prevalence of diabetes: an ecological analysis. *Nutrition, Metabolism, and Cardiovascular Diseases* 24, 1105–1111.

Owen, N. (2012) Sedentary behavior: understanding and influencing adults' prolonged sitting time. *Preventive Medicine* 55, 535–539.

Patterson, F., Mitchell, J.A., Dominick, G., Lozano, A.J., Huang, L. and Hanlon, A.L. (2020) Does meeting physical activity recommendations ameliorate association between television viewing with cardiovascular disease risk? A cross-sectional, population-based analysis. *BMJ Open* 10, e036507. https://doi.org/10.1136/bmjopen-2019-036507

Prince, S.A., Blanchard, C.M., Grace, S.L. and Reid, R.D. (2015) Objectively-measured sedentary time and its association with markers of cardiometabolic health and fitness among cardiac rehabilitation graduates. *European Journal of Preventive Cardiology* 23(8), 818–825. https://doi.org/10.1177/2047487315617101

Prince, S.A., Elliott, C.G., Scott, K., Visintini, S. and Reed, J.L. (2019) Device-measured physical activity, sedentary behaviour and cardiometabolic health and fitness across occupational groups: a systematic review and meta-analysis. *International Journal of Behavioral Nutrition and Physical Activity* 16, 30. https://doi.org/10.1186/s12966-019-0790-9

Ussery, E.N., Fulton, J.E., Galuska, D.J., Katzmarzyk, P.T. and Carlson, S.A. (2018) Joint prevalence of sitting time and leisure-time physical activity among US adults, 2015–2016. *JAMA* 320, 2036–2038. https://doi.org/10.1001/jama.2018.17797

Yoo, J.-I., Cho, J., Baek, K.-W., Kim, M.-H. and Kim, J.-S. (2020) Relationship between smartphone use time, sitting time, and fitness level in university students. *Exercise Science* 29(2), 170–177. https://doi.org/10.15857/ksep.2020.29.2.170

30 Complications of Exercise

Despite the concerns expressed by some, exercise is extremely safe. Even strenuous and prolonged exercise rarely produces more than muscle or joint strains and sprains. Not exercising is far more dangerous than exercising. However, no physical activity can be entirely free from risk. This chapter starts with the most significant (also the rarest) and works backwards.

Sudden Death

The best known – but also the rarest – complication of exercise is literally dropping dead. The incidence is about one per 50,000 in professional athletes in whom the usual cause is a congenital abnormality of the heart (Maron *et al.*, 2009). Sudden death is nearly always caused by a disturbance of heart rhythm known as ventricular fibrillation (VF). The muscle fibres of the main heart chambers, the ventricles, lose their rhythmic coordinated control. Consequently, each muscle fibre contracts and relaxes independently of all the other fibres. As a result, the ventricles stop pumping and death follows swiftly if normal heart rhythm is not restored. Definitive treatment is 'defibrillation'. If a defibrillator is not immediately available, the victim can be kept alive by external cardiac massage until one can be acquired. Automatic external defibrillators (AEDs) are carried by all emergency ambulances and by many 'first responders'. They are also widely available in community facilities and public places. It is not unreasonable for all concerned citizens to learn how to perform external cardiac massage and acquaint themselves with the way to use an AED. The instructions for their use do make it easy enough to allow completely untrained individuals to apply the defibrillation successfully. St John Ambulance Brigades offer resuscitation courses across the country.

The most common cause of VF in young people is a congenital abnormality of the heart – hypertrophic cardiomyopathy (HCM). This is inherited as an autosomal dominant gene, which means that on average half the offspring of a sufferer will have the condition. All the children of HCM patients should be screened. If found to be positive, they will usually be fitted with an implanted defibrillator which delivers a defibrillating shock if the heart goes into VF. It has been suggested that all professional sports people should be screened for HCM. Unfortunately, screening has a high false negative rate – six out of eight in one study of sudden death in young footballers had previously had normal screening results (Malhotra *et al.*, 2018). So screening is generally not thought to be a cost-effective endeavour and may also lead to a range of psychological, ethical and legal problems (Semsarian *et al.*, 2015).

In middle and later life sudden death from VF is usually caused by CHD, either at the onset of a heart attack or as a result of severe heart damage from previous heart attacks. There is a widespread belief that sudden death from a heart attack is a result of 'massive' cardiac damage. In fact, VF at the onset of a heart attack is an electrical accident unrelated to the extent of cardiac injury. Those who are successfully resuscitated have the same prognosis as those who have not suffered this complication.

VF can be triggered by exercise – the rate of VF during competitive sports is about one per 130,000 person-years (Landry *et al.*, 2017), during triathlons about one per 60,000 person-years (mostly during the swimming section) (Harris *et al.*, 2017), and during marathon running about one per 50,000 person-years (James *et al.*, 2013). The risk of exercise-related VF in fit exercisers is far lower than in unfit non-exercisers. When the risk of sudden death during exercise is compared with the benefits of being a regular exerciser, the regular exerciser is by far the less susceptible. There is always a small risk with vigorous exercise, but the reduction in the death rate resulting from being physically fit easily outweighs the dangers of vigorous exercise.

© H.J.N. Bethell and D. Brodie 2023. *Exercise: A Scientific and Clinical Overview*
(H.J.N. Bethell and D. Brodie)
DOI: 10.1079/9781800621855.0030

Other Cardiac Arrhythmias

Atrial fibrillation (AF) is a very common condition of later life. AF is similar to VF but involving the 'antechambers' of the heart. Since the atria are not necessary for the heart to pump out blood, AF is not fatal, but it does reduce the heart's efficiency. The heart beats more rapidly and irregularly. The main complication is the development of blood clots in the atria. These can be dislodged and end up in the brain, causing a stroke. It is important that people with AF take blood thinners to prevent this.

AF affects about seven in 100 people over the age of 65 and becomes gradually more common with increasing age. CVD risk factors such as obesity, hypertension and diabetes all increase AF risk. High levels of physical fitness are protective (Abdulla and Nielsen, 2009) – the fitter the individual, the lower the risk (Franklin et al., 2020). Increasing physical fitness also lessens the risk associated with other factors, particularly obesity (Kamil-Rosenberg et al., 2020). However, it has been suggested that excessive exercise can reverse this effect in men. In an analysis derived from the UK Biobank study, Elliott et al. (2020) found that women showed a more pronounced risk reduction with activity than men, as well as a protective effect over the entire range of physical activity levels examined. The results showed a statistically significant reduction in AF risk up to 2500 MET minutes per week. For men, however, increasing physical activity was only protective against AF to a level of 1500 MET minutes per week. Beyond that the protective effect was lost, with a progressive increase in AF risk with greater amounts of vigorous physical activity and a statistically significant 12% risk enhancement at 5000 MET minutes per week. This possible ill effect of very intense physical training was denied by a subsequent study of 460,000 hypertensive US veterans given a symptom-limited treadmill test (Faselis et al., 2016). During follow-up of a mean of 9.8 years, 42,639 individuals developed AF. Exercise capacity was inversely related to AF risk through the full range of fitness levels, the risk being 11% lower for each 1-MET increase in exercise capacity.

Other Cardiac Problems

It has been suggested that excessive exercise, particularly in older athletes, may damage heart muscle. There is no good evidence for this (George et al., 2011). Towards the end of a very long bout of exercise there may be some fall-off in left ventricular performance. This is the so-called 'exercise-induced cardiac fatigue', but it reverses itself within 48 hours. Some electrographic changes are also found in endurance athletes, such as evidence of a thicker-than-normal heart-muscle wall, but again there is no evidence that this is harmful.

Older athletes do have a higher prevalence of calcium in their coronary arteries, but this is not associated with an increased risk of heart attacks. One study of 'extreme exercise' examined 22,000 healthy men aged 40–80 and compared their activity levels with their risk of death during the period of study (DeFina et al., 2019). The most active men had half the risk of death of the least active, and those taking 8 hours or more per week at 10 METs or more were 23% less likely to die than their less-active peers. Other studies have confirmed the direct relationship of very high levels of both physical activity and CRF with high coronary artery calcification. There was, however, no increase in ischaemic outcomes (Jafar et al., 2019; Kermott et al., 2019). It has been postulated that high-intensity physical activity or high levels of CRF may promote more calcific coronary atherosclerosis. This may be more stable than soft, non-calcified plaque, and less likely to rupture and cause acute, morbid CVD events.

Musculoskeletal Injuries

Physically active adults (not necessarily older adults) tend to experience a higher incidence of leisure-time and sports-related injuries than their less-active counterparts (Haskell et al., 2007). However, healthy adults who meet the usual governmental activity recommendations have an overall musculoskeletal injury rate that is not much different from that of inactive adults. Active men and women have a higher injury rate during sport and leisure-time activity, while inactive adults report more injuries during non-sport and non-leisure time. A possible reason for this lower injury incidence during non-leisure time is the increased fitness levels (endurance, strength, balance) of the more active adults. Inevitably, more vigorous exercise with its greater benefits does bring a higher risk of musculoskeletal injuries as the intensity and amount of activity increase. It seems that the benefits of a vigorous exercise regimen greatly outweigh the temporary inconvenience and discomfort of these minor injuries.

The common belief that it is exercise that causes chronic joint problems and osteoarthritis is wrong. Regular physical activity may even reduce the risk of developing painful osteoarthritis (Heesch et al., 2007) by improving cartilage resilience and by increasing the strength of the muscles that support the joints. High levels of walking are associated with reduced need for hip-replacement surgery (Ageberg et al., 2012) and it has been suggested that cycling can also be an effective way of delaying hip surgery. Activities, such as jogging, that place greater strain on joints appear to be more protective than lower-impact activities and it is a myth that recreational running leads to osteoarthritis of the knees (Hootman et al., 2003).

It is probably true, however, that excessive exercise such as that taken by ultra-marathon runners and the like may bring increased levels of musculo-skeletal injury. A study of runners training for a half-marathon in Sweden found that one-third suffered such problems during the year before the event (Jungmalm et al., 2020). Half were related to knees, calves or Achilles tendons but were mostly minor and short-lived. Surprisingly, the incidence of injuries was not related to gender, age, BMI or running experience.

Studies on injuries in adults aged 65 and over are scarce. The rate of injuries occurring during physical activity in advanced age, based on existing data, is very low compared to other ages. Based on current available research, there is no substantial evidence to justify the fear of getting injured through purposeful physical activity or in sports in advanced age (Dunsky and Netz, 2012). Indeed, strengthening bones and improving balance by exercise training programmes reduces the risk of injurious falls in the elderly (Uusi-Rasi et al., 2015).

The long-term effects of strenuous exercise at international level may be greater. A study of 3300 retired Olympians found that 63% reported at least one injury and about a third suffered ongoing pain and/or functional limitations (Palmer et al., 2021). Sports students, who often train for many hours per week, are also at risk of painful injuries with resulting psychological problems (Bumann et al., 2020).

Stress Fractures

Stress fractures are small cracks in the bone, usually in the foot or lower leg, brought on by overuse and repetitive activity. High-impact or prolonged exercises are most often involved – running, football and basketball in particular. Sudden increase in activity or changes in exercise pattern are the most likely causes. Other possible sites include the pelvis and vertebrae.

Women athletes are twice as likely as men to sustain stress fractures and postmenopausal women are at even greater risk. In premenopausal women, stress fractures are more common in those whose athletic endeavours have provoked menstrual irregularities or infrequency (Johnston et al., 2020). The symptoms include pain and tenderness at the site of the injury. An X-ray may not initially show the fracture, but within a week the repair mechanisms can be seen. Treatment is rest and avoidance of further impact until healing has taken place – usually about 8 weeks.

Exercise and Trauma

Some sports, like cycling, carry an increased risk of trauma, mainly as a result of impact injuries from other road users. Despite this, the cyclists are the ultimate winners. A study of 230,390 commuters identified 5704 who travelled to work by bicycle. The cyclists were 3.4 times as likely to sustain transport-related injuries as the other travellers. However, the overall mortality over the period of study was still lower in the cyclists (Welsh et al., 2020).

Contact sports often result in head injuries. Boxing is the obvious example, but soccer, rugby, hockey and American football can all involve repetitive head impacts, which can eventually result in 'chronic traumatic encephalopathy' (Jildeh et al., 2020; Stewart, 2021). This causes brain damage and accounts for up to 15% of cases of dementia. Recent media reports of high-profile former soccer and rugby players with diagnoses of neurodegenerative disease have raised concerns about the dangers of contact sports and led to threats of litigation against sports organizations over perceived failures in duty of care. Wisely, the government has banned primary-school children in the UK from heading the ball in football training – but not in matches.

Another outcome of repeated head trauma is lowered testosterone production with resultant erectile dysfunction (Abbasi, 2020).

Extreme Endurance Exercise

Excessive physical activity produces its own problems. A number of cardiac indicators are worse in those undertaking very high levels of exercise, including enzymes released by heart-muscle damage and calcification of the coronary arteries (Lavie *et al.*, 2019). Physical performance can also decline with excessive training. With extreme exercise mitochondrial function may diminish substantially, with reduced generation of ATP from glycolysis and reduced glucose tolerance (Flockhart *et al.*, 2021).

Electrolyte imbalance – including hyponatraemia, hypernatraemia and fluid overload – is all found in long-distance runners whose choice of rehydration fluid may not be appropriate (Rehrer, 2001). Extreme endurance activity may impair normal inflammatory and immune responses, resulting in an increased susceptibility to respiratory infections (Ihalainen *et al.*, 2016).

Exercise Addiction

People with exercise addiction experience loss of control to the extent that exercise becomes obligatory and excessive (Hausenblas *et al.*, 2017). This is very similar to the obsession seen in some eating disorders when the excessive exercise is part of the strategy to maintain weight control. Exercise addiction is not common, occurring in about 0.3% of the general population and about 2% of regular exercisers. In some sports it is much more common – up to about 25% in runners (Slay *et al.*, 1998). It is seen about equally in men and women, though in women it is more often associated with eating disorders. Some of the characteristics include continuing to exercise despite injury and illness, and giving up social, occupational and family interests which might interfere with the exercise programme. Sufferers may report withdrawal effects when their exercise schedule is disrupted. The most effective treatment is probably CBT with the aim not of stopping the subject from exercising but of helping them to recognize the addictive behaviour and adapt to a less rigid exercise routine.

Summary

Minor ill effects of exercise include muscle and joint strains and sprains, which are seldom serious.

Life-threatening effects are extremely rare. It is much safer to be an exerciser than an idler.

References

Abbasi, J. (2020) Concussions linked with erectile dysfunction in football player study. *JAMA* 323(7), 597–598. https://doi.org/10.1001/jama.2019.21883

Abdulla, J. and Nielsen, J.R. (2009) Is the risk of atrial fibrillation higher in athletes than in the general population? A systematic review and meta-analysis. *Europace* 11, 1156–1159.

Ageberg, E., Engström, G., Gerhardsson de Verdier, M., Rollof, J., Roos, E.M. and Lohmander, L.S. (2012) Effect of leisure time physical activity on severe knee or hip osteoarthritis leading to total joint replacement: a population-based prospective cohort study. *BMC Musculoskeletal Disorders* 3, 73.

Bumann, A., Banzer, W. and Fleckenstein, J. (2020) Prevalence of biopsychosocial factors of pain in 865 sports students of the DACH (Germany, Austria, Switzerland) region – a cross-sectional survey. *Journal of Sports Science and Medicine* 19(2), 323–336.

DeFina, L.F., Radford, N.B., Barlow, C.E., Willis, B.L., Leonard, D., *et al.* (2019) Association of all-cause and cardiovascular mortality with high levels of physical activity and concurrent coronary artery calcification. *JAMA Cardiology* 4(2), 174–181. https://doi.org/10.1001/jamacardio.2018.4628

Dunsky, A. and Netz, Y. (2012) Physical activity and sport in advanced age: is it risky? – A summary of data from articles published between 2000–2009. *Current Aging Science* 5, 66–71.

Elliott, A.D., Linz, D., Mishima, R., Kadhim, K., Gallagher, C., *et al.* (2020) Association between physical activity and risk of incident arrhythmias in 402 406 individuals: evidence from the UK Biobank cohort. *European Heart Journal* 41, 1479–1486. https://doi.org/10.1093/eurheartj/ehz897

Faselis, C., Kokkinos, P., Tsimploulis, A., Pittaras, A., Myers, J., *et al.* (2016) Exercise capacity and atrial fibrillation risk in veterans: a cohort study. *Mayo Clinic Proceedings* 91(5), 558–566. https://doi.org/10.1016/j.mayocp.2016.03.002

Flockhart, M., Nilsson, L.C., Tais, S., Ekblom, B., Apró, W. and Larsen, F.J. (2021) Excessive exercise training causes mitochondrial functional impairment and decreases glucose tolerance in healthy volunteers. *Cell Metabolism* 33(5), 957–970.e6. https://doi.org/10.1016/j.cmet.2021.02.017

Franklin, B.A., Thompson, P.D., Al-Zaiti, S.S., Albert, C.M., Hivert, M.F., *et al.* (2020) Exercise-related acute cardiovascular events and potential deleterious adaptations following long-term exercise training: placing the risks into perspective – an update: a scientific statement from the American Heart Association. *Circulation* 141(13), e705–e736. https://doi.org/10.1161/CIR.0000000000000749

George, K., Spence, A., Naylor, L.H., Whyte, G.P. and Green, D.J. (2011) Cardiac adaptation to acute and chronic participation in endurance sports. *Heart* 97, 1999–2004.

Harris, K.M., Creswell, L.L., Haas, T.S., Thomas, T., Tung, M., *et al.* (2017) Death and cardiac arrest in US triathlon participants, 1985 to 2016: a case series. *Annals of Internal Medicine* 167(8), 529–535.

Haskell, W., Lee, I.-M., Pate, R.R., Powell, K.E., Blair, S.N., *et al.* (2007) Physical activity and public health: updated recommendations for adults from the American College for Sports Medicine and the American Heart Association. *Circulation* 116, 1081–1093.

Hausenblas, H.A., Schreiber, K. and Smoliga, J.M. (2017) Addiction to exercise. *BMJ* 375, j1745.

Heesch, K.C., Miller, Y.D. and Brown, W.J. (2007) Relationship between physical activity and stiff or painful joints in mid-aged women and older women: a 3-year prospective study. *Arthritis Research & Therapy* 9(2), R34.

Hootman, J.M., Macera, C.A., Helmick, C.G. and Blair, S.N. (2003) Influence of physical activity-related joint stress on the risk of self-reported hip/knee osteoarthritis: a new method to quantify physical activity. *Preventive Medicine* 36, 636–644.

Ihalainen, J.K., Schumann, M., Häkkinen, K. and Mero, A.A. (2016) Mucosal immunity and upper respiratory tract symptoms in recreational endurance runners. *Applied Physiology, Nutrition, and Metabolism* 41(1), 96–102.

Jafar, O., Friedman, J., Bogdanovicz, I., Muneer, A., Thompson, P.D., *et al.* (2019) Assessment of coronary atherosclerosis using calcium scores in short- and long-distance runners. *Mayo Clinic Proceedings: Innovations, Quality & Outcomes* 3(2), 116–121.

James, J., Merghani, A. and Sharma, S. (2013) Sudden death in marathon runners. *Cardiac Electrophysiology Clinics* 5, 43–51.

Jildeh, T.R., Okoroha, K.R., Denha, E., Eyers, C., Johnson, A., *et al.* (2020) Return to sport following adolescent concussion: epidemiologic findings from a high school population. *Orthopedics* 43(4), e306–e310. https://doi.org/10.3928/01477447-20200521-03

Johnston, T.E., Dempsey, C., Gilman, F., Tomlinson, R., Jacketti, A.-K. and Close, J. (2020) Physiological factors of female runners with and without stress fracture histories: a pilot study. *Sports Health* 12(4), 334–340. https://doi.org/10.1177/1941738120919331

Jungmalm, J., Nielsen, R.Ø., Desai, P., Karlsson, J., Hein, T. and Grau, S. (2020) Associations between biomechanical and clinical/anthropometrical factors and running-related injuries among recreational runners: a 52-week prospective cohort study. *Injury Epidemiology* 7(1), 10. https://doi.org/10.1186/s40621-020-00237-2

Kamil-Rosenberg, S., Kokkinos, P., de Sousa e Silva, C.G., Yee, W.L.S., Abella, J., *et al.* (2020) Association between cardiorespiratory fitness, obesity, and incidence of atrial fibrillation. *International Journal of Cardiology: Heart & Vasculature* 31, 100663.

Kermott, C., Schroeder, D., Kopecky, S. and Behrenbeck, T. (2019) Cardiorespiratory fitness and coronary artery calcification in a primary prevention population. *Mayo Clinic Proceedings: Innovations, Quality & Outcomes* 3(2), 122–130.

Landry, C.H., Allan, K.S., Connelly, K.A., Cunningham, K., Morrison, L.J. and Dorian, P. (2017) Sudden cardiac arrest during participation in competitive sports. *New England Journal of Medicine* 377, 1943–1953.

Lavie, C., Hecht, H.F. and Wisloff, U. (2019) Extreme physical activity may increase coronary calcification, but fitness still prevails. *Mayo Clinic Proceedings: Innovations, Quality & Outcomes* 3(2), 103–105.

Malhotra, A., Dhutia, H., Finocchario, G., Gati, S., Beasley, I., *et al.* (2018) Outcomes of screening in adolescent soccer players. *New England Journal of Medicine* 379, 524–534.

Maron, B.J., Doerer, J.J., Haas, T.S., Tierney, D.M. and Mueller, F.O. (2009) Sudden deaths in young competitive athletes: analysis of 1866 deaths in the United States, 1980–2006. *Circulation* 119, 1085–1092.

Palmer, D., Cooper, D.J., Emery, C., Batt, M.E., Engebretsen, L., *et al.* (2021) Self-reported sports injuries and later-life health status in 3357 retired Olympians from 131 countries: a cross-sectional survey among those competing in the games between London 1948 and PyeongChang 2018. *British Journal of Sports Medicine* 55, 46–53.

Rehrer, N.J. (2001) Fluid and electrolyte balance in ultra-endurance sport. *Sports Medicine* 31(10), 701–715. https://doi.org/10.2165/00007256-200131100-00001

Semsarian, C., Sweeting, J. and Ackerman, M. (2015) Sudden cardiac death in athletes. *BMJ* 350, h1218.

Slay, H.A., Hayaki, J., Napolitano, M.A. and Brownell, K.D. (1998) Motivations for running and eating attitudes in obligatory versus nonobligatory runners. *International Journal of Eating Disorders* 357, 267–275.

Stewart, W. (2021) Sport associated dementia. *BMJ* 372, n168. https://doi.org/10.1136/bmj.n168

Uusi-Rasi, K., Patil, R., Karinkanta, S., Kannus, P., Tokola, K., *et al.* (2015) Exercise and vitamin D in fall prevention among older women: a randomized clinical trial. *JAMA Internal Medicine* 175, 703–711.

Welsh, C., Celis-Morales, C., Ho, F., Lyall, D.M., Mackay, D., *et al.* (2020) Association of injury related hospital admissions with commuting by bicycle in the UK: prospective population based study. *BMJ* 368, m336. https://doi.org/10.1136/bmj.m336

31 Excuses to Avoid Exercise

This text has provided clinicians and exercise professionals with convincing arguments for the benefits of exercise and for the disadvantages of failing to exercise on a regular basis. In spite of these entreaties, there will be many members of the public who will remain resistant. They provide a rich variety of excuses for not adopting exercise as part of their natural lifestyle. Genetically, perhaps there is a predisposition to do very little unless engaged in hunter-gathering. Unfortunately there is no longer a need to hunt or gather as life has changed so that these pursuits are largely automated or made considerably less demanding. There is an island called Taquile in Lake Titicaca, Peru, where the moral code includes the statement *do not be lazy*. The Taquileans embody this, starting with over 500 steps to reach the main town from the beach. This culture is unfamiliar to many in the Western world, where a pizza in front of the TV is more likely the recreational option. There are numerous excuses for avoiding exercise and health professionals need to be prepared to respond to them. The following suggests a few excuses and possible responses.

'I am not fit enough.'

This may initially be the case when someone has been sedentary for any length of time. Everyone starts from a very low base, but a properly planned, progressive exercise schedule can make a substantial difference in a very short time. Clearly it would be inadvisable for anyone who is genuinely unfit to start to train at a high intensity. It could be both physiologically and psychologically damaging and should be avoided. Fortunately there are many strategies to ensure that a seriously unfit person can seek the correct approach to improve. A properly organized gym will provide a full fitness assessment and set a programme appropriate to the needs of the individual, however unfit they are. For those who would be initially embarrassed by exercising in front of people who are much fitter, there are a variety of options. These include the *Healthy Walks* schemes, the *Couch to 5K* programme, and many online videos which can be accessed in the privacy of their own homes. For those who fancy rekindling a sport which they might have done when much younger, there are opportunities to engage in walking football, walking cricket and the like, which are structured to be fun, yet less demanding.

'I am too fat.'

One can sympathize with this excuse because being overweight, as discussed in Chapter 10 (this volume), can undoubtedly be perceived as a barrier to exercise. However, there is much an overweight person can achieve as they combine sensible eating with exercise. In a country like France, where cycling is part of the national culture, overweight people can enjoy that particular exercise, and do so in large numbers. Activities that avoid shifting one's body weight, such as cycling, rowing and swimming, are tolerated well by overweight people. Appropriate weight training is also an option. As with many activities, one of the obstacles is the person's appearance compared with others. Wearing loose clothing, finding a group of similar people and exercising as part of a weight-reduction class can help. Some running events, such as the ubiquitous parkruns, especially welcome people of all shapes and sizes.

'I have a long-standing injury.'

Some injuries clearly prevent exercise until they are resolved, but quite a number of problems such as chronic backache, arthritis and sinus problems can be improved dramatically as a result of exercise. The interest shown in the Paralympic Games, where people of all sorts of permanent disabilities perform, is testimony to injury being no bar to sports performance. These athletes train to an

DOI: 10.1079/9781800621855.0031

extremely high level and clearly do not see their disability as a reason for avoiding exercise.

'I am too busy.'

The expression 'I am too busy' should really read, 'My priorities are different'. Most people engage in activities that, on reflection, could have been spent in more productive ways. It is not always necessary to watch numerous TV news broadcasts. The news does not change that much during the day. The time the average person spends watching soap operas is probably the same as the government's recommended weekly allocation to exercise. Many senior statesmen, including several recent US Presidents, commit themselves to exercising regularly. If they, with their level of responsibility and time pressures, can find time for exercise, then so can the majority of other people. Usually it is simply a case of organizing the available time differently. One strategy is to fill one's diary with the exercise sessions *first* and then let other commitments fit around them.

'I might get cold and uncomfortable.'

Modern sports clothing reduces this possibility and layers of clothing that can be taken off or put on work well for most people. Thirty minutes is probably the average time to exercise and even if individuals get cold in that time, the warming shower beckons soon afterwards. If the conditions are unbearable outdoors, then it is useful to have an indoor circuit available, either at home or in a local gym. It takes relatively little time to adapt to cold and discomfort. Getting into cold water, even in a swimming bath, can be temporarily uncomfortable, but soon the pleasure of the swim makes it worthwhile. Many hardy souls actually enjoy exercising in extreme temperatures. Wild swimming is one example, as is participating in the *Marathon des Sables* or *Tough Mudder* races.

'I am too old.'

There is no evidence to show that elderly people cannot exercise. They may have to make certain modifications, but a trawl of YouTube will show hundreds of cases of older people engaging in a variety of physical exercises and activities. Of growing interest are seated exercises, specifically for people who have more difficulty with balance. Exercise is a common option in good care homes and the physical and psychological benefits are well documented. In China, elderly people will often be seen in the outdoors engaging in ballroom dancing or tai chi. In Western countries, most towns offer lessons in dancing, which are often populated by the elderly. Membership of the University of the Third Age (U3A) will open opportunities for retired people to enjoy a range of physical activities.

'I might look stupid.'

When observing a group of exercisers, there is the temptation to notice a few people who look out of place. Their clothes may be garish; they may appear too fat, too old, too slow or too red in the face. The important thing is *they are doing it* and the observer is not. If looking stupid is a concern, then watch the average marathon and see the range of ridiculous costumes that people wear. It may not be normal to run dressed like a nun or a ballet dancer, but this is far more extreme than anything the average runner will look like. The ones looking stupid are the ones not participating.

'I have children to look after.'

Many pushchairs or strollers are ideally designed for runners. Children will enjoy the outing and the participant will get considerable exercise benefit from pushing a child. The average parkrun will have a number of people pushing their children round the course, some faster than a few of the runners without one. Joining a running group with other young people with children is another option, so that the caring arrangements can be shared. As children get older, they can be introduced to exercise along with their parents or carers. It is important, however, to remember that quite a short distance seems like a marathon to a young child, so distances and speed need to be adjusted accordingly.

'I have no one to exercise with.'

This is a common concern or excuse, but the truth is that there will be someone out there who feels the same and would welcome the company. There is strong evidence that exercising with someone else is a strong motivator, so it is very worthwhile to find someone who will become involved. Social media, such as Meta or Nextdoor, are possible vehicles to find people who would also welcome an exercising partner. Many towns have *Running*

Sisters groups and this could be a start to find a partner with whom to exercise. A further option is to offer to take a neighbour's dog for a walk. The true altruist could explore the options of exercising with someone who is unable to do so without help. One example would be a blind person who needs help, perhaps to run or cycle a tandem. The RNIB will be able to provide contacts for individuals who need such support.

The Role of Health Professionals

The person who provides a list of excuses is clearly reluctant to exercise but is often the one who needs it most. A health professional should try to connect such people with others who have or had the same issues. Fortunately most exercising organizations, whether they are gyms or sports clubs or recreational groups, will recognize the need to introduce those who have a limited exercise experience to their structure. It is important to realize that for many, exercise is a new or long-forgotten experience. Local authorities are increasingly recognizing this need and are providing a range of professionals to satisfy it. Any health professional reading this book should take the trouble to become familiar with the options available for the sort of person who is likely to make excuses. Helping people to overcome these barriers to exercise may be the biggest contribution a health professional can make.

Summary

Those engaged in promoting exercise regularly hear a variety of excuses. These can include people considering themselves insufficiently fit, being too fat, being injured, being too busy, the risk of getting cold or wet, being too old, having to look after children, looking stupid, and having no one with whom to exercise. Health professionals need to be aware of these excuses and counter them appropriately.

32 Conclusions

Regular exercise is the most effective 'treatment' available for the prevention and treatment of a wide range of diseases. It maintains physical fitness, muscular strength and activity in old age. It is especially beneficial for improving quality of life. Indeed, a positive relationship has been demonstrated between the amount of exercise taken and quality of life (Byberg *et al.*, 2009).

In his Annual Report in 2009, England's Chief Medical Officer stated that the benefits of regular physical activity on health, longevity and well-being 'easily surpass the effectiveness of any drugs or other medical treatment' (Department of Health, 2010). This fact is gradually being recognized by the medical profession, yet promoting exercise remains a major challenge in a world that seems to reduce or eliminate physical activity at every opportunity.

As has been seen so often in the preceding chapters, there is a dose response for the amount of exercise taken and the resulting beneficial effects. Relatively speaking, however, the greatest return on a person's efforts comes from increasing from a low level of exercise to the next level above. The greatest relative benefit is gained by those who go from doing nothing to doing a little (though the benefits are still well below those that can be attained by doing even more).

The dose-response associations between total physical activity and risks of some cancers, diabetes and CHD have been assessed in large meta-analyses. The quickest reductions in risk were achieved at between 600 MET minutes per week and 4000 MET minutes per week, but this included all physical activities undertaken.

It is still appreciated that the majority of people are unable to maintain the higher beneficial exercise doses. This presents a real challenge for the clinical and health professional.

The levels of exercise recommended by governments across the world reflect this reality. They are set at a level that has definite benefits but are not high enough to discourage most would-be exercisers from becoming involved. The choice of exercise is highly individual. The messages to take from this book include:

- if a person does nothing, encourage them to start exercising a little; and
- if a person exercises a little, encourage them to increase it incrementally.

Health professionals and clinicians should aim to encourage people to exercise as much as is practical for them as individuals. Any recommendation to increase the physical activity should be enjoyable. If not, the prospect of failure is high.

It is never too late to begin exercising. If exercise is maintained for a decade, starting later in life can become as effective as longer-term exercise (Byberg *et al.*, 2009). However, the benefits of physical activity can only be gained by those who are physically able to do it and also able to continue it. Once disability has become established, taking up exercise is much less likely to be successful (Miller *et al.*, 2000).

Despite the recognized benefits of physical activity, less than 10% of the population take enough regular exercise to improve their health. Political action is needed to achieve public awareness of these facts and to encourage everyone, and particularly older age groups, to increase their exercising habits.

Perhaps the best target group would be the recently retired, who are still young enough and also have the time to be able to start exercising. The gains will be great. Not only will they remain well, live longer and enjoy life more, but the period of ill health at the end of life will be reduced, with huge financial benefits for the whole population (Brown *et al.*, 2004).

© H.J.N. Bethell and D. Brodie 2023. *Exercise: A Scientific and Clinical Overview* (H.J.N. Bethell and D. Brodie)
DOI: 10.1079/9781800621855.0032

Summary

Exercise is hugely effective to prevent and treat a wide range of diseases. It will improve the quality of life right up to old age. There is often a dose-response relationship between the amount of exercise and the benefits. However, the most benefit often occurs at the lowest level, with less-fit people gaining more through exercise. The critical advice is to increase the level of exercise to the next level for each individual. Encouragement to exercise by politicians, by the NHS, by other health professionals, by local communities, by employers and through TV and the Internet is essential to increase the current level of involvement. The benefit to the nation's health from increased involvement in exercise is assured.

References

Brown, D.W., Brown, D.R., Heath, G.W., Balluz, L., Giles, W.H., *et al.* (2004) Associations between physical activity dose and health-related quality of life. *Medicine and Science in Sports and Exercise* 36, 890–896.

Byberg, L., Melhus, H., Gedeborg, R., Sundström, J., Ahlbom, A., *et al.* (2009) Total mortality after changes in leisure time physical activity in 50 year old men: 35 year follow-up of population based cohort. *British Journal of Sports Medicine* 43(7), 482.

Department of Health (2010) On the state of public health: Annual report of the Chief Medical Officer 2009. Available at: https://webarchive.nationalarchives.gov.uk/ukgwa/20130105021742/http://www.dh.gov.uk/en/Publicationsandstatistics/Publications/AnnualReports/DH_113912 (accessed 27 January 2023).

Miller, M.E., Rejeski, W.J., Reboussin, B.A., Ten Have, T.R. and Ettinger, W.H. (2000) Physical activity, functional limitations and disability in older adults. *Journal of the American Geriatric Society* 48, 1264–1272.

Glossary

accelerometer Device worn to record movement, similar to a pedometer but providing information on other activities.

activities of daily living (ADL) Refers to someone's daily self-care activities. Often used as a measure of a person's functional status.

aerobic Requiring oxygen. Usually describing a type of exercise.

anaerobic Not using oxygen. Usually describing a type of exercise.

arteriovenous oxygen difference The difference between the oxygen content of arterial blood as it reaches its target and the oxygen content of the venous blood as it returns to the heart.

atheroma Patchy narrowing of arteries, or 'hardening' of the arteries, responsible for heart attacks, strokes and peripheral vascular disease.

atrial fibrillation (AF) A common rhythm disturbance of the heart.

automatic external defibrillator (AED) Device which passes an electric shock to the chest – used after sudden death in attempt to revive the victim.

blood doping Technique for increasing oxygen-carrying capacity of blood by transfusing an athlete with red blood cells previously extracted and stored. Illegal in competitive sport.

body mass index (BMI) The most popular way of assessing 'fatness' – calculated by dividing weight in kilograms by height in metres squared.

Borg scale Also known as rate of perceived exertion (RPE). A way for exercisers to express how hard they find a particular exercise on a scale of 0 to 10 or the original scale of 6–20.

calorie A unit of energy. One calorie is the energy required to heat 1 ml water by 1°C. One thousand calories = 1 kilocalorie (kcal), sometimes written as Calorie. This is the usual unit used to express the energy content of food.

cardiac output (CO) The volume of blood pumped out by the heart in unit time, usually expressed as litres per minute (l/min).

cognitive behavioural therapy (CBT) A talking therapy for psychological problems such as anxiety or depression.

Cooper test A method for measuring physical fitness based on the distance that can be covered on foot in 12 minutes.

coronary heart disease (CHD) A narrowing of one or more of the coronary arteries, causing a reduction of blood flow to the heart muscle.

diastolic pressure The lowest pressure reached in the arterial system between heartbeats. In a blood pressure reading it is the second figure, as in 120 over 80 (120/80).

dyslipidaemia An abnormal amount of lipids in the blood.

epidemiology The science of study of how often diseases occur in different populations and why.

Gaussian curve The bell-shaped curve which shows the usual distribution of physical characteristics.

glycogen A compound made up of multiple glucose molecules. Provides glucose storage and, when needed, is broken down into glucose for use in energy production.

hippocampus A region of the brain concerned with memory and spatial awareness.

hypertrophic cardiomyopathy (HCM) An inherited abnormality of heart muscle, which becomes abnormally thickened and is prone to causing dangerous disturbances of heart rhythm.

joule (J) A unit of energy. One kilojoule is approximately one quarter of a kilocalorie.

lipoprotein A complex of protein and lipid circulating in the bloodstream, transporting fats around the body, including cholesterol.

meta-analysis A summation of a number of different clinical trials to confirm or disprove the effectiveness of a treatment.

metabolic equivalent (MET) The rate of energy production by an adult human at rest. It is equivalent to 3.5 ml of oxygen per minute per kilogram of body weight (3.5 ml/min/kg).

metabolic syndrome (MetSyn) A cluster of at least three of the following five medical conditions: abdominal obesity, high blood pressure, high blood sugar, high serum triglycerides and low serum high-density lipoprotein cholesterol.

mitochondria Bundles of protein and enzymes inside cells. Their main function is energy production.

mortality The death rate, usually expressed as the rate of death over a particular period or by a certain age. It is used to compare the effectiveness of treatments in lengthening or shortening life.

myocardium Heart muscle.

peripheral vascular disease (PVD) The disease of any of the peripheral arteries except those supplying the heart or brain. Caused by a build-up of fatty deposits in the arteries, most common is the restriction of blood supply to the legs.

Q-Risk The risk of developing cardiovascular disease over the following years, expressed as a percentage.

retinopathy Any disease of the retina of the eye. A particular feature of long-standing diabetes.

sarcopenia Loss of muscle tissue. It is the most important element of frailty of old age.

sleep apnoea Episodes of cessation of breathing while asleep. The typical sufferer is overweight and snores.

stroke volume (SV) The volume of blood pumped out by the heart with each beat.

sympathetic tone The background activity of the sympathetic nervous system, which controls such functions as heart rate and constriction of small arteries.

systematic review A collection and summary of all the papers and research aiming to answer a particular question. When all the evidence is gathered the meta-analysis is the application of statistics to quantify the results.

systolic pressure The highest pressure reached in the arterial system after contraction of the left ventricle. In the blood pressure reading, it is the first figure, as in 120 over 80 (120/80).

type 2 diabetes mellitus (T2DM) This is the so-called maturity onset diabetes. The body still produces insulin but not in sufficient quantities to keep the blood sugar level under control.

ventricular fibrillation (VF) A disturbance in heart rhythm, with each individual muscle fibre of the ventricles (the pumping engine of the heart) contracting independently of the rest. The heart stops pumping blood and death ensues rapidly unless the heart can be restarted by defibrillation.

VO_2 The rate of use of oxygen by the body, expressed either as litres per minute (l/min) or related to body weight as millilitres per minute per kilogram of body weight (ml/min/kg).

VO_{2max} The greatest rate at which the body can use oxygen to fuel maximal effort. This is the standard measure of physical fitness.

watts (W) A unit of energy expenditure (power) equivalent to 1 joule per second.

Index

Note: Page numbers in bold type refer to figures
Page numbers in italic type refer to tables